Cardio-Oncology

Gretchen G. Kimmick • Daniel J. Lenihan
Douglas B. Sawyer • Erica L. Mayer
Dawn L. Hershman

Editors

Cardio-Oncology

The Clinical Overlap of Cancer and Heart Disease

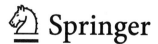 Springer

Editors
Gretchen G. Kimmick, MD, MS
Duke Cancer Institute
Duke University Medical Center
Durham, NC, USA

Douglas B. Sawyer, MD
Maine Medical Center
Cardiovascular Institute
Portland, ME, USA

Dawn L. Hershman, MD, MS
Herbert Irving Comprehensive Cancer Center
Columbia University Medical Center
New York, NY, USA

Daniel J. Lenihan, MD
Vanderbilt Heart and Vascular Institute
Vanderbilt University Medical Center
Nashville, TN, USA

Erica L. Mayer, MD, MPH
Dana-Farber Cancer Institute
Harvard Medical School
Boston, MA, USA

Additional material to this book can be downloaded from http://www.springerlink.com/ 978-3-319-43096-6

© 2016 Genevieve Kimmick, "Rhythm in Nature", Watercolor on paper (photographed by Rodger D. Israel)

ISBN 978-3-319-43094-2   ISBN 978-3-319-43096-6   (eBook)
DOI 10.1007/978-3-319-43096-6

Library of Congress Control Number: 2017932686

Printed on acid-free paper

This Springer imprint is published by Springer Nature
The registered company is Springer International Publishing AG
The registered company address is: Gewerbestrasse 11, 6330 Cham, Switzerland

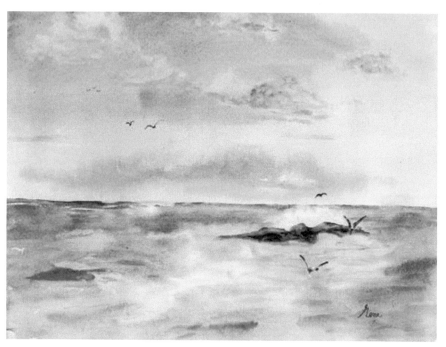

For the inspiration and support to write this truly collaborative book, we thank our families and loved ones, those for whom we have the honor of providing care, our colleagues/collaborators, mentors, and students.

Preface

As we see the explosion of new treatment approaches for many diseases, medicine becomes more and more subspecialized, and subsequently there is increased fragmentation. As a result of this progressive partitioning of medical care, close collaboration between medical subspecialties becomes an essential component to effective health care. The emerging medical discipline of cardio-oncology is a prime instance when such cooperation is paramount. In adults, cancer and heart disease have remarkable similarities in epidemiology. These two diseases, cardiovascular disease and cancer, account for at least half of the reasons for death in developed countries. It is no surprise that these diseases may coexist in many patients, emphasizing the need for there to be close collaboration between oncology and cardiology specialists.

With this textbook, we hope to provide a clinically useful volume containing knowledge about cardiac complications of cancer therapy, treatment of cancer in patients with cardiovascular disease, and treatment of cardiovascular disease in patients with cancer for practicing cardiologists, medical and radiation oncologists, and trainees in these fields. The book has been edited by three oncologists and two cardiologists with the purpose of integrating the two medicine subspecialties to be clinically useful to the oncologist and the cardiologist in caring for these patients. Each chapter is coauthored by at least one oncologist and one cardiologist, in order to include the perspective of each discipline and make the text user-friendly and clinically applicable to both specialties as well as others. We believe that this is the first textbook of cardio-oncology to provide this comprehensive coverage from a truly multidisciplinary standpoint. Combined, the chapters provide a clinically relevant overview of the epidemiology, basic science, and clinical knowledge in the ever-expanding space in which cardiology and oncology overlap.

This textbook adds to available learning resources in that it expands the topic from one focused only on heart failure caused by cancer therapies to a more inclusive one, where multiple cardiovascular issues, including coronary artery disease, hypertension, and vascular complications, among others, are thoroughly considered. We also asked the authors to generally include practical management approaches to common clinical problems in order be a useful guide to clinicians encountering these potentially difficult decisions. We hope that you find this text engaging and informative, but we also recognize this is a rapidly changing discipline. Perhaps by reading this text, a practitioner will be stimulated to contribute to our combined knowledge and advance the research in this invigorating discipline to continuously improve patient care.

Durham, NC, USA   Gretchen G. Kimmick, MD, MS
Nashville, TN, USA   Daniel J. Lenihan, MD
Portland, ME, USA   Douglas B. Sawyer, MD
Boston, MA, USA   Erica L. Mayer, MD, MPH
New York, NY, USA   Dawn L. Hershman, MD, MS

Acknowledgements

Great thanks to the leadership and staff at the American Society of Clinical Oncology for their enthusiasm about this field. Particular thanks to Teresa Gilewski, MD, who led the Education Committee for the Patient and Survivorship Care Track during 2012, when the idea for the book was conceived.

We acknowledge Julie Hughes at the Duke Cancer Institute, whose administrative assistance was invaluable in completing this work.

We also would like to thank the publisher, Springer, and our project coordinator in book production, Susan Westendorf, for their patience and guidance through the publication process.

Contents

Contributors

Monica Ahluwalia, MD Department of Internal Medicine, Perelman School of Medicine, University of Pennsylvania, Philadelphia, PA, USA

Ana Barac, MD MedStar Heart and Vascular Institute, Medstar Washington Hospital Center, Washington, DC, USA

Joshua A. Beckman, MD Vanderbilt Heart and Vascular Institute, Vanderbilt University Medical Center, Nashville, TN, USA

Anne Blaes, MD Division of Hematology, Oncology and Transplantation, Department of Medicine, University of Minnesota, Minneapolis, MN, USA

Joseph R. Carver, MD, FACC Abramson Cancer Center, University of Pennsylvania, Philadelphia, PA, USA

Anna Catino, MD Division of Cardiovascular Medicine, Department of Medicine, University of Utah, Salt Lake City, UT, USA

Robert Frank Cornell, MD, MS Division of Hematology and Oncology, Vanderbilt University Medical Center, Nashville, TN, USA

Carmen Criscitiello, MD Division of Early Drug Development for Innovative Therapies, Istituto Europeo di Oncologia, Milano, Italy

Giuseppe Curigliano, MD, PhD Division of Early Drug Development for Innovative Therapies, Istituto Europeo di Oncologia, Milano, Italy

Susan F. Dent, MD Division of Medical Oncology, Department of Medicine, University of Ottawa, Ottawa, ON, Canada

Angela Esposito, MD Division of Early Drug Development for Innovative Therapies, Istituto Europeo di Oncologia, Milano, Italy

Lauren Gilstrap, MD Newton-Wesley Hospital, Newton, MA, USA

Cardiovascular Medicine, Brigham and Women's Hospital, Boston, MA, USA

Stacey Goodman, MD Vanderbilt Blood Disorders, Vanderbilt University Medical Center, Nashville, TN, USA

Mike Harrison, MD Duke Cancer Institute, Duke University Medical Center, Durham, NC, USA

Michel G. Khouri, MD Division of Cardiology, Department of Medicine, Duke University Medical Center, Durham, NC, USA

Gretchen G. Kimmick, MD, MS Department of Medicine, Duke University Medical Center, Durham, NC, USA

David G. Kirsch, MD, PhD Department of Radiation Oncology, Duke University Medical Center, Durham, NC, USA

Aaron P. Kithcart, MD, PhD Cardiology, Brigham and Women's Hospital, Boston, MA, USA

Igor Klem, MD Division of Cardiology, Department of Medicine, Duke University Medical Center, Durham, NC, USA

Ronald J. Krone, MD Cardiovascular Division, John T Milliken Department of Internal Medicine, Washington University Medical School, Saint Louis, MO, USA

Bonnie Ky, MD Division of Cardiology, Department of Medicine, University of Pennsylvania, Philadelphia, PA, USA

Chang-Lung Lee, MD, PhD Department of Radiation Oncology, Duke University Medical Center, Durham, NC, USA

Daniel J. Lenihan, MD Vanderbilt Heart and Vascular Institute, Vanderbilt University Medical Center, Nashville, TN, USA

Carrie Geisberg Lenneman, MD, MSCI Divistion of Cardiology, Department of Medicine, University of Louisville, Louisville, KY, USA

Gary H. Lyman, MD, MPH, FASCO, FACP, FRCP(Edin) Hutchinson Institute for Cancer Outcomes Research, Fred Hutchinson Cancer Research Center, Seattle, WA, USA

University of Washington, Seattle, WA, USA

Erica L. Mayer, MD, MPH Dana-Farber Cancer Institute, Harvard Medical School, Boston, MA, USA

Chiara Melloni, MD, MHS Duke Clinical Research Institute, Durham, NC, USA

Myles Nickolich, MD Department of Internal Medicine, Duke University Medical Center, Durham, NC, USA

Anju Nohria, MD Brigham and Womens Hospital, Brigham and Womens Cardiology, Boston, MA, USA

Daniel S. O'Connor, MD, PhD Division of Cardiology, Columbia College of Physicians & Surgeons, New York Presbyterian Hospital, New York, NY, USA

Manisha Palta, MD Department of Radiation Oncology, Duke University Medical Center, Durham, NC, USA

Gregg F. Rosner, MD, MFS Cardiology & Cardiac Intensive Care, Columbia University Medical Center, New York, NY, USA

Rabih Said, MD, MPH Division of Cancer Medicine, Department of Investigational Cancer Therapeutics, The University of Texas MD Anderson Cancer Center, Houston, TX, USA

Division of Oncology, Department of Internal Medicine, The University of Texas Health Science Center at Houston, Houston, TX, USA

Douglas B. Sawyer, MD Maine Medical Center, Cardiovascular Institute, Portland, ME, USA

Chetan Shenoy, MD, MBBS Division of Cardiology, Department of Medicine, University of Minnesota Medical Center, Minneapolis, MN, USA

Preet Paul Singh, MD Siteman Cancer Center, Saint Louis, MO, USA

Jeffrey Sulpher, MD Division of Medical Oncology, Department of Medicine, University of Ottawa, Ottawa, ON, Canada

Dava Szalda, MD, MSHP Abramson Cancer Center, Cancer Survivorship Program, Pediatric Oncology, The Children's Hospital of Philadelphia, Phialdelphia, PA, USA

Apostolia M. Tsimberidou, MD, PhD Division of Cancer Medicine, Department of Investigational Cancer Therapeutics, The University of Texas MD Anderson Cancer Center, Houston, TX, USA

Syed Wamique Yusuf, MBBS, MRCPI, FACC Department of Cardiology, University of Texas MD Anderson Cancer Center, Houston, TX, USA

Chapter 1
Epidemiology of Cardio-Oncology

Carrie Geisberg Lenneman, Gretchen G. Kimmick, and Douglas B. Sawyer

Introduction

Heart disease and cancer are the first and second leading causes of death, accounting for 47 % of all mortality in the United States in 2010 [1, 2]. In adults, cancer and heart disease have remarkable similarities in epidemiology, explaining why many adult patients require the care of both oncology and cardiology specialists. This is augmented by the fact that patients with cardiovascular disease (CVD) and cancer are living longer due to improved screening, earlier detection, and increasingly successful treatments, as demonstrated in Fig. 1.1. New insights into the biology of inflammation and senescence may help understand why these have become the dominant diseases of aging. Many breast cancer patients, for instance, have multiple risk factors for cardiac disease, such as cigarette smoking, diabetes, dyslipidemia, alcohol consumption, obesity, and sedentary lifestyle [3–5]. These risk factors also increase the likelihood of adverse cardiovascular effects of some cancer therapies. For a newly diagnosed cancer patient, preexisting cardiovascular

Electronic supplementary material: The online version of this chapter (doi:10.1007/978-3-319-43096-6_1) contains supplementary material, which is available to authorized users.

C.G. Lenneman, M.D., MSCI (✉)
Division of Cardiology, Department of Medicine, University of Louisville,
Louisville, KY, USA
e-mail: carrie.lenneman@louisville.edu

G.G. Kimmick
Department of Medicine, Duke University Medical Center, Durham, NC, USA
e-mail: Gretchen.kimmick@duke.edu

D.B. Sawyer
Maine Medical Center, Cardiovascular Institute, Portland, ME, USA
e-mail: DSawyer@mmc.org

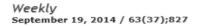
Weekly
September 19, 2014 / 63(37);827

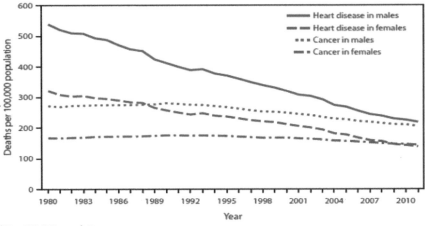

* Per 100,000 population.

Fig. 1.1 Age-adjusted death rates for heart disease and cancer in the United States, 1980–2011

disease may significantly limit the diagnosis, staging, and therapy offered. This is a particularly common problem in the older patient. The purpose of this chapter is to summarize the current state of knowledge of the shared epidemiology between common cancers and cardiovascular diseases and discuss the potential biological explanations as well as the clinical implications.

Cancer and Cardiovascular Disease: Convergent Epidemiology

Many of the risk factors for cardiovascular disease (e.g., tobacco use) are also well-known risk factors for cancer development. This is demonstrated by the similarity of geographic clustering of heart disease deaths and cancer deaths in the United States (Fig. 1.2). Genetic predisposition and age are strong determinants of risk for both classes of disease, but the majority of cancer and cardiovascular diseases are caused by modifiable risk factors. A multinational study of the epidemiology of heart disease (INTERHEART) revealed that nine risk factors, including abnormal lipids, smoking, hypertension, diabetes, abdominal obesity, psychosocial factors, physical activity, and consumption of fruits, vegetables, and alcohol, account for 90 % of population attributable risk of myocardial infarction in men and 94 % in women [6]. Similarly, several epidemiologic studies have demonstrated association between these same modifiable risk factors and development of cancer. Lung, breast, prostate, and colon cancers have been linked to obesity, high-fat diets, and smoking [7, 8].

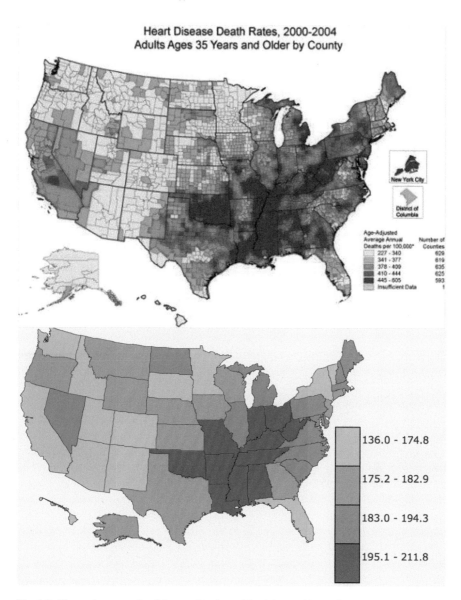

Fig. 1.2 Illustrative example of the overlapping epidemiology of heart disease and cancer, drawn from the US Center for Disease Control and Prevention data

Obesity. Defined as a body mass index (BMI) greater than 30, obesity is a known risk factor for CVD and is now a well-established risk factor for cancer and is highly prevalent with estimates that 35 % of populations in developed countries are obese [9]. In addition to its association with known risk factors for cardiovascular disease, including hypertension and reduced HDL cholesterol, in multivariate analysis, including traditional risk factors for cardiovascular disease, obesity was significantly and independently predictive of cardiovascular disease [10, 11].

Studies have also shown that obesity is a risk factor for certain cancers and may have an adverse effect on outcome. The data is very strong for the adverse association of breast cancer risk and outcome and obesity. A higher BMI and/or perimenopausal weight gain is consistently associated with increased risk of breast cancer [12–16]. Since 1976, when Abe et al. first reported the association between obesity and breast cancer recurrence, there have been more than 50 studies examining the relationship between body weight and breast cancer prognosis [17, 18]. In a prospective cohort of 14,709 patients, obesity was linked to adverse breast cancer prognosis [8]. Other population-based studies have demonstrated that both premenopausal and postmenopausal women who gained 16 kg and 12.7 kg, respectively, increased risk of breast cancer-related death by at least twofold [19]. Similarly, prostate and colon cancer studies show a positive correlation between body mass index (BMI) and cancer incidence [20, 21]. Visceral adipose tissue which is not reflected by measurements of BMI, waist circumference, and subcutaneous adipose tissue may play an important role in inflammation and oxidative stress [22]. Epidemiologic-based cancer studies have more recently been performed and show similar associations between overall obesity and central obesity and risk of colorectal cancer (CRC) [23] and mortality from pancreatic cancer [24].

Diabetes Similarly, diabetes mellitus (DM) has an adverse effect on risk and outcome in cancer and heart disease. The presence of DM at the age of 50 years, in the Framingham Heart Study (FHS), conferred the highest lifetime risk of CVD and mortality of any single risk factor [25]. Type II DM is also associated with risk of malignancy [26]. In patients with DM, high insulin levels and insulin-like growth factor have been associated with worse breast and colon cancer outcomes [27–30]. Interestingly, a series of observational studies reported decreased cancer incidence and mortality among type 2 diabetics who were treated with high doses or long duration of metformin [31]. Retrospective clinical data of 2529 women receiving neoadjuvant chemotherapy for breast cancer reported increased pathologic complete response (pCR) by 24 % in diabetics on metformin versus 8 % in diabetics not receiving metformin [32]. Metformin use during adjuvant chemotherapy, however, has not been shown to significantly impact survival outcomes in diabetic patients with hormone receptor and HER2-negative breast cancer. In a retrospective study from MD Anderson Cancer Center, at a median follow-up of 62 months, there were no significant differences among diabetics receiving metformin, diabetics not receiving metformin, and nondiabetic patients, with regard to 5-year distant metastasis-free survival (0.73 vs 0.66 vs 0.60; $p = 0.23$), recurrence-free survival (0.65 vs 0.64 vs 0.54; $p = 0.38$), and overall survival (0.67 vs 0.69 vs 0.66; $p = 0.58$) [33]. Higher risk of distant metastases was seen in patients who did not receive metformin (HR, 1.63; 95 % CI 0.87–3.06) and nondiabetic patients (HR, 1.62; 95 % CI 0.97–2.71), compared to diabetic patients taking metformin. Likewise, a phase II study of metformin in 44 men with chemotherapy-naïve castration-resistant prostate cancer found limited evidence of antitumor activity with two cases of >50 % decrease in serum PSA, although approximately one-half of men showed a prolongation in the PSA doubling time [34]. These observational studies generated a biologically plausible link between breast cancer and insulin receptor activity. For example, insulin receptors are overexpressed in breast cancer cells and can bind insulin and insulin-like growth factors (IGF1 and IGF2). When IGFs bind to the insulin receptors instead of insulin, this predominately activates a proliferative rather than metabolic pathway [35]. Additional phase II studies are underway in men with advanced prostate cancer. In addition, a phase III study is comparing metformin with placebo in men being managed with active surveillance for low-risk prostate cancer (NCT01864096).

Smoking Another common risk factor for heart disease and cancer is smoking. Smoking increases inflammation, thrombosis, and endothelial dysfunction [36, 37]. Tobacco smoking strongly increased the risk of lung cancer for current smokers (4.4 for men and 2.8 for females) compared to never smokers. In a comprehensive meta-analysis, tobacco smoking also increased the risk of colorectal cancer (CRC) incidence and mortality [38]. The mechanism linking smoking to colon cancer remains incomplete; however, animal studies have demonstrated that smoking exposure promoted inflammation-associated adenoma formation with increased expression in 5-lipoxygenase, upregulation of matrix metalloproteinase-2 (MMP-2), and vascular endothelial growth factor (VEGF) [39]. There is also an association between smoking and higher cancer stage at diagnosis [40] and the development of lung metastases [41].

While our understanding of the mechanistic link between tobacco exposure and pathogenesis of atherosclerosis and cancer is incomplete, it is very clear that reducing tobacco consumption has health benefits to individuals and society in general. Former smokers reduce their risk of heart disease and cancer within a year of quitting [42]. Similarly, communities that invest in comprehensive tobacco control programs are experiencing a reduction in smoking and smoking-related health costs due to cancer and cardiovascular disease, as well as pulmonary disease [43].

Mechanistic Theories Regarding the Common Epidemiology of CVD and Cancer

Inflammation is one of the common links between obesity, metabolic syndrome, smoking, diabetes, and the pathogenesis of atherosclerosis, heart failure, and cancer (Fig. 1.3). It has long been known that chronic inflammation from conditions such as hepatitis, inflammatory bowel disease, HPV, and *Helicobacter pylori* can lead to increased risk of cancer [44, 45]. Recent studies also demonstrate increased cytokine levels (TNF-α, IL-2, IL-6) or cytokine genetic alterations can lead to increased risk of breast cancer and a worse prognosis [46]. Similarly, elevated inflammatory biomarkers are associated with coronary disease and heart failure [47, 48]. Increased

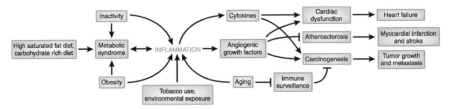

Fig. 1.3 Model for how modifiable risk factors promote development of both cardiovascular disease as well as tumorigenesis

levels of high-sensitivity C-reactive protein (hs-CRP) are associated with cardio-vascular events. Elevated plasma levels of CRP are also associated with increased risk of cancer with worse survival [49, 50].

Use of Nonsteroidal Anti-inflammatories Aspirin is recommended for primary and secondary prevention of CVD [51]. It reduces the total morality (RR 0.94, 95 % CI 0.88–1.00) and risk of myocardial infarction (0.80, 0.67–0.96) and stroke (0.95, 0.85–1.06) [52, 53]. The rate of major extracranial bleeding was higher (1.54, 1.30–1.82) [54].

With regard to cancers, the data for a relationship between aspirin and nonste-roidal anti-inflammatory drugs (NSAIDs) is strongest for colon cancers [55–64]. Aspirin lowers risk of mortality from colon cancer risk. In a study that combined data from four randomized trials of aspirin versus control (mean duration of scheduled treatment 6.0 years), in which 391 (2.8 %) of 14,033 patients had colorectal cancer during a median follow-up of 18.3 years, risk and mortality of colon cancer were lower in those randomized to aspirin [65]. Allocation to aspirin reduced the 20-year risk of colon cancer incidence (HR 0.76, 0.60–0.96; $p = 0.02$) and mortality (HR 0.65, 0.48–0.88; $p = 0.005$). Randomized trials have also shown reduced incidence of colorectal adenomas and cancer with aspirin use [66, 67], presumed to be through its actions as an inhibitor of the cyclooxygenase-2 (COX-2) pathway, which is overexpressed in 80–85 % of colon cancers. In a study that combined information from the Nurses' Health Study and the Health Professionals Follow-up Study, at a median follow-up of 11.8 years, aspirin users had a signif-icant 29 % (95 % CI, 0.53–0.95) lower cancer-specific mortality and a 21 % (95 % CI, 0.65–0.97) lower overall mortality than nonusers [57]. Reduction in risk was 61 % (95 % CI, 0.20–0.76) in those whose tumors overexpressed COX-2 when aspirin was initiated after diagnosis, but aspirin use was not associated with lower risk in those where COX-2 was not overexpressed (multivariate HR, 1.22; 95 % CI, 0.36–4.18). Studies have also shown that the beneficial effect of aspirin in colon cancer patients may vary by other mutations, including *PIK3CA* (phosphatidylinositol-4,5-bisphosphate 3-kinase, catalytic subunit alpha polypep-tide) gene status [68, 69], PTGS2 expression [64], BRAF mutations [70], expres-sion of human leukocyte antigen (HLA) class I antigens [61], and potentially other factors that have not yet been determined. The 2013 ASCO guidelines for follow-up care, surveillance, and secondary prevention measures for survivors of CRC do not, however, endorse the routine use of aspirin or a cyclooxygenase inhibitor [62]. These encouraging reports led to the development of two prospective randomized trials to study aspirin use in colorectal cancer patients: the phase III Alliance trial 80,702 and the Aspirin for Dukes C and High Risk Dukes B Colorectal Cancers (ASCOLT) study.

Regular aspirin use may also decrease risk of breast cancer. In the prospective Women's Health Initiative (WHI) study, which included 80,741 postmenopausal women between 50 and 79 years of age who reported no history of breast cancer or other cancers, regular (two or more tablets/week for 10 or more years) use of aspirin, ibuprofen, and other nonsteroidal anti-inflammatory drugs (NSAIDs) was associated with a 28 % reduction in the incidence of breast cancer (95 % CI, 0.56–0.91) [71]. The estimated risk reduction for long-term use of ibuprofen (RR, 0.51; CI, 0.28–0.96) was greater than for aspirin (RR, 0.79; CI, 0.60–1.03). Other meta-analyses of aspirin use have confirmed the reduced risk of breast cancer [72, 73]. The US Preventive Services Task Force (USPSTF), therefore, recommends that adults 50–69 years of age should take daily low-dose aspirin for at least 10 years to reduce their risk for cardiovascular disease (CVD) and colorectal cancer [74–77].

Changing modifiable lifestyle risk factors, such as weight loss, regular physical exercise, and diet rich in fruits and vegetables, improves prognosis and survival in many patients with cardiovascular disease and lung, breast, prostate, and colon cancers. Age, however, is a nonmodifiable risk factor, which influences both cardiovascular disease and cancer. The longitudinal Physicians' Health Study demonstrated that both cardiovascular disease and cancer rose dramatically in the sixth to seventh decade of life and that commonly both conditions were coexistent in a substantial number of patients [78]. With the rise in an aging population, and the overlap in risk factors between cancer and cardiovascular disease, there is an opportunity that presents itself to physicians and investigators to define common biology, mechanisms, and clinical treatments which optimize cardio-oncology patient outcomes.

Cancer Survivors: Cardiovascular vs Cancer Mortality

In cancer survivors, the risk of death from cardiovascular disease may be greater than the risk of death from cancer. Mortality rates from cancer have declined over the past 30 years, due to more effective methods of early detection and more effective management strategies [79, 80]. As a result, there are a growing number of cancer survivors [81]. According to 2015 estimates, the cancers with the largest differential in incident cases and estimated deaths are breast cancer, with 231,840 new cases and 40,290 deaths; prostate cancer, with 20,800 new cases and 27,540 deaths; and colon and rectal cancer, with 132,700 new cases and 49,700 deaths [82]. From 2014 to 2024, the number of survivors of female breast cancer is estimated to rise from 3,131,400 to 3,951,930, of prostate cancer from 2,975,970 to 4,194,190, and of colon and rectal from 1,246,320 to 1,561,020[83]. In breast cancer survivors, especially those who are elderly, cardiovascular disease is the predominant cause of mortality [84–88]. This is also true of childhood cancer survivors, of whom over 80 % are cured of their cancer and are at risk of cardiovascular death. The Childhood Cancer Survivor Study, which is the largest and most complete cohort study of childhood cancer survivors, showed that childhood cancer survivors suffer from chronic conditions at an alarmingly high rate, and cardiovascular disease is a major cause of morbidity and mortality in this group [89–91].

Adult cancer survivors are at risk for cardiovascular diseases on several levels. First, the diagnosis of cardiovascular disease may predate the cancer diagnosis. In one population-based study of 6439 women, with a mean age of 58.7 years, who were diagnosed with incident breast cancer in 2004, 45.8 % had preexisting cardiovascular disease [92].

Second, coexisting cardiovascular risk factors may lead to the development of cardiovascular disease and/or the manifestation of symptoms of cardiovascular disease after the cancer is diagnosed. This is demonstrated in a study of 2542 breast cancer survivors, in whom 11 % had cardiovascular disease diagnoses before the diagnosis of cancer, and an additional 10 % were diagnosed with cardiovascular disease after diagnosis [4]. Among cardiovascular diagnoses, angina pectoris was the most common, followed by myocardial infarction, stroke, and arterial occlusive disease. Hypertension was also present in 37 % at diagnosis and diagnosed in an additional 12 % after diagnosis.

Interestingly, there may be associations between hypertension or its treatment and cancer outcomes. Epidemiologic studies have described better outcomes in breast cancer patients with hypertension [93]. Beta-blocker use is associated with reduced mortality in cancer patients [94]. Anticancer effects of antihypertensive medications, such as beta-blockers, have been speculated [95–97]. Although beta-blocker use was not associated with reduced mortality in melanoma [98], beta-blockers and angiotensin-converting enzyme inhibitors [99–101] have been linked to reduced breast cancer mortality. In another population-based case-control study of women 65–79 years old, the use of immediate-release calcium channel blockers, thiazide diuretics, and potassium-sparing diuretics was associated with increased risk of breast cancer (OR 1.5, 95 % CI, 1.0–2.1; OR 1.4, 95 % CI, 1.1–1.8; and OR 1.6, 95 % CI, 1.2–2.1, respectively). One large epidemiologic study, however, showed that women with breast cancer were more likely to receive guideline-concordant care [92] leading to better outcomes. Better access to healthcare in general, there, may be a confounder in studies of the relationship between hypertension and cancer outcomes.

Third, cardiotoxicity of cancer therapies, including hypertension, cardiomyopathy, QT prolongation, arrhythmias, thrombosis, and metabolic abnormalities, may lead to cardiovascular disease. Cardiotoxicities of cancer therapies will be covered in greater depth in other chapters of this book.

References

1. Siegel R, Naishadham D, Jemal A. Cancer statistics, 2012. CA Cancer J Clin. 2012;62 (1):10–29.
2. Murphy SL, Jiaquan X, Kochanek KD. National Vital Statistics Reports: Deaths Preliminary Report for 2010. 2012.
3. Weaver KE, Foraker RE, Alfano CM, Rowland JH, Arora NK, Bellizzi KM, et al. Cardio-vascular risk factors among long-term survivors of breast, prostate, colorectal, and gyneco-logic cancers: a gap in survivorship care? J Cancer Surviv. 2013;7(2):253–61.
4. Obi N, Gornyk D, Heinz J, Vrieling A, Seibold P, Chang-Claude J, et al. Determinants of newly diagnosed comorbidities among breast cancer survivors. J Cancer Surviv. 2014;8 (3):384–93.
5. Lakoski SG, Willis BL, Barlow CE, Leonard D, Gao A, Radford NB, et. al. Midlife cardiorespiratory fitness, incident cancer, and survival after cancer in men: The Cooper Center Longitudinal Study. JAMA Oncol. 2015;1(2):231–7.
6. Yusuf S, Hawken S, Ounpuu S, Dans T, Avezum A, Lanas F, et al. Effect of potentially modifiable risk factors associated with myocardial infarction in 52 countries (the INTERHEART study): case-control study. Lancet. 2004;364(9438):937–52.
7. Khan N, Afaq F, Mukhtar H. Lifestyle as risk factor for cancer: evidence from human studies. Cancer Lett. 2010;293(2):133–43.
8. Majed B, Moreau T, Senouci K, Salmon RJ, Fourquet A, Asselain B. Is obesity an indepen-dent prognosis factor in woman breast cancer? Breast Cancer Res Treat. 2008;111(2):329–42.
9. Ogden CL, Carroll MD, Kit BK, Flegal KM. Prevalence of childhood and adult obesity in the United States, 2011–2012. JAMA. 2014;311(8):806–14.
10. Wilson PW, Bozeman SR, Burton TM, Hoaglin DC, Ben-Joseph R, Pashos CL. Prediction of first events of coronary heart disease and stroke with consideration of adiposity. Circulation. 2008;118(2):124–30.
11. Twig G, Yaniv G, Levine H, Leiba A, Goldberger N, Derazne E, et al. Body-mass index in 2.3 million adolescents and cardiovascular death in adulthood. N Engl J Med. 2016;374:2430–40.
12. Lahmann PH, Hoffmann K, Allen N, van Gils CH, Khaw KT, Tehard B, et al. Body size and breast cancer risk: findings from the European Prospective Investigation into Cancer and Nutrition (EPIC). Int J Cancer. 2004;111(5):762–71.
13. Eliassen AH, Colditz GA, Rosner B, Willett WC, Hankinson SE. Adult weight change and risk of postmenopausal breast cancer. JAMA. 2006;296(2):193–201.
14. Ahn J, Schatzkin A, Lacey Jr JV, Albanes D, Ballard-Barbash R, Adams KF, et al. Adiposity, adult weight change, and postmenopausal breast cancer risk. Arch Intern Med. 2007;167 (19):2091–102.
15. Alsaker MD, Janszky I, Opdahl S, Vatten LJ, Romundstad PR. Weight change in adulthood and risk of postmenopausal breast cancer: the HUNT study of Norway. Br J Cancer. 2013;109 (5):1310–7.
16. Emaus MJ, van Gils CH, Bakker MF, Bisschop CN, Monninkhof EM, Bueno-de-Mesquita HB, et al. Weight change in middle adulthood and breast cancer risk in the EPIC-PANACEA study. Int J Cancer. 2014;135(12):2887–99.
17. Abe R, Kumagai N, Kimura M, Hirosaki A, Nakamura T. Biological characteristics of breast cancer in obesity. Tohoku J Exp Med. 1976;120(4):351–9.
18. Protani M, Coory M, Martin JH. Effect of obesity on survival of women with breast cancer: systematic review and meta-analysis. Breast Cancer Res Treat. 2010;123(3):627–35.
19. Cleveland RJ, Eng SM, Abrahamson PE, Britton JA, Teitelbaum SL, Neugut AI, et al. Weight gain prior to diagnosis and survival from breast cancer. Cancer Epidemiol Biomarkers Prev. 2007;16(9):1803–11.

20. Andersson SO, Wolk A, Bergstrom R, Adami HO, Engholm G, Englund A, et al. Body size and prostate cancer: a 20-year follow-up study among 135006 Swedish construction workers. J Natl Cancer Inst. 1997;89(5):385–9.
21. Tamakoshi K, Wakai K, Kojima M, Watanabe Y, Hayakawa N, Toyoshima H, et al. A prospective study of body size and colon cancer mortality in Japan: the JACC Study. Int J Obes Relat Metab Disord. 2004;28(4):551–8.
22. Pou KM, Massaro JM, Hoffmann U, Vasan RS, Maurovich-Horvat P, Larson MG, et al. Visceral and subcutaneous adipose tissue volumes are cross-sectionally related to markers of inflammation and oxidative stress: the Framingham Heart Study. Circulation. 2007;116 (11):1234–41.
23. Song M, Hu FB, Spiegelman D, Chan AT, Wu K, Ogino S, et al. Long-term status and change of body fat distribution, and risk of colorectal cancer: a prospective cohort study. Int J Epidemiol. 2015.
24. Genkinger JM, Kitahara CM, Bernstein L, Berrington de Gonzalez A, Brotzman M, Elena JW, et al. Central adiposity, obesity during early adulthood, and pancreatic cancer mortality in a pooled analysis of cohort studies. Ann Oncol. 2015;26(11):2257–66.
25. Lloyd-Jones DM, Leip EP, Larson MG, D'Agostino RB, Beiser A, Wilson PW, et al. Prediction of lifetime risk for cardiovascular disease by risk factor burden at 50 years of age. Circulation. 2006;113(6):791–8.
26. Gallagher EJ, LeRoith D. Obesity and diabetes: the increased risk of cancer and cancer-related mortality. Physiol Rev. 2015;95(3):727–48.
27. Chlebowski RT, Aiello E, McTiernan A. Weight loss in breast cancer patient management. J Clin Oncol. 2002;20(4):1128–43.
28. Rollison DE, Newschaffer CJ, Tao Y, Pollak M, Helzlsouer KJ. Premenopausal levels of circulating insulin-like growth factor I and the risk of postmenopausal breast cancer. Int J Cancer. 2006;118(5):1279–84.
29. Goodwin PJ, Ennis M, Bahl M, Fantus IG, Pritchard KI, Trudeau ME, et al. High insulin levels in newly diagnosed breast cancer patients reflect underlying insulin resistance and are associated with components of the insulin resistance syndrome. Breast Cancer Res Treat. 2009;114(3):517–25.
30. Yeh HC, Platz EA, Wang NY, Visvanathan K, Helzlsouer KJ, Brancati FL. A prospective study of the associations between treated diabetes and cancer outcomes. Diabetes Care. 2012;35(1):113–8.
31. Monami M, Lamanna C, Balzi D, Marchionni N, Mannucci E. Sulphonylureas and cancer: a case-control study. Acta Diabetol. 2009;46(4):279–84.
32. Jiralerspong S, Palla SL, Giordano SH, Meric-Bernstam F, Liedtke C, Barnett CM, et al. Metformin and pathologic complete responses to neoadjuvant chemotherapy in diabetic patients with breast cancer. J Clin Oncol. 2009;27(20):3297–302.
33. Bayraktar S, Hernadez-Aya LF, Lei X, Meric-Bernstam F, Litton JK, Hsu L, et al. Effect of metformin on survival outcomes in diabetic patients with triple receptor-negative breast cancer. Cancer. 2012;118(5):1202–11.
34. Rothermundt C, Hayoz S, Templeton AJ, Winterhalder R, Strebel RT, Bartschi D, et al. Metformin in chemotherapy-naive castration-resistant prostate cancer: a multicenter phase 2 trial (SAKK 08/09). Eur Urol. 2014;66(3):468–74.
35. Belfiore A, Frasca F. IGF and insulin receptor signaling in breast cancer. J Mammary Gland Biol Neoplasia. 2008;13(4):381–406.
36. Zieske AW, McMahan CA, McGill Jr HC, Homma S, Takei H, Malcom GT, et al. Smoking is associated with advanced coronary atherosclerosis in youth. Atherosclerosis. 2005;180 (1):87–92.
37. Chia S, Newby DE. Atherosclerosis, cigarette smoking, and endogenous fibrinolysis: is there a direct link? Curr Atheroscler Rep. 2002;4(2):143–8.
38. Botteri E, Iodice S, Bagnardi V, Raimondi S, Lowenfels AB, Maisonneuve P. Smoking and colorectal cancer: a meta-analysis. JAMA. 2008;300(23):2765–78.

39. Ye YN, Liu ES, Shin VY, Wu WK, Cho CH. Contributory role of 5-lipoxygenase and its association with angiogenesis in the promotion of inflammation-associated colonic tumorigenesis by cigarette smoking. Toxicology. 2004;203(1-3):179–88.
40. Kobrinsky NL, Klug MG, Hokanson PJ, Sjolander DE, Burd L. Impact of smoking on cancer stage at diagnosis. J Clin Oncol. 2003;21(5):907–13.
41. Abrams JA, Lee PC, Port JL, Altorki NK, Neugut AI. Cigarette smoking and risk of lung metastasis from esophageal cancer. Cancer Epidemiol Biomarkers Prev. 2008;17 (10):2707–13.
42. Health Benefits of Smoking Cessation. A report of the Surgeon General. DHHS Publication No. (CDC) 90-8416. In: Department of Health and Human Services NCfHS, editor. Washington, DC1990.
43. Atusingwize E, Lewis S, Langley T. Economic evaluations of tobacco control mass media campaigns: a systematic review. Tob Control. 2015;24(4):320–7.
44. Lin WW, Karin M. A cytokine-mediated link between innate immunity, inflammation, and cancer. J Clin Invest. 2007;117(5):1175–83.
45. Coussens LM, Werb Z. Inflammation and cancer. Nature. 2002;420(6917):860–7.
46. Berger FG. The interleukin-6 gene: a susceptibility factor that may contribute to racial and ethnic disparities in breast cancer mortality. Breast Cancer Res Treat. 2004;88(3):281–5.
47. Vasan RS, Sullivan LM, Roubenoff R, Dinarello CA, Harris T, Benjamin EJ, et al. Inflammatory markers and risk of heart failure in elderly subjects without prior myocardial infarction: the Framingham Heart Study. Circulation. 2003;107(11):1486–91.
48. Pai JK, Pischon T, Ma J, Manson JE, Hankinson SE, Joshipura K, et al. Inflammatory markers and the risk of coronary heart disease in men and women. N Engl J Med. 2004;351 (25):2599–610.
49. Allin KH, Bojesen SE, Nordestgaard BG. Baseline C-reactive protein is associated with incident cancer and survival in patients with cancer. J Clin Oncol. 2009;27(13):2217–24.
50. Erlinger TP, Platz EA, Rifai N, Helzlsouer KJ. C-reactive protein and the risk of incident colorectal cancer. JAMA. 2004;291(5):585–90.
51. Hennekens CH, Dyken ML, Fuster V. Aspirin as a therapeutic agent in cardiovascular disease: a statement for healthcare professionals from the American Heart Association. Circulation. 1997;96(8):2751–3.
52. Seshasai SR, Wijesuriya S, Sivakumaran R, Nethercott S, Erqou S, Sattar N, et al. Effect of aspirin on vascular and nonvascular outcomes: meta-analysis of randomized controlled trials. Arch Intern Med. 2012;172(3):209–16.
53. Baigent C, Blackwell L, Collins R, Emberson J, Godwin J, Peto R, et al. Aspirin in the primary and secondary prevention of vascular disease: collaborative meta-analysis of individual participant data from randomised trials. Lancet. 2009;373(9678):1849–60.
54. Raju N, Sobieraj-Teague M, Hirsh J, O'Donnell M, Eikelboom J. Effect of aspirin on mortality in the primary prevention of cardiovascular disease. Am J Med. 2011;124 (7):621–9.
55. Cardwell CR, Kunzmann AT, Cantwell MM, Hughes C, Baron JA, Powe DG, et al. Low-dose aspirin use after diagnosis of colorectal cancer does not increase survival: a case-control analysis of a population-based cohort. Gastroenterology. 2014;146(3):700–8.
56. Walker AJ, Grainge MJ, Card TR. Aspirin and other non-steroidal anti-inflammatory drug use and colorectal cancer survival: a cohort study. Br J Cancer. 2012;107(9):1602–7.
57. Chan AT, Ogino S, Fuchs CS. Aspirin use and survival after diagnosis of colorectal cancer. JAMA. 2009;302(6):649–58.
58. Zell JA, Ziogas A, Bernstein L, Clarke CA, Deapen D, Largent JA, et al. Nonsteroidal anti-inflammatory drugs: effects on mortality after colorectal cancer diagnosis. Cancer. 2009;115 (24):5662–71.
59. Coghill AE, Newcomb PA, Campbell PT, Burnett-Hartman AN, Adams SV, Poole EM, et al. Prediagnostic non-steroidal anti-inflammatory drug use and survival after diagnosis of colorectal cancer. Gut. 2011;60(4):491–8.

60. Bastiaannet E, Sampieri K, Dekkers OM, de Craen AJ, van Herk-Sukel MP, Lemmens V, et al. Use of aspirin postdiagnosis improves survival for colon cancer patients. Br J Cancer. 2012;106(9):1564–70.
61. Reimers MS, Bastiaannet E, Langley RE, van Eijk R, van Vlierberghe RL, Lemmens VE, et al. Expression of HLA class I antigen, aspirin use, and survival after a diagnosis of colon cancer. JAMA Intern Med. 2014;174(5):732–9.
62. Ng K, Meyerhardt JA, Chan AT, Sato K, Chan JA, Niedzwiecki D, et al. Aspirin and COX-2 inhibitor use in patients with stage III colon cancer. J Natl Cancer Inst. 2015;107(1):345.
63. McCowan C, Munro AJ, Donnan PT, Steele RJ. Use of aspirin post-diagnosis in a cohort of patients with colorectal cancer and its association with all-cause and colorectal cancer specific mortality. Eur J Cancer. 2013;49(5):1049–57.
64. Li P, Wu H, Zhang H, Shi Y, Xu J, Ye Y, et al. Aspirin use after diagnosis but not prediagnosis improves established colorectal cancer survival: a meta-analysis. Gut. 2015;64 (9):1419–25.
65. Rothwell PM, Wilson M, Elwin CE, Norrving B, Algra A, Warlow CP, et al. Long-term effect of aspirin on colorectal cancer incidence and mortality: 20-year follow-up of five randomised trials. Lancet. 2010;376(9754):1741–50.
66. Baron JA, Cole BF, Sandler RS, Haile RW, Ahnen D, Bresalier R, et al. A randomized trial of aspirin to prevent colorectal adenomas. N Engl J Med. 2003;348(10):891–9.
67. Sandler RS, Halabi S, Baron JA, Budinger S, Paskett E, Keresztes R, et al. A randomized trial of aspirin to prevent colorectal adenomas in patients with previous colorectal cancer. N Engl J Med. 2003;348(10):883–90.
68. Liao X, Lochhead P, Nishihara R, Morikawa T, Kuchiba A, Yamauchi M, et al. Aspirin use, tumor PIK3CA mutation, and colorectal-cancer survival. N Engl J Med. 2012;367 (17):1596–606.
69. Paleari L, Puntoni M, Clavarezza M, DeCensi M, Cuzick J, DeCensi A. PIK3CA mutation, aspirin use after diagnosis and survival of colorectal cancer. A systematic review and meta-analysis of epidemiological studies. Clin Oncol (R Coll Radiol). 2016;28(5):317–26.
70. Nishihara R, Lochhead P, Kuchiba A, Jung S, Yamauchi M, Liao X, et al. Aspirin use and risk of colorectal cancer according to BRAF mutation status. JAMA. 2013;309(24):2563–71.
71. Harris RE, Chlebowski RT, Jackson RD, Frid DJ, Ascenseo JL, Anderson G, et al. Breast cancer and nonsteroidal anti-inflammatory drugs: prospective results from the women's health initiative. Cancer Res. 2003;63(18):6096.
72. Luo T, Yan HM, He P, Luo Y, Yang YF, Zheng H. Aspirin use and breast cancer risk: a meta-analysis. Breast Cancer Res Treat. 2012;131(2):581–7.
73. Zhong S, Chen L, Zhang X, Yu D, Tang J, Zhao J. Aspirin use and risk of breast cancer: systematic review and meta-analysis of observational studies. Cancer Epidemiol Biomarkers Prev. 2015;24(11):1645–55.
74. Michaud TL, Abraham J, Jalal H, Luepker RV, Duval S, Hirsch AT. Cost-effectiveness of a statewide campaign to promote aspirin use for primary prevention of cardiovascular disease. J Am Heart Assoc. 2015;4(12).
75. Guirguis-Blake JM, Evans CV, Senger CA, et al. Aspirin for the primary prevention of cardiovascular events: a systematic evidence review for the U.S. Preventive Services Task Force [Internet]. Rockville: Agency for Healthcare Research and Quality (US); 2015. (Evidence Syntheses, No. 131). Available from https://www.ncbi.nlm.nih.gov/books/ NBK321623/.
76. Chubak J, Kamineni A, Buist DSM, et al. Aspirin use for the prevention of colorectal cancer: an updated systematic evidence review for the U.S. Preventive Services Task Force [Internet]. Rockville: Agency for Healthcare Research and Quality (US); 2015. (Evidence Syntheses, No. 133). Available from https://www.ncbi.nlm.nih.gov/books/NBK321661/.
77. Whitlock EP, Williams SB, Burda BU, et al. Aspirin use in adults: cancer, all-cause mortality, and harms: a systematic evidence review for the U.S. Preventive Services Task Force [Internet]. Rockville: Agency for Healthcare Research and Quality (US); 2015. (Evidence Syntheses, No. 132). Available from https://www.ncbi.nlm.nih.gov/books/NBK321643/.

78. Driver JA, Djousse L, Logroscino G, Gaziano JM, Kurth T. Incidence of cardiovascular disease and cancer in advanced age: prospective cohort study. BMJ. 2008;337:a2467.
79. Jemal A, Siegel R, Xu J, Ward E. Cancer statistics, 2010. CA Cancer J Clin. 2010;60 (5):277–300.
80. Howlader N, Ries LAG, Mariotto AB, Reichman ME, Ruhl J, Cronin KA. Improved estimates of cancer-specific survival rates from population-based data. J Natl Cancer Inst. 2010;102(20):1584–98.
81. Parry C, Kent EE, Mariotto AB, Alfano CM, Rowland JH. Cancer survivors: a booming population. Cancer Epidemiol Biomarkers Prev. 2011;20(10):1996–2005.
82. Siegel RL, Miller KD, Jemal A. Cancer statistics, 2016. CA Cancer J Clin. 2016;66(1):7–30.
83. DeSantis CE, Lin CC, Mariotto AB, Siegel RL, Stein KD, Kramer JL, et al. Cancer treatment and survivorship statistics, 2014. CA Cancer J Clin. 2014;64(4):252–71.
84. Chapman JA, Meng D, Shepherd L, Parulekar W, Ingle JN, Muss HB, et al. Competing causes of death from a randomized trial of extended adjuvant endocrine therapy for breast cancer. J Natl Cancer Inst. 2008;100(4):252–60.
85. Hanrahan EO, Gonzalez-Angulo AM, Giordano SH, Rouzier R, Broglio KR, Hortobagyi GN, et al. Overall survival and cause-specific mortality of patients with stage T1a, bN0M0 breast carcinoma. J Clin Oncol. 2007;25(31):4952–60.
86. Schairer C, Mink PJ, Carroll L, Devesa SS. Probabilities of death from breast cancer and other causes among female breast cancer patients. J Natl Cancer Inst. 2004;96(17):1311–21.
87. Patnaik JL, Byers T, Diguiseppi C, Dabelea D, Denberg TD. Cardiovascular disease competes with breast cancer as the leading cause of death for older females diagnosed with breast cancer: a retrospective cohort study. Breast Cancer Res. 2011;13(3):R64.
88. Colzani E, Liljegren A, Johansson AL, Adolfsson J, Hellborg H, Hall PF, et al. Prognosis of patients with breast cancer: causes of death and effects of time since diagnosis, age, and tumor characteristics. J Clin Oncol. 2011;29(30):4014–21.
89. Smith MA, Altekruse SF, Adamson PC, Reaman GH, Seibel NL. Declining childhood and adolescent cancer mortality. Cancer. 2014;120(16):2497–506.
90. Oeffinger KC, Mertens AC, Sklar CA, Kawashima T, Hudson MM, Meadows AT, et al. Chronic health conditions in adult survivors of childhood cancer. N Engl J Med. 2006;355 (15):1572–82.
91. Armstrong GT, Kawashima T, Leisenring W, Stratton K, Stovall M, Hudson MM, et al. Aging and risk of severe, disabling, life-threatening, and fatal events in the childhood cancer survivor study. J Clin Oncol. 2014;32(12):1218–27.
92. Kimmick G, Fleming ST, Sabatino SA, Wu XC, Hwang W, Wilson JF, et al. Comorbidity burden and guideline-concordant care for breast cancer. J Am Geriatr Soc. 2014;62(3):482–8.
93. Braithwaite D, Tammemagi CM, Moore DH, Ozanne EM, Hiatt RA, Belkora J, et al. Hypertension is an independent predictor of survival disparity between African-American and white breast cancer patients. Int J Cancer. 2009;124(5):1213–9.
94. Zhong S, Yu D, Zhang X, Chen X, Yang S, Tang J, et al. beta-Blocker use and mortality in cancer patients: systematic review and meta-analysis of observational studies. Eur J Cancer Prev. 2015. Epub 2015/09/05.
95. Drell TL, Joseph J, Lang K, Niggemann B, Zaenker KS, Entschladen F. Effects of neurotransmitters on the chemokinesis and chemotaxis of MDA-MB-468 human breast carcinoma cells. Breast Cancer Res Treat. 2003;80(1):63–70.
96. Lang K, Drell TL, Lindecke A, Niggemann B, Kaltschmidt C, Zaenker KS, et al. Induction of a metastatogenic tumor cell type by neurotransmitters and its pharmacological inhibition by established drugs. Int J Cancer. 2004;112(2):231–8.
97. Sloan EK, Priceman SJ, Cox BF, Yu S, Pimentel MA, Tangkanangnukul V, et al. The sympathetic nervous system induces a metastatic switch in primary breast cancer. Cancer Res. 2010;70(18):7042–52.

98. McCourt C, Coleman HG, Murray LJ, Cantwell MM, Dolan O, Powe DG, et al. Beta-blocker usage after malignant melanoma diagnosis and survival: a population-based nested case-control study. Br J Dermatol. 2014;170(4):930–8.

99. Powe DG, Voss MJ, Zanker KS, Habashy HO, Green AR, Ellis IO, et al. Beta-blocker drug therapy reduces secondary cancer formation in breast cancer and improves cancer specific survival. Oncotarget. 2010;1(7):628–38.

100. Ganz PA, Habel LA, Weltzien EK, Caan BJ, Cole SW. Examining the influence of beta blockers and ACE inhibitors on the risk for breast cancer recurrence: results from the LACE cohort. Breast Cancer Res Treat. 2011;129(2):549–56.

101. Barron TI, Connolly RM, Sharp L, Bennett K, Visvanathan K. Beta blockers and breast cancer mortality: a population- based study. J Clin Oncol. 2011;29(19):2635–44.

Chapter 2
Cardiotoxicity of Anticancer Therapies

**Rabih Said, Myles Nickolich, Daniel J. Lenihan,
and Apostolia M. Tsimberidou**

Introduction

Cardiotoxicity associated with anticancer therapies represents a complex clinical challenge, as well as a major economic and health burden, given the increasing number of cancer survivors [1, 2]. In Western countries, a large number of cancer survivors are at a higher risk of cardiotoxicity-related death than of cancer recurrence [2]. Cardiac impairment due to cancer therapy may require the discontinuation of anticancer agents, including chemotherapeutic, targeted, and biologic

Electronic supplementary material: The online version of this chapter (doi:10.1007/978-3-319-43096-6_2) contains supplementary material, which is available to authorized users.

R. Said
Division of Cancer Medicine, Department of Investigational Cancer Therapeutics,
The University of Texas MD Anderson Cancer Center, Houston, TX 77030, USA

Division of Oncology, Department of Internal Medicine, The University of Texas Health Science Center at Houston, Houston, TX 77030, USA
e-mail: Rabih.Said@uth.tmc.edu

M. Nickolich
Department of Internal Medicine, Duke University Medical Center, Durham, NC, USA
e-mail: myles.nickolich@dm.duke.edu

D.J. Lenihan
Vanderbilt Heart and Vascular Institute, Vanderbilt University Medical Center, Nashville, TN 37232, USA
e-mail: daniel.lenihan@Vanderbilt.Edu

A.M. Tsimberidou (✉)
Division of Cancer Medicine, Department of Investigational Cancer Therapeutics,
The University of Texas MD Anderson Cancer Center, Houston, TX 77030, USA
e-mail: atsimber@mdanderson.org

treatments [3]. The risk of cardiotoxicity during cancer therapy varies by therapeutic class and agent as well as by coexisting cardiac disease and concomitant use of other cardiotoxic agents [3]. The use of various cardioprotective agents (e.g., angiotensin-converting enzyme inhibitors/angiotensin receptor blockers and beta-blockers) is critical in preventing and/or reversing cardiac injury related to anti-cancer therapy [4, 5]. The emergence and rapid adoption of "Cardio-oncology"—a multidisciplinary, integrative clinical approach involving general practitioners, oncologists, and cardiologists to prevent and treat cardiotoxicity in patients being treated for cancer—aims to increase awareness of cardiotoxicity caused by cancer therapy and cardiac risk factors and to optimize the monitoring and treatment of patients with these conditions [3, 6].

This chapter focuses on anticancer agents with potential cardiotoxicity (Table 2.1 and Fig. 2.1). The incidence and type of cardiotoxicity and the most common preventive and therapeutic approaches are summarized in Fig. 2.2.

Chemotherapy

Anthracyclines

Doxorubicin

Anthracycline-induced cardiotoxicity was initially reported more than four decades ago during the early clinical development of doxorubicin [7, 8]. The incidence of anthracycline-induced heart failure (HF), based on clinical signs and symptoms, was reported to be less than 3 % [8]. However, the development of noninvasive monitoring techniques enabled the detection of a higher incidence of cardiac dysfunction [9]. The key mechanisms involved in the pathogenesis of cardiac dysfunction are increased reactive oxygen species and alteration of topoisomerase IIb, which are both associated with damage to cardiomyocytes [10, 11]. Acute cardiac dysfunction is reported in 3.2 % of patients receiving anthracyclines [12], and it occurs within several weeks of the initiation of therapy. Acute cardiac dysfunction presents with electrocardiographic abnormalities, including arrhythmias (supraventricular and ventricular), heart block, ventricular dysfunction, increased cardiac filling pressures, HF, and pericarditis-myocarditis syndrome [13–17]. Cardiac dysfunction may present as a reduction in left ventricular ejection fraction (LVEF) in up to 20 % of patients and may not become evident until after the completion of chemotherapy [18–20].

These late-occurring complications are serious and consist of HF that develops within a few months to several years (most frequently within 3 months) after anthracycline therapy [8, 21–23]. However, symptomatic HF can occur more than a decade after treatment, which represents a major clinical concern, especially among survivors of childhood malignancies [22]. Chronic cardiomyopathy can present as asymptomatic diastolic or systolic dysfunction, which frequently

Table 2.1 Selected anticancer agents with potential cardiotoxicity

Agents	Drug class	Cancer clinical use	Type of cardiotoxicity	Frequency
Chemotherapeutic agents				
Doxorubicin	Anthracyclines	Breast, sarcoma, lung, bladder, gastric, prostate, leukemia, lymphoma, others	LV dysfunction	Common
Epirubicin	Anthracyclines	Breast, esophageal, gastric	Arrhythmia	Uncommon
Cyclophosphamide	Alkylating agents	Sarcoma, SCT, lymphoma, myeloma, breast	Myopericarditis, arrhythmias	Common
Ifosfamide	Alkylating agents	Testicular, sarcoma, lymphoma	Arrhythmias, LV dysfunction	Common
Cisplatin	Alkylating agents	Lung, bladder, testicular, sarcoma, breast, esophageal, head and neck	Arrhythmias, ischemia, vascular toxicity	Uncommon
5-Fluorouracil	Antimetabolites	Colon, pancreatic, breast, head and neck	Coronary vasospasm, ischemia, arrhythmias	Common
Capecitabine	Antimetabolites	Breast, colon, gastric, pancreatic	Chest pain, ischemia, arrhythmias	Uncommon
Fludarabine	Antimetabolites	Lymphoma, leukemia, stem cell transplant	Chest pain	Rare
Vinblastine	Antimicrotubule	Lymphoma, testicular, lung, melanoma	Ischemia, hypertension	Common
Paclitaxel	Antimicrotubule	Breast, ovarian, lung, sarcoma, bladder, cervical, gastric, esophageal, head and neck	Arrhythmias	Rare
Docetaxel	Antimicrotubule	Breast, lung, prostate, gastric, head and neck	Arrhythmias, LV dysfunction	Uncommon
Biologic agents				
Bevacizumab	Antibody (VEGF)	Colon, rectal, cervical, glioblastoma, ovarian, renal, endometrial, sarcoma	Hypertension, LV dysfunction	Common
Trastuzumab	Antibody (HER-2)	Breast, gastric, gastro-esophageal	LV dysfunction	Common

(continued)

Table 2.1 (continued)

Agents	Drug class	Cancer clinical use	Type of cardiotoxicity	Frequency
Pertuzumab	Antibody (HER-2)	Breast	LV dysfunction	Uncommon
Alemtuzumab	Antibody (CD-52)	Leukemia, stem cell transplant	Arrhythmias	Rare
Cetuximab	Antibody (EGFR)	Colon, rectal, head and neck, lung, squamous skin	Ischemia, cardiorespiratory	Uncommon
Ramucirumab	Antibody (VEGFR-2)	Colon, rectal, gastric, lung	Hypertension, thromboembolism	Common
IL-2	Immune agent	Melanoma, renal	Capillary leak syndrome, hypotension, myocardial toxicity	Common
INF	Immune agent	Melanoma, renal, lymphoma	Arrhythmias, ischemia	Common
Tyrosine kinase inhibitors				
Sunitinib	VEGFR, PDGFR, c-Kit	Renal, thyroid, sarcoma, GIST, PNET	Hypertension, LV dysfunction, thrombosis	Common
Sorafenib	VEGFR-2, PDGFR, RAF-1, c-Kit	Hepatocellular, renal, thyroid, angiosarcoma, GIST	Hypertension, ischemia, LV dysfunction	Common
Pazopanib	VEGFR-1–3, PDGFR, FGFR-1, FGFR-3, c-Kit	Renal, sarcoma, thyroid	Hypertension, LV dysfunction, arrhythmias, ischemia, thromboembolism	Common
Axitinib	VEGFR-1–3	Renal	Hypertension, thromboembolism	Common
Lapatinib	EGFR1, HER2	Breast	LV dysfunction	Uncommon
Imatinib	BCR/ABL, PDGF, c-Kit	Leukemia, GIST, MDS, melanoma, mastocytosis, sarcoma	LV dysfunction, edema	Rare
Dasatinib	BCR/ABL, Src, c-Kit	Leukemia, GIST	Pleural effusion, LV dysfunction, arrhythmias	Uncommon
Trametinib	MEK1/MEK2	Melanoma	Hypertension, LV dysfunction	Common
Vandetanib	VEGFR-2, EGFR, RET	Thyroid	Hypertension, prolonged QT	Common
Ponatinib	BCR/ABL	Leukemia	LV dysfunction Vascular events	Rare Common

(continued)

Table 2.1 (continued)

Agents	Drug class	Cancer clinical use	Type of cardiotoxicity	Frequency
Regorafenib	VEGFR-1–3, KIT, PDGFR-α, PDGFR-β, RET, FGFR-1 and FGFR-2	Colon, rectal, GIST	Hypertension	Common
Cediranib	VEGFR-1–3, PDGFR-α/β, FGFR-1, c-Kit	Various solid tumors	Hypertension	Common
Proteasome inhibitors				
Bortezomib	26S	Multiple myeloma, mantle cell lymphoma	LV dysfunction, hypotension	Uncommon
Carfilzomib	26S	Multiple myeloma	LV dysfunction Vascular events	Uncommon Common
Decoy receptors				
Aflibercept	VEGFR-1, VEGFR-2	Colon, rectal	Hypertension	Common

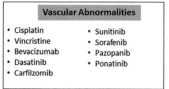

Potential Cardiotoxic Neoplastic Agents

Electrical Abnormalities
- 5-Fluorouracil
- Capecitabine
- Pentostatin
- Interferon
- Dasatinib
- Sunitinib
- Pazopanib
- Bortezomib
- Vandetanib
- Carfilzomib

Vascular Abnormalities
- Cisplatin
- Vincristine
- Bevacizumab
- Dasatinib
- Carfilzomib
- Sunitinib
- Sorafenib
- Pazopanib
- Ponatinib

Pericardial Abnormalities
- Cyclophosphamide
- Busulfan
- Clofarabine
- Cytarabine
- Dasatinib
- Imatinib
- All-trans-retinoic
- Radiation therapy

Myocardial Dysfunction
- Anthracyclins
- Cyclophosphamide
- Mitoxantrone
- Sorafenib
- Pazopanib
- Trastuzumab
- Tramatenib
- Bortezomib
- Carfilzomib

Fig. 2.1 Manifestations of cardiotoxicity with selected anticancer agents

progresses to HF. The incidence of cardiac dysfunction is directly related to the cumulative dose of anthracyclines, but it may also occur at low doses [24]. Other risk factors for the development of cardiac dysfunction include being elderly or a child at the time of drug exposure, concomitant administration of other cardiotoxic agents (such as trastuzumab), radiation therapy to the chest, and preexisting cardiovascular disease. Awareness of these risks for cardiac dysfunction may lead to the early identification and treatment of HF [25].

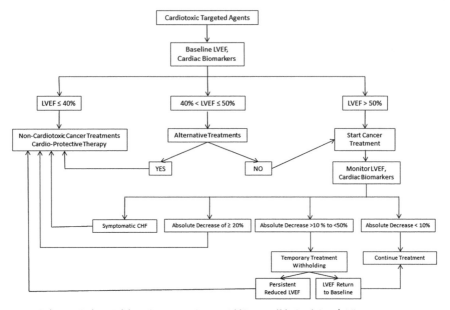

Fig. 2.2 Proposed therapeutic management of patients with anticancer therapy—induced left ventricular dysfunction

The encapsulation of doxorubicin in a liposomal moiety (pegylated liposomal doxorubicin) allows for the administration of higher cumulative doses with similar efficacy and a lower rate of HF and myocardial damage compared to doxorubicin [26]. Despite the better cardiac safety profile of liposomal doxorubicin compared to doxorubicin [clinical cardiotoxicity (odds ratio [OR] 0.18) and subclinical cardiotoxicity (relative risk [RR] 0.31)] [27], the US Food and Drug Administration (FDA) recommends routine surveillance of LVEF with the use of liposomal doxorubicin.

Dexrazoxane is an ethylenediaminetetraacetic acid (EDTA)-like chelator that binds iron and protects cardiomyocytes from the effects of doxorubicin [28]. The cardioprotective efficacy of dexrazoxane with the use with either doxorubicin or epirubicin has been clinically confirmed [27]; however, some concerns about lower response rate to chemotherapy and secondary leukemia in childhood cancer survivors have arisen [29].

Epirubicin

Epirubicin is less cardiotoxic than doxorubicin, and it is sometimes considered the preferred anthracycline [30, 31]. In comparison to doxorubicin, epirubicin significantly decreased the risks of both clinical (OR 0.39, 95 % CI [0.2–0.78]) and subclinical (OR 0.30, 95 % CI [0.16–0.57]) cardiotoxicity [27]. According to the FDA, the cumulative dose of epirubicin should be limited to 900 mg/m [2].

Alkylating Agents

Cyclophosphamide

Cyclophosphamide, which has been associated with reduced cardiac function, pericardial effusion, and decreased electrocardiographic (ECG) voltage (even without pericardial effusion) [32–34], is used in high-dose regimens that accompany stem cell transplantation [35]. The incidence of cyclophosphamide-associated cardiotoxicity is not clearly dose dependent [32, 33]. Cyclophosphamide also causes hemorrhagic myopericarditis with pericardial effusion that is attributed to endothelial capillary damage [32, 36]. These cardiac complications are mostly conservatively managed, but they can in rare instances lead to tamponade and death [32]. Factors that increase the risk of cyclophosphamide-associated cardiotoxicity include prior radiation therapy to the mediastinum or left chest wall, older age, and prior reduced LVEF.

Ifosfamide

Cardiotoxicity is infrequently reported with ifosfamide and includes cardiac arrhythmias, ST-T wave changes, and HF (dose related) [37, 38]. Most of these complications are reversible with medical management.

Cisplatin

Cisplatin-induced cardiotoxicity includes supraventricular tachycardia, bradycardia, ST-T wave changes, bundle branch block, acute ischemia with or without myocardial infarction, and cardiomyopathy [39, 40]. Cisplatin is also associated with vascular toxicities, including Raynaud's phenomenon, hypertension, and cerebral ischemic events. Electrolyte abnormalities, commonly seen with cisplatin-induced nephrotoxicity, can also contribute to cardiotoxicity.

Antimetabolite Agents

5-Fluorouracil

5-Fluorouracil (5-FU)-induced cardiotoxicity can occur in 8–20 % of treated patients [41–43]. Chest pain associated with ECG changes is the most common symptom. Other more significant manifestations include myocardial infarction and arrhythmia. Pericarditis and cardiac arrest are less common. The main pathophysiologic mechanism causing these symptoms is likely coronary artery vasospasm. Other mechanisms include endothelial cytotoxicity, myocarditis, and takotsubo cardiomyopathy [44]. Risk factors include infusion of 5-FU (vs. bolus), preexisting coronary artery disease, and concurrent use of radiation therapy or anthracyclines.

The majority of patients respond to the termination of 5-FU treatment or concurrent antianginal therapy with nitrates; however, death has been reported in a small percentage of patients [45]. Restarting therapy is usually not recommended, unless no other effective therapeutic regimens are available. The available data on calcium channel blockers or nitrates as preventative agents are conflicting [41, 46–49].

Capecitabine

Capecitabine is a prodrug that is metabolized to its active moiety, 5-FU, and has cardiotoxicity similar to that of infusional 5-FU [50]. Patients with a history of 5-FU-induced vasospasm will likely experience recurrent symptoms with capecitabine [51]. The incidence of vasospasm, including chest pain/angina, myocardial infarction, and arrhythmia, in patients receiving capecitabine ranges from 3 to 9 % [50, 52, 53]. The management of capecitabine-induced cardiotoxicity is similar to that of 5-FU-induced cardiotoxicity.

Fludarabine

Chest pain and hypotension have been reported with the use of fludarabine [54]. The combination of fludarabine and melphalan as a conditioning regimen for stem cell transplantation has been associated with cardiac dysfunction [55]. Other antimetabolite agents (cladribine, methotrexate, and cytarabine) have been rarely associated with cardiotoxicity in case reports [56–58].

Antimicrotubule Agents

Vinca Alkaloids

Cardiotoxicity is uncommon with all vinca alkaloids but may be more frequent with vinblastine than with vincristine and vinorelbine [59]; symptoms include hypertension, myocardial ischemia, infarction, and other vaso-occlusive complications [59–61].

Paclitaxel

Paclitaxel is associated with a low incidence of cardiotoxicity that includes asymptomatic bradycardia and heart block [62, 63]. Routine cardiac monitoring is not required during administration of this agent [62]. Nanoparticle albumin-bound paclitaxel (nab-paclitaxel) has the same cardiotoxicity profile as paclitaxel.

Docetaxel

Abnormal ECG and angina have been described in patients treated with docetaxel [64, 65]. Docetaxel appears to potentiate the cardiotoxicity of anthracyclines [66].

Biologic Therapy

Bevacizumab

Bevacizumab, a monoclonal antibody that binds and inactivates vascular endothelial growth factor (VEGF), exerts its anti-tumor effect by preventing microvascular angiogenesis. The most common cardiac adverse event associated with anti-VEGF therapy is hypertension [67]. Preexisting hypertension may predispose patients to worsened hypertension with bevacizumab [68]. While there has been controversy regarding the cardiotoxicity of bevacizumab [69–71], several studies and meta-analyses have identified an increased incidence of HF and decreased LVEF [71]. Early cardiotoxicity manifests as takotsubo cardiomyopathy-like events [72]. However, the pathophysiology of these events is poorly understood [73]. - Bevacizumab-induced cardiotoxicity has been noted in patients with renal cell carcinoma (RCC) [70], breast cancer [71, 74], and glioma [75]. In a meta-analysis, the risk of high-grade congestive HF in patients with breast cancer was higher in those receiving bevacizumab than in those receiving placebo (RR 4.74, 95 % CI [1.66–11.18]; $P = 0.001$), without a dose-related effect [74]. The risk of cardiotoxicity is increased when bevacizumab is combined with docetaxel or anthracycline [74, 76].

Trastuzumab

Trastuzumab is a monoclonal antibody targeting the human epidermal growth factor receptor-2 (HER2 or ErbB2) and is used for tumors that overexpress HER2 protein, including breast and gastric cancers [77–79]. One meta-analysis demonstrated that trastuzumab significantly increased the incidence of congestive HF (RR 5.11, 90 % CI [3.00–8.72]; $P < 0.00001$) and that the LVEF significantly declined after trastuzumab administration (RR 1.83, 90 % CI [1.36–2.47]; $P = 0.0008$) [80]. Trastuzumab cardiotoxicity is thought to arise from a loss of contractility (rather than from cardiomyocyte death) and thus may be reversible

[81, 82]. Risk factors for trastuzumab-induced cardiotoxicity include prior anthracycline use (worse with doxorubicin >300 mg/m^2) [24, 83], preexisting decreased LVEF, hypertension, elevated body mass index, and older age [84].

Pertuzumab

Similar to trastuzumab, pertuzumab targets HER2 (ErbB2) receptors through prevention of HER2 homodimerization [85–87]. Recent studies show a clinical benefit with the use of pertuzumab and trastuzumab combination regimens [87, 88]. The addition of pertuzumab to therapy with trastuzumab and docetaxel was not associated with increased cardiotoxicity in the CLEOPATRA trial [89], and a cardiac safety analysis of early-phase trials showed no increase in cardiotoxicity above that of trastuzumab [90]. In one study with trastuzumab and pertuzumab, one of 64 patients developed an LVEF below 40 % following the completion of therapy [91], and in another study with the same combination, 3.9 % of patients had a decrease of >10 % in their pretreatment LVEF assessment following therapy [92]. The FDA recommends assessment of LVEF prior to initiating anti-HER2 therapies such as trastuzumab and pertuzumab followed by reassessment at regular intervals (every 3 months and 6 months after discontinuation of therapy).

The general consensus is to discontinue trastuzumab plus pertuzumab therapy and reassess LVEF while considering cardioprotective treatment with accepted HF-based therapies in the event of a decrease in LVEF to <45 % or to 45–49 % with a 10 % or greater decrease from pretreatment LVEF values.

Alemtuzumab

Alemtuzumab is a monoclonal antibody targeting CD52, a cell-surface antigen present on B and T cells that, after binding, leads to antibody-dependent cell lysis. This agent is currently approved for the treatment of B-cell chronic lymphocytic leukemia and relapsing multiple sclerosis [93–95]. One study reported the development of decreased LVEF and/or arrhythmia, including atrial fibrillation and ventricular tachycardia, with the use of alemtuzumab in four of eight patients with mycosis fungoides/Sezary syndrome [96]. Recovery of decreased LVEF was seen after discontinuation of therapy in most patients [96].

Cetuximab

Cetuximab is a human/mouse chimeric monoclonal antibody that targets epidermal growth factor receptor (EGFR), resulting in the inhibition of cell growth, apoptosis, cellular VEGF production, and wild-type *KRAS* activation [97]. Cetuximab is approved for use in *KRAS* mutation-negative colorectal cancer in combination with FOLFIRI (irinotecan, 5-FU, and leucovorin) or as a single agent in refractory disease. Cetuximab-associated cardiotoxicity events observed in patients with colorectal cancer are limited. One sudden cardiac death was reported in a study of 128 patients undergoing therapy with cetuximab, oxaliplatin, and 5-FU followed by capecitabine [98]. Cetuximab is also approved for the treatment of squamous cell carcinoma of the head and neck, but an FDA black box warning exists for cardiopulmonary arrest, which has been observed in 2 % of patients treated with cetuximab and radiation and is thought to be associated with electrolyte abnormalities [99].

Ramucirumab

Ramucirumab is an antiangiogenic monoclonal antibody that targets the VEGF pathway by binding and blocking ligand-mediated activation of VEGF receptor-2 (VEGFR-2) [100–102]. In the REGARD trial, the use of ramucirumab was associated with a higher incidence of hypertension in patients treated with best supportive care plus ramucirumab compared to patients who received best supportive care plus placebo (16 % vs. 8 %, respectively). The respective rates of arterial thromboembolism were 2 % and 1 %. One patient treated with ramucirumab developed a myocardial infarction leading to death [100].

Interleukin-2

Interleukin-2 is associated with direct myocardial toxicity [103] and with capillary leak syndrome. These events result in increased cardiac output and decreased systemic vascular resistance with a systemic inflammatory response-like syndrome [104, 105], which can be managed with supportive care [106].

Interferon-Alpha

The use of interferon-alpha is associated with cardiotoxicity, mainly arrhythmias (atrial and ventricular tachycardias and heart block), which are reported in 8–20 % of cases [107–109]. One study in melanoma and RCC reported cardiomyopathy in patients treated with interferon-alpha [67, 110]. By contrast, another study demonstrated that only 1 % of patients had a decrease in LVEF [111].

Targeted Therapy

Sunitinib

Sunitinib is an oral tyrosine kinase inhibitor (TKI) targeting VEGFR, platelet-derived growth factor receptor (PDGFR), c-Kit, and fms-like tyrosine kinase-3. Sunitinib is approved by the FDA for use in RCC, advanced pancreatic neuroendocrine tumors, and imatinib-refractory gastrointestinal stromal tumor (GIST) [112]. A retrospective analysis of patients with GIST treated with sunitinib demonstrated that up to 8 % of patients developed clinically significant HF exacerbations, 28 % of patients had at least a 10 % decrease in LVEF, 9 % of patients had a 15 % or greater decrease in LVEF, and 47 % of patients developed hypertension (>150/100 mmHg) [113–115]. Additionally, hypertension preceded the development of life-threatening HF in selected patients treated with sunitinib, which emphasizes the need for the management of hypertension to prevent HF [116]. As hypertension is a common adverse event of anti-VEGF agents, blood pressure should be closely monitored and aggressively managed during all cycles of anti-VEGF-containing therapy. The decrease in LVEF is likely mediated by direct mitochondrial injury and cardiac myocyte apoptosis through inhibition of rapidly accelerated fibrosarcoma (RAF-1) kinase [113, 117] and inhibition of PDGFR coupled with systemic vasoconstriction, leading to cardiac dysfunction [118]. Sunitinib is also associated with QT prolongation and arrhythmias [119]. Preexisting HF, coronary artery disease, and lower BMI may predispose patients to these adverse cardiovascular effects related to sunitinib [120].

Sorafenib

Sorafenib is a small-molecule TKI that inhibits VEGF through inhibition of VEGFR-2, PDGFR, RAF-1, proto-oncogene B-Raf, fms-like tyrosine kinase-3, and c-Kit. Sorafenib is FDA approved for use in RCC, hepatocellular carcinoma, and well-differentiated thyroid cancer [117]. The cardiotoxicity of sorafenib is less well defined than that of sunitinib. In one study, 2.9 % of patients with RCC treated with sorafenib developed myocardial ischemia compared with 0.4 % of those treated with placebo [121]. In patients with hepatocellular carcinoma, myocardial ischemia was noted in 2.7 % of patients treated with sorafenib compared to 1.3 % of those treated with placebo [122]. One meta-analysis suggested an RR of 1.78 (95 % CI [1.09–2.92]) for the development of hypertension with the use of sorafenib [123].

Pazopanib

Pazopanib, a TKI approved for use in soft-tissue sarcoma and RCC, is thought to act through inhibition of surface VEGF receptors 1, 2, and 3, PDGF receptors, fibroblast growth factor receptor (FGFR)-1 and FGFR-3, c-Kit, transmembrane glycoprotein receptor tyrosine kinase, and interleukin-2 receptor-inducible T-cell kinase [124]. One study showed that 49 % of patients developed hypertension with pazopanib use and 6.6 % of patients showed a decrease in LVEF with therapy compared to 2.4 % of control subjects [125]. Patients receiving pazopanib also showed a concentration-independent QT prolongation [126].

Axitinib

Axitinib is a specific TKI for VEGFR-1, VEGFR-2, and VEGFR-3 and is used to treat advanced RCC. Like other VEGF-targeted TKIs, axitinib is associated with an increased risk of hypertension (all grades up to 40 %; grade 3/4, 16 %), thrombotic events, and left ventricular dysfunction [127–130].

Lapatinib

Lapatinib is an oral TKI approved for use in HER2-overexpressing breast cancer. Lapatinib inhibits EGFR (ErbB1) and HER2 (ErbB2) [79, 131] and has thus raised concerns that is has a cardiotoxic effect similar to that of trastuzumab [132]. Recent studies, including one phase III trial investigating the use of lapatinib and trastuzumab in HER2-positive breast cancer, have shown that this theoretical risk may not be a reality [133]. An additional study examining pooled data from 44 trials involving lapatinib alone or in combination with trastuzumab or anthracycline-based regimens found that fewer than 5 % of patients experienced clinically significant cardiac events and that 88 % of patients recovered to pretreatment levels (when an LVEF reduction was noted) following discontinuation of drug therapy [132]. Despite these findings, current FDA labeling recommends pretreatment LVEF evaluation, as well as discontinuation of lapatinib in the event of a decrease in LVEF to <50 %.

Imatinib

Imatinib is a BCR-ABL TKI and an inhibitor of PDGFR stem cell factor and c-Kit [134]. Shortly after its release, an initial concern about LV contractile dysfunction arose due to a suspected loss in mitochondrial membrane potential thought to be secondary to a cellular stress response induced by imatinib [135]. However, subsequent retrospective studies reviewing toxicities in 1276 patients undergoing therapy for chronic myelogenous leukemia (CML) found that imatinib-associated systolic heart failure was observed in only 0.6 % of patients and that adverse cardiovascular events were seen primarily in elderly patients who had preexisting cardiovascular disease or coronary artery disease [136, 137]. Similar findings were observed in patients receiving imatinib for GIST [138–140].

Dasatinib

Dasatinib is a small-molecule TKI that inhibits imatinib-resistant BRC-ABL kinase [141, 142]. Pleural and pericardial effusions occur with the use of dasatinib, but their mechanisms are unknown. One phase III trial comparing once- with twice-daily dosing of dasatinib in accelerated-phase CML observed 0 and 3 % incidences of congestive HF and 12.7 and 24.5 % incidences of pleural effusion, respectively [143]. Dasatinib use has also been associated with QT prolongation [144].

Trametinib

Trametinib is a selective and potent inhibitor of MEK1/MEK2 that is commonly used for the treatment of advanced melanoma with documented BRAF V600E or V600K mutations. In a phase III clinical trial of patients with melanoma, trametinib was associated with decreased LVEF or ventricular dysfunction in 7 % of patients [145]. In 1 % of the patients, these events were grade 3 cardiotoxicities, leading to the permanent discontinuation of trametinib [145]. In addition, hypertension was reported in 15 % of patients (grade 3, 12 %) [145].

Vandetanib

Vandetanib, a multi-kinase inhibitor targeting VEGFR-2, EGFR, and RET, is an effective and FDA-approved treatment for medullary thyroid carcinoma [146]. In a phase III clinical trial, vandetanib was associated with a higher risk of hypertension than placebo (32 % vs. 5 %, respectively). Grade 3/4 hypertension was noted in 9 % of patients. In addition, vandetanib was found to be associated with prolonged QTc (all grades, 14 %; grade 3/4, 8 %) [146].

Bortezomib

Bortezomib is a first-generation reversible 26S proteasome inhibitor that leads to cell cycle arrest and apoptosis and is approved for use in mantle cell lymphoma and multiple myeloma [147, 148]. An increased incidence of HF and associated symptoms has been seen with bortezomib use; however, one study suggested similar rates of HF in patients undergoing therapy for relapsed multiple myeloma with bortezomib or high-dose dexamethasone [149] and found that the effects, if present, did not appear to be dose dependent [148].

Carfilzomib

Carfilzomib is a second-generation 26S proteasome inhibitor that causes cell cycle arrest and apoptosis and is approved for use in multiple myeloma [150, 151]. Carfilzomib has been implicated in LVEF reduction, instigation of new-onset HF or exacerbation of preexisting HF, and, in limited cases, myocardial infarction. One study demonstrated that 2 of 257 patients had a myocardial infarction shortly after initiation of carfilzomib therapy and 9 (3.4 %) developed grade 3/4 dyspnea; however, the vast majority of patients in this trial had previously been treated with bortezomib [152]. Another study suggested an 11 % incidence of HF-associated symptoms following carfilzomib initiation [153]. It is likely that, similar to that with anthracyclines, the cardiac adverse events seen with carfilzomib are not limited to LV systolic dysfunction but include an increase in thrombotic events as well [154].

Ponatinib

A BCR-ABL tyrosine kinase inhibitor, ponatinib is approved for use in Philadelphia chromosome-positive acute lymphoblastic leukemia and CML [155]. One phase I study demonstrated that 1 % of patients exhibited grade 3/4 HF-like symptoms and 2 % of patients exhibited a prolonged QTc during therapy [155]. Another study suggested serious adverse vascular events, with 3 % of patients having ponatinib-associated arterial thrombotic events and 9 % of patients having arterial thrombotic events observed during therapy (although these were not necessarily considered treatment associated) [156]. Understanding the nature of these events is crucial for the future of this therapy [157].

Regorafenib

Regorafenib is a multi-kinase inhibitor approved for use in metastatic colorectal cancer and GIST that targets VEGF receptors 1–3, KIT, PDGFR-alpha, PDGFR-beta, RET, FGFR-1 and FGFR-2, TIE2, DDR2, TrkA, Eph2A, RAF-1, BRAF, $BRAF^{V600E}$, SAPK2, PTK5, and ABL [158, 159]. Although HF has not been reported with regorafenib, grade 3/4 hypertension is a frequently reported toxicity [158, 160–162].

Cediranib

Cediranib is a multi-kinase inhibitor targeting the VEGF pathway and angiogenesis through VEGFR-1, VEGFR-2, and VEGFR-3, PDGFR-alpha/PDGFR-beta, FGFR-1, and c-Kit [163]. As with other inhibitors of the VEGF pathway, hypertension is a primary toxicity of cediranib and has been identified in several studies [163–166], with one phase II study showing that 46 % of patients enrolled exhibited hypertension with grade 3 or higher toxicity [167].

Aflibercept

Aflibercept is an antiangiogenic agent acting as a decoy receptor for VEGF-A and VEGF-B and placental growth factor composed of components of VEGFR-1 and VEGFR-2 binding domains attached to the Fc portion of a human IgG-1 [168]. One trial showed a significantly increased incidence of hypertension with aflibercept treatment, with grade 3 adverse events occurring in 19 % of patients compared to 1.5 % of control subjects as well as an increased incidence of arterial-thromboembolic events (1.8 % of patients vs. 0.5 % of control subjects) and venous-thromboembolic events (7.9 % of patients vs. 6.3 % of control subjects) [168]. Other studies have also found an increased incidence of hypertension and thromboembolic events in patients receiving aflibercept [169–171].

Conclusions

The exponential development of novel therapeutics for the treatment of cancer has prompted extensive research to recognize cardiotoxicity associated with the use of these agents. Early detection and effective therapeutic management of adverse events associated with the use of anticancer drugs have led to the safe and successful development of several breakthrough FDA-approved drugs, which have improved the clinical outcomes of patients with cancer. As cardiotoxicity is a major challenge—associated with severe complications and comorbidities—in the development of novel therapeutic agents [172], rigorous monitoring for adverse events has been successful in eliminating antineoplastic agents with severe cardiotoxicity [173].

In the current review, as expected, results from clinical trials in select patient populations were not always similar to the results derived from observational studies. This difference may be attributed to patient heterogeneity and the innate differences between these types of studies. Interestingly, in many instances case reports and case series raised awareness, thereby emphasizing the need to encourage clinical investigators to publish case reports.

In conclusion, collaborative efforts between cardiologists and oncologists have decreased the incidence of severe cardiotoxicity in patients treated with potentially cardiotoxic or novel anticancer agents and promise to eliminate cardiotoxicity associated with the use of new drugs (Fig. 2.2).

References

1. Thakur A, Witteles RM. Cancer therapy-induced left ventricular dysfunction: interventions and prognosis. J Card Fail. 2014;20:155–8.
2. Cardinale D, Colombo A, Torrisi R, Sandri MT, Civelli M, Salvatici M, Lamantia G, Colombo N, Cortinovis S, Dessanai MA, Nole F, Veglia F, Cipolla CM. Trastuzumab-induced cardiotoxicity: clinical and prognostic implications of troponin I evaluation. J Clin Oncol. 2010;28:3910–6.
3. Herrmann J, Lerman A, Sandhu NP, Villarraga HR, Mulvagh SL, Kohli M. Evaluation and management of patients with heart disease and cancer: cardio-oncology. Mayo Clin Proc. 2014;89:1287–306.
4. Nakamae H, Tsumura K, Terada Y, Nakane T, Nakamae M, Ohta K, Yamane T, Hino M. Notable effects of angiotensin II receptor blocker, valsartan, on acute cardiotoxic changes after standard chemotherapy with cyclophosphamide, doxorubicin, vincristine, and prednisolone. Cancer. 2005;104:2492–8.
5. Wells QS, Lenihan DJ. Reversibility of left ventricular dysfunction resulting from chemotherapy: can this be expected? Prog Cardiovasc Dis. 2010;53:140–8.
6. Albini A, Pennesi G, Donatelli F, Cammarota R, De Flora S, Noonan DM. Cardiotoxicity of anticancer drugs: the need for cardio-oncology and cardio-oncological prevention. J Natl Cancer Inst. 2010;102:14–25.
7. Lefrak EA, Pitha J, Rosenheim S, Gottlieb JA. A clinicopathologic analysis of adriamycin cardiotoxicity. Cancer. 1973;32:302–14.
8. Von Hoff DD, Layard MW, Basa P, Davis Jr HL, Von Hoff AL, Rozencweig M, Muggia FM. Risk factors for doxorubicin-induced congestive heart failure. Ann Intern Med. 1979;91:710–7.
9. Swain SM, Whaley FS, Ewer MS. Congestive heart failure in patients treated with doxorubicin: a retrospective analysis of three trials. Cancer. 2003;97:2869–79.
10. Gianni L, Herman EH, Lipshultz SE, Minotti G, Sarvazyan N, Sawyer DB. Anthracycline cardiotoxicity: from bench to bedside. J Clin Oncol. 2008;26:3777–84.
11. Zhang S, Liu X, Bawa-Khalfe T, Lu LS, Lyu YL, Liu LF, Yeh ET. Identification of the molecular basis of doxorubicin-induced cardiotoxicity. Nat Med. 2012;18:1639–42.
12. Wojnowski L, Kulle B, Schirmer M, Schluter G, Schmidt A, Rosenberger A, Vonhof S, Bickeboller H, Toliat MR, Suk EK, Tzvetkov M, Kruger A, Seifert S, Kloess M, Hahn H, Loeffler M, Nurnberg P, Pfreundschuh M, Trumper L, Brockmoller J, Hasenfuss G. NAD(P) H oxidase and multidrug resistance protein genetic polymorphisms are associated with doxorubicin-induced cardiotoxicity. Circulation. 2005;112:3754–62.
13. Singal PK, Iliskovic N. Doxorubicin-induced cardiomyopathy. N Engl J Med. 1998;339:900–5.
14. Isner JM, Ferrans VJ, Cohen SR, Witkind BG, Virmani R, Gottdiener JS, Beck JR, Roberts WC. Clinical and morphologic cardiac findings after anthracycline chemotherapy. Analysis of 64 patients studied at necropsy. Am J Cardiol. 1983;51:1167–74.
15. Guglin M, Aljayeh M, Saiyad S, Ali R, Curtis AB. Introducing a new entity: chemotherapy-induced arrhythmia. Europace. 2009;11:1579–86.
16. Shan K, Lincoff AM, Young JB. Anthracycline-induced cardiotoxicity. Ann Intern Med. 1996;125:47–58.

17. Steinberg JS, Cohen AJ, Wasserman AG, Cohen P, Ross AM. Acute arrhythmogenicity of doxorubicin administration. Cancer. 1987;60:1213–8.

18. Tirelli U, Errante D, Van Glabbeke M, Teodorovic I, Kluin-Nelemans JC, Thomas J, Bron D, Rosti G, Somers R, Zagonel V, Noordijk EM. CHOP is the standard regimen in patients > or = 70 years of age with intermediate-grade and high-grade non-Hodgkin's lymphoma: results of a randomized study of the European Organization for Research and Treatment of Cancer Lymphoma Cooperative Study Group. J Clin Oncol. 1998;16:27–34.

19. Luminari S, Montanini A, Caballero D, Bologna S, Notter M, Dyer MJ, Chiappella A, Briones J, Petrini M, Barbato A, Kayitalire L, Federico M. Nonpegylated liposomal doxorubicin (MyocetTM) combination (R-COMP) chemotherapy in elderly patients with diffuse large B-cell lymphoma (DLBCL): results from the phase II EUR018 trial. Ann Oncol. 2010;21:1492–9.

20. Cardinale D, Sandri MT, Martinoni A, Tricca A, Civelli M, Lamantia G, Cinieri S, Martinelli G, Cipolla CM, Fiorentini C. Left ventricular dysfunction predicted by early troponin I release after high-dose chemotherapy. J Am Coll Cardiol. 2000;36:517–22.

21. Von Hoff DD, Rozencweig M, Layard M, Slavik M, Muggia FM. Daunomycin-induced cardiotoxicity in children and adults. A review of 110 cases. Am J Med. 1977;62:200–8.

22. Lipshultz SE, Colan SD, Gelber RD, Perez-Atayde AR, Sallan SE, Sanders SP. Late cardiac effects of doxorubicin therapy for acute lymphoblastic leukemia in childhood. N Engl J Med. 1991;324:808–15.

23. van der Pal HJ, van Dalen EC, Hauptmann M, Kok WE, Caron HN, van den Bos C, Oldenburger F, Koning CC, van Leeuwen FE, Kremer LC. Cardiac function in 5-year survivors of childhood cancer: a long-term follow-up study. Arch Intern Med. 2010;170:1247–55.

24. Bowles EJ, Wellman R, Feigelson HS, Onitilo AA, Freedman AN, Delate T, Allen LA, Nekhlyudov L, Goddard KA, Davis RL, Habel LA, Yood MU, McCarty C, Magid DJ, Wagner EH, Pharmacovigilance ST. Risk of heart failure in breast cancer patients after anthracycline and trastuzumab treatment: a retrospective cohort study. J Natl Cancer Inst. 2012;104:1293–305.

25. Cardinale D, Colombo A, Lamantia G, Colombo N, Civelli M, De Giacomi G, Rubino M, Veglia F, Fiorentini C, Cipolla CM. Anthracycline-induced cardiomyopathy: clinical relevance and response to pharmacologic therapy. J Am Coll Cardiol. 2010;55:213–20.

26. Safra T, Muggia F, Jeffers S, Tsao-Wei DD, Groshen S, Lyass O, Henderson R, Berry G, Gabizon A. Pegylated liposomal doxorubicin (doxil): reduced clinical cardiotoxicity in patients reaching or exceeding cumulative doses of 500 mg/m2. Ann Oncol. 2000;11:1029–33.

27. Smith LA, Cornelius VR, Plummer CJ, Levitt G, Verrill M, Canney P, Jones A. Cardiotoxicity of anthracycline agents for the treatment of cancer: systematic review and meta-analysis of randomised controlled trials. BMC Cancer. 2010;10:337.

28. Seifert CF, Nesser ME, Thompson DF. Dexrazoxane in the prevention of doxorubicin-induced cardiotoxicity. Ann Pharmacother. 1994;28:1063–72.

29. Meadows AT, Friedman DL, Neglia JP, Mertens AC, Donaldson SS, Stovall M, Hammond S, Yasui Y, Inskip PD. Second neoplasms in survivors of childhood cancer: findings from the Childhood Cancer Survivor Study cohort. J Clin Oncol. 2009;27:2356–62.

30. Nair R, Ramakrishnan G, Nair NN, Saikia TK, Parikh PM, Joshi SR, Soman CS, Mukhadan M, Dinshaw KT, Advani SH. A randomized comparison of the efficacy and toxicity of epirubicin and doxorubicin in the treatment of patients with non-Hodgkin's lymphoma. Cancer. 1998;82:2282–8.

31. Ryberg M, Nielsen D, Skovsgaard T, Hansen J, Jensen BV, Dombernowsky P. Epirubicin cardiotoxicity: an analysis of 469 patients with metastatic breast cancer. J Clin Oncol. 1998;16:3502–8.

32. Gottdiener JS, Appelbaum FR, Ferrans VJ, Deisseroth A, Ziegler J. Cardiotoxicity associated with high-dose cyclophosphamide therapy. Arch Intern Med. 1981;141:758–63.

33. Braverman AC, Antin JH, Plappert MT, Cook EF, Lee RT. Cyclophosphamide cardiotoxicity in bone marrow transplantation: a prospective evaluation of new dosing regimens. J Clin Oncol. 1991;9:1215–23.
34. Lichtman SM, Ratain MJ, Van Echo DA, Rosner G, Egorin MJ, Budman DR, Vogelzang NJ, Norton L, Schilsky RL. Phase I trial of granulocyte-macrophage colony-stimulating factor plus high-dose cyclophosphamide given every 2 weeks: a Cancer and Leukemia Group B study. J Natl Cancer Inst. 1993;85:1319–26.
35. Zver S, Zadnik V, Bunc M, Rogel P, Cernelc P, Kozelj M. Cardiac toxicity of high-dose cyclophosphamide in patients with multiple myeloma undergoing autologous hematopoietic stem cell transplantation. Int J Hematol. 2007;85:408–14.
36. Appelbaum F, Strauchen JA, Graw Jr RG, Savage DD, Kent KM, Ferrans VJ, Herzig GP. Acute lethal carditis caused by high-dose combination chemotherapy. A unique clinical and pathological entity. Lancet. 1976;1:58–62.
37. Quezado ZM, Wilson WH, Cunnion RE, Parker MM, Reda D, Bryant G, Ognibene FP. High-dose ifosfamide is associated with severe, reversible cardiac dysfunction. Ann Intern Med. 1993;118:31–6.
38. Kandylis K, Vassilomanolakis M, Tsoussis S, Efremidis AP. Ifosfamide cardiotoxicity in humans. Cancer Chemother Pharmacol. 1989;24:395–6.
39. Tomirotti M, Riundi R, Pulici S, Ungaro A, Pedretti D, Villa S, Scanni A. Ischemic cardiopathy from cis-diamminedichloroplatinum (CDDP). Tumori. 1984;70:235–6.
40. Mortimer JE, Crowley J, Eyre H, Weiden P, Eltringham J, Stuckey WJ. A phase II randomized study comparing sequential and combined intraarterial cisplatin and radiation therapy in primary brain tumors. A southwest oncology group study. Cancer. 1992;69:1220–3.
41. Anand AJ. Fluorouracil cardiotoxicity. Ann Pharmacother. 1994;28:374–8.
42. de Forni M, Malet-Martino MC, Jaillais P, Shubinski RE, Bachaud JM, Lemaire L, Canal P, Chevreau C, Carrie D, Soulie P, et al. Cardiotoxicity of high-dose continuous infusion fluorouracil: a prospective clinical study. J Clin Oncol. 1992;10:1795–801.
43. Wacker A, Lersch C, Scherpinski U, Reindl L, Seyfarth M. High incidence of angina pectoris in patients treated with 5-fluorouracil. A planned surveillance study with 102 patients. Oncology. 2003;65:108–12.
44. Grunwald MR, Howie L, Diaz Jr LA. Takotsubo cardiomyopathy and Fluorouracil: case report and review of the literature. J Clin Oncol. 2012;30:e11–4.
45. Saif MW, Shah MM, Shah AR. Fluoropyrimidine-associated cardiotoxicity: revisited. Expert Opin Drug Saf. 2009;8:191–202.
46. Cianci G, Morelli MF, Cannita K, Morese R, Ricevuto E, Di Rocco ZC, Porzio G, Lanfiuti Baldi P, Ficorella C. Prophylactic options in patients with 5-fluorouracil-associated cardiotoxicity. Br J Cancer. 2003;88:1507–9.
47. Akpek G, Hartshorn KL. Failure of oral nitrate and calcium channel blocker therapy to prevent 5-fluorouracil-related myocardial ischemia: a case report. Cancer Chemother Pharmacol. 1999;43:157–61.
48. Oleksowicz L, Bruckner HW. Prophylaxis of 5-fluorouracil-induced coronary vasospasm with calcium channel blockers. Am J Med. 1988;85:750–1.
49. Kleiman NS, Lehane DE, Geyer Jr CE, Pratt CM, Young JB. Prinzmetal's angina during 5-fluorouracil chemotherapy. Am J Med. 1987;82:566–8.
50. Ng M, Cunningham D, Norman AR. The frequency and pattern of cardiotoxicity observed with capecitabine used in conjunction with oxaliplatin in patients treated for advanced colorectal cancer (CRC). Eur J Cancer. 2005;41:1542–6.
51. Frickhofen N, Beck FJ, Jung B, Fuhr HG, Andrasch H, Sigmund M. Capecitabine can induce acute coronary syndrome similar to 5-fluorouracil. Ann Oncol. 2002;13:797–801.
52. Van Cutsem E, Hoff PM, Blum JL, Abt M, Osterwalder B. Incidence of cardiotoxicity with the oral fluoropyrimidine capecitabine is typical of that reported with 5-fluorouracil. Ann Oncol. 2002;13:484–5.

53. Saif MW, Tomita M, Ledbetter L, Diasio RB. Capecitabine-related cardiotoxicity: recognition and management. J Support Oncol. 2008;6:41–8.
54. Gutheil JFD. Antimetabolites. In: Perry MC editor. The chemotherapy sourcebook, 3rd edn. Lippincott, Williams and Wilkins, Philadelphia.
55. Van Besien K, Devine S, Wickrema A, Jessop E, Amin K, Yassine M, Maynard V, Stock W, Peace D, Ravandi F, Chen YH, Hoffman R, Sossman J. Regimen-related toxicity after fludarabine-melphalan conditioning: a prospective study of 31 patients with hematologic malignancies. Bone Marrow Transplant. 2003;32:471–6.
56. Grem JL, King SA, Chun HG, Grever MR. Cardiac complications observed in elderly patients following 2'-deoxycoformycin therapy. Am J Hematol. 1991;38:245–7.
57. Perez-Verdia A, Angulo F, Hardwicke FL, Nugent KM. Acute cardiac toxicity associated with high-dose intravenous methotrexate therapy: case report and review of the literature. Pharmacotherapy. 2005;25:1271–6.
58. Hermans C, Straetmans N, Michaux JL, Ferrant A. Pericarditis induced by high-dose cytosine arabinoside chemotherapy. Ann Hematol. 1997;75:55–7.
59. Kantor AF, Greene MH, Boice JD, Fraumeni Jr JF, Flannery JT. Are vinca alkaloids associated with myocardial infarction? Lancet. 1981;1:1111.
60. Zabernigg A, Gattringer C. Myocardial infarction associated with vinorelbine (Navelbine). Eur J Cancer. 1996;32A:1618–9.
61. Mandel EM, Lewinski U, Djaldetti M. Vincristine-induced myocardial infarction. Cancer. 1975;36:1979–82.
62. Arbuck SG, Strauss H, Rowinsky E, Christian M, Suffness M, Adams J, Oakes M, McGuire W, Reed E, Gibbs H, et al. A reassessment of cardiac toxicity associated with Taxol. J Natl Cancer Inst Monogr. 1993:117–30.
63. Rowinsky EK, McGuire WP, Guarnieri T, Fisherman JS, Christian MC, Donehower RC. Cardiac disturbances during the administration of taxol. J Clin Oncol. 1991;9:1704–12.
64. Fossella FV, Lee JS, Murphy WK, Lippman SM, Calayag M, Pang A, Chasen M, Shin DM, Glisson B, Benner S, et al. Phase II study of docetaxel for recurrent or metastatic non-small-cell lung cancer. J Clin Oncol. 1994;12:1238–44.
65. Francis P, Schneider J, Hann L, Balmaceda C, Barakat R, Phillips M, Hakes T. Phase II trial of docetaxel in patients with platinum-refractory advanced ovarian cancer. J Clin Oncol. 1994;12:2301–8.
66. Malhotra V, Dorr VJ, Lyss AP, Anderson CM, Westgate S, Reynolds M, Barrett B, Perry MC. Neoadjuvant and adjuvant chemotherapy with doxorubicin and docetaxel in locally advanced breast cancer. Clin Breast Cancer. 2004;5:377–84.
67. des Guetz G, Uzzan B, Chouahnia K, Morere JF. Cardiovascular toxicity of anti-angiogenic drugs. Target Oncol. 2011;6:197–202.
68. Wicki A, Hermann F, Pretre V, Winterhalder R, Kueng M, von Moos R, Rochlitz C, Herrmann R. Pre-existing antihypertensive treatment predicts early increase in blood pressure during bevacizumab therapy: the prospective AVALUE cohort study. Oncol Res Treat. 2014;37:230–6.
69. Hurvitz SA, Bosserman LD, Chan D, Hagenstad CT, Kass FC, Smith FP, Rodriguez GI, Childs BH, Slamon DJ. Cardiac safety results from a phase II, open-label, multicenter, pilot study of two docetaxel-based regimens plus bevacizumab for the adjuvant treatment of subjects with node-positive or high-risk node-negative breast cancer. Springerplus. 2014;3:244.
70. Hall PS, Harshman LC, Srinivas S, Witteles RM. The frequency and severity of cardiovascular toxicity from targeted therapy in advanced renal cell carcinoma patients. JACC Heart Failure. 2013;1:72–8.
71. Qi WX, Fu S, Zhang Q, Guo XM. Bevacizumab increases the risk of severe congestive heart failure in cancer patients: an up-to-date meta-analysis with a focus on different subgroups. Clin Drug Investig. 2014;34:681–90.

72. Franco TH, Khan A, Joshi V, Thomas B. Takotsubo cardiomyopathy in two men receiving bevacizumab for metastatic cancer. Ther Clin Risk Manag. 2008;4:1367–70.
73. Groarke JD, Choueiri TK, Slosky D, Cheng S, Moslehi J. Recognizing and managing left ventricular dysfunction associated with therapeutic inhibition of the vascular endothelial growth factor signaling pathway. Curr Treat Options Cardiovasc Med. 2014;16:335.
74. Choueiri TK, Mayer EL, Je Y, Rosenberg JE, Nguyen PL, Azzi GR, Bellmunt J, Burstein HJ, Schutz FA. Congestive heart failure risk in patients with breast cancer treated with bevacizumab. J Clin Oncol. 2011;29:632–8.
75. Nagane M, Nishikawa R, Narita Y, Kobayashi H, Takano S, Shinoura N, Aoki T, Sugiyama K, Kuratsu J, Muragaki Y, Sawamura Y, Matsutani M. Phase II study of single-agent bevacizumab in Japanese patients with recurrent malignant glioma. Jpn J Clin Oncol. 2012;42:887–95.
76. Yardley DA, Hart L, Waterhouse D, Whorf R, Drosick DR, Murphy P, Badarinath S, Daniel BR, Childs BH, Burris H. Addition of bevacizumab to three docetaxel regimens as adjuvant therapy for early stage breast cancer. Breast Cancer Res Treat. 2013;142:655–65.
77. Andersson M, Lidbrink E, Bjerre K, Wist E, Enevoldsen K, Jensen AB, Karlsson P, Tange UB, Sorensen PG, Moller S, Bergh J, Langkjer ST. Phase III randomized study comparing docetaxel plus trastuzumab with vinorelbine plus trastuzumab as first-line therapy of metastatic or locally advanced human epidermal growth factor receptor 2-positive breast cancer: the HERNATA study. J Clin Oncol. 2011;29:264–71.
78. Bang YJ, Van Cutsem E, Feyereislova A, Chung HC, Shen L, Sawaki A, Lordick F, Ohtsu A, Omuro Y, Satoh T, Aprile G, Kulikov E, Hill J, Lehle M, Ruschoff J, Kang YK. Trastuzumab in combination with chemotherapy versus chemotherapy alone for treatment of HER2-positive advanced gastric or gastro-oesophageal junction cancer (ToGA): a phase 3, open-label, randomised controlled trial. Lancet. 2010;376:687–97.
79. Blackwell KL, Burstein HJ, Storniolo AM, Rugo HS, Sledge G, Aktan G, Ellis C, Florance A, Vukelja S, Bischoff J, Baselga J, O'Shaughnessy J. Overall survival benefit with lapatinib in combination with trastuzumab for patients with human epidermal growth factor receptor 2-positive metastatic breast cancer: final results from the EGF104900 Study. J Clin Oncol. 2012;30:2585–92.
80. Moja L, Tagliabue L, Balduzzi S, Parmelli E, Pistotti V, Guarneri V, D'Amico R. Trastuzumab containing regimens for early breast cancer. Cochrane Datab Syst Rev. 2012;4:Cd006243.
81. Ewer MS, Lippman SM. Type II chemotherapy-related cardiac dysfunction: time to recognize a new entity. J Clin Oncol. 2005;23:2900–2.
82. Romond EH, Jeong JH, Rastogi P, Swain SM, Geyer CE, Jr., Ewer MS, Rathi V, Fehrenbacher L, Brufsky A, Azar CA, Flynn PJ, Zapas JL, Polikoff J, Gross HM, Biggs DD, Atkins JN, Tan-Chiu E, Zheng P, Yothers G, Mamounas EP, Wolmark N. Seven-year follow-up assessment of cardiac function in NSABP B-31, a randomized trial comparing doxorubicin and cyclophosphamide followed by paclitaxel (ACP) with ACP plus trastuzumab as adjuvant therapy for patients with node-positive, human epidermal growth factor receptor 2-positive breast cancer. J Clin Oncol. 2012;30:3792–9.
83. Russell SD, Blackwell KL, Lawrence J, Pippen JE Jr., Roe MT, Wood F, Paton V, Holmgren E, Mahaffey KW. Independent adjudication of symptomatic heart failure with the use of doxorubicin and cyclophosphamide followed by trastuzumab adjuvant therapy: a combined review of cardiac data from the National Surgical Adjuvant breast and Bowel Project B-31 and the North Central Cancer Treatment Group N9831 clinical trials. J Clin Oncol. 2010;28:3416–21.
84. Perez EA, Suman VJ, Davidson NE, Sledge GW, Kaufman PA, Hudis CA, Martino S, Gralow JR, Dakhil SR, Ingle JN, Winer EP, Gelmon KA, Gersh BJ, Jaffe AS, Rodeheffer RJ. Cardiac safety analysis of doxorubicin and cyclophosphamide followed by paclitaxel with or without trastuzumab in the North Central Cancer Treatment Group N9831 adjuvant breast cancer trial. J Clin Oncol. 2008;26:1231–8.

85. Agus DB, Gordon MS, Taylor C, Natale RB, Karlan B, Mendelson DS, Press MF, Allison DE, Sliwkowski MX, Lieberman G, Kelsey SM, Fyfe G. Phase I clinical study of pertuzumab, a novel HER dimerization inhibitor, in patients with advanced cancer. J Clin Oncol. 2005;23:2534–43.
86. Baselga J, Cortes J, Kim SB, Im SA, Hegg R, Im YH, Roman L, Pedrini JL, Pienkowski T, Knott A, Clark E, Benyunes MC, Ross G, Swain SM. Pertuzumab plus trastuzumab plus docetaxel for metastatic breast cancer. N Engl J Med. 2012;366:109–19.
87. Baselga J, Gelmon KA, Verma S, Wardley A, Conte P, Miles D, Bianchi G, Cortes J, McNally VA, Ross GA, Fumoleau P, Gianni L. Phase II trial of pertuzumab and trastuzumab in patients with human epidermal growth factor receptor 2-positive metastatic breast cancer that progressed during prior trastuzumab therapy. J Clin Oncol. 2010;28:1138–44.
88. Swain SM, Baselga J, Kim SB, Ro J, Semiglazov V, Campone M, Ciruelos E, Ferrero JM, Schneeweiss A, Heeson S, Clark E, Ross G, Benyunes MC, Cortes J. Pertuzumab, trastuzumab, and docetaxel in HER2-positive metastatic breast cancer. N Engl J Med. 2015;372:724–34.
89. Swain SM, Ewer MS, Cortes J, Amadori D, Miles D, Knott A, Clark E, Benyunes MC, Ross G, Baselga J. Cardiac tolerability of pertuzumab plus trastuzumab plus docetaxel in patients with HER2-positive metastatic breast cancer in CLEOPATRA: a randomized, double-blind, placebo-controlled phase III study. Oncologist. 2013;18:257–64.
90. Lenihan D, Suter T, Brammer M, Neate C, Ross G, Baselga J. Pooled analysis of cardiac safety in patients with cancer treated with pertuzumab. Ann Oncol. 2012;23:791–800.
91. Miller KD, Dieras V, Harbeck N, Andre F, Mahtani RL, Gianni L, Albain KS, Crivellari D, Fang L, Michelson G, de Haas SL, Burris HA. Phase IIa trial of trastuzumab emtansine with pertuzumab for patients with human epidermal growth factor receptor 2-positive, locally advanced, or metastatic breast cancer. J Clin Oncol. 2014;32:1437–44.
92. Schneeweiss A, Chia S, Hickish T, Harvey V, Eniu A, Hegg R, Tausch C, Seo JH, Tsai YF, Ratnayake J, McNally V, Ross G, Cortes J. Pertuzumab plus trastuzumab in combination with standard neoadjuvant anthracycline-containing and anthracycline-free chemotherapy regimens in patients with HER2-positive early breast cancer: a randomized phase II cardiac safety study (TRYPHAENA). Ann Oncol. 2013;24:2278–84.
93. Dearden CE, Johnson R, Pettengell R, Devereux S, Cwynarski K, Whittaker S, McMillan A. Guidelines for the management of mature T-cell and NK-cell neoplasms (excluding cutaneous T-cell lymphoma). Br J Haematol. 2011;153:451–85.
94. Coles AJ, Compston DA, Selmaj KW, Lake SL, Moran S, Margolin DH, Norris K, Tandon PK. Alemtuzumab vs. interferon beta-1a in early multiple sclerosis. N Engl J Med. 2008;359:1786–801.
95. Ferrajoli A, O'Brien SM, Cortes JE, Giles FJ, Thomas DA, Faderl S, Kurzrock R, Lerner S, Kontoyiannis DP, Keating MJ. Phase II study of alemtuzumab in chronic lymphoproliferative disorders. Cancer. 2003;98:773–8.
96. Lenihan DJ, Alencar AJ, Yang D, Kurzrock R, Keating MJ, Duvic M. Cardiac toxicity of alemtuzumab in patients with mycosis fungoides/Sezary syndrome. Blood. 2004;104:655–8.
97. Jonker DJ, O'Callaghan CJ, Karapetis CS, Zalcberg JR, Tu D, Au HJ, Berry SR, Krahn M, Price T, Simes RJ, Tebbutt NC, van Hazel G, Wierzbicki R, Langer C, Moore MJ. Cetuximab for the treatment of colorectal cancer. N Engl J Med. 2007;357:2040–8.
98. Primrose J, Falk S, Finch-Jones M, Valle J, O'Reilly D, Siriwardena A, Hornbuckle J, Peterson M, Rees M, Iveson T, Hickish T, Butler R, Stanton L, Dixon E, Little L, Bowers M, Pugh S, Garden OJ, Cunningham D, Maughan T, Bridgewater J. Systemic chemotherapy with or without cetuximab in patients with resectable colorectal liver metastasis: the New EPOC randomised controlled trial. Lancet Oncol. 2014;15:601–11.
99. Bonner JA, Harari PM, Giralt J, Azarnia N, Shin DM, Cohen RB, Jones CU, Sur R, Raben D, Jassem J, Ove R, Kies MS, Baselga J, Youssoufian H, Amellal N, Rowinsky EK, Ang KK. Radiotherapy plus cetuximab for squamous-cell carcinoma of the head and neck. N Engl J Med. 2006;354:567–78.

100. Fuchs CS, Tomasek J, Yong CJ, Dumitru F, Passalacqua R, Goswami C, Safran H, dos Santos LV, Aprile G, Ferry DR, Melichar B, Tehfe M, Topuzov E, Zalcberg JR, Chau I, Campbell W, Sivan andan C, Pikiel J, Koshiji M, Hsu Y, Liepa AM, Gao L, Schwartz JD, Tabernero J. Ramucirumab monotherapy for previously treated advanced gastric or gastro-oesophageal junction adenocarcinoma (REGARD): an international, randomised, multicentre, placebo-controlled, phase 3 trial. Lancet. 2014;383:31–9.
101. Wilke H, Muro K, Van Cutsem E, Oh SC, Bodoky G, Shimada Y, Hironaka S, Sugimoto N, Lipatov O, Kim TY, Cunningham D, Rougier P, Komatsu Y, Ajani J, Emig M, Carlesi R, Ferry D, Chandrawansa K, Schwartz JD, Ohtsu A. Ramucirumab plus paclitaxel versus placebo plus paclitaxel in patients with previously treated advanced gastric or gastro-oesophageal junction adenocarcinoma (RAINBOW): a double-blind, randomised phase 3 trial. Lancet Oncol. 2014;15:1224–35.
102. Garon EB, Ciuleanu TE, Arrieta O, Prabhash K, Syrigos KN, Goksel T, Park K, Gorbunova V, Kowalyszyn RD, Pikiel J, Czyzewicz G, Orlov SV, Lewanski CR, Thomas M, Bidoli P, Dakhil S, Gans S, Kim JH, Grigorescu A, Karaseva N, Reck M, Cappuzzo F, Alexandris E, Sashegyi A, Yurasov S, Perol M. Ramucirumab plus docetaxel versus placebo plus docetaxel for second-line treatment of stage IV non-small-cell lung cancer after disease progression on platinum-based therapy (REVEL): a multicentre, double-blind, randomised phase 3 trial. Lancet. 2014;384:665–73.
103. Margolin KA, Rayner AA, Hawkins MJ, Atkins MB, Dutcher JP, Fisher RI, Weiss GR, Doroshow JH, Jaffe HS, Roper M, et al. Interleukin-2 and lymphokine-activated killer cell therapy of solid tumors: analysis of toxicity and management guidelines. J Clin Oncol. 1989;7:486–98.
104. Lee RE, Lotze MT, Skibber JM, Tucker E, Bonow RO, Ognibene FP, Carrasquillo JA, Shelhamer JH, Parrillo JE, Rosenberg SA. Cardiorespiratory effects of immunotherapy with interleukin-2. J Clin Oncol. 1989;7:7–20.
105. Weiss GR, Margolin KA, Aronson FR, Sznol M, Atkins MB, Dutcher JP, Gaynor ER, Boldt DH, Doroshow JH, Bar MH, et al. A randomized phase II trial of continuous infusion interleukin-2 or bolus injection interleukin-2 plus lymphokine-activated killer cells for advanced renal cell carcinoma. J Clin Oncol. 1992;10:275–81.
106. White Jr RL, Schwartzentruber DJ, Guleria A, MacFarlane MP, White DE, Tucker E, Rosenberg SA. Cardiopulmonary toxicity of treatment with high dose interleukin-2 in 199 consecutive patients with metastatic melanoma or renal cell carcinoma. Cancer. 1994;74:3212–22.
107. Atkins MB, Hsu J, Lee S, Cohen GI, Flaherty LE, Sosman JA, Sondak VK, Kirkwood JM. Phase III trial comparing concurrent biochemotherapy with cisplatin, vinblastine, dacarbazine, interleukin-2, and interferon alfa-2b with cisplatin, vinblastine, and dacarbazine alone in patients with metastatic malignant melanoma (E3695): a trial coordinated by the Eastern Cooperative Oncology Group. J Clin Oncol. 2008;26:5748–54.
108. Kruit WH, Punt KJ, Goey SH, de Mulder PH, van Hoogenhuyze DC, Henzen-Logmans SC, Stoter G. Cardiotoxicity as a dose-limiting factor in a schedule of high dose bolus therapy with interleukin-2 and alpha-interferon. An unexpectedly frequent complication. Cancer. 1994;74:2850–6.
109. Kruit WH, Goey SH, Lamers CH, Gratama JW, Visser B, Schmitz PI, Eggermont AM, Bolhuis RL, Stoter G. High-dose regimen of interleukin-2 and interferon-alpha in combination with lymphokine-activated killer cells in patients with metastatic renal cell cancer. J Immunother. 1997;20:312–20.
110. Khakoo AY, Halushka MK, Rame JE, Rodriguez ER, Kasper EK, Judge DP. Reversible cardiomyopathy caused by administration of interferon alpha. Nat Clin Pract Cardiovasc Med. 2005;2:53–7.
111. Motzer RJ, Hutson TE, Tomczak P, Michaelson MD, Bukowski RM, Rixe O, Oudard S, Negrier S, Szczylik C, Kim ST, Chen I, Bycott PW, Baum CM, Figlin RA. Sunitinib versus interferon alfa in metastatic renal-cell carcinoma. N Engl J Med. 2007;356:115–24.

112. Force T, Kolaja KL. Cardiotoxicity of kinase inhibitors: the prediction and translation of preclinical models to clinical outcomes. Nat Rev Drug Discov. 2011;10:111–26.
113. Chu TF, Rupnick MA, Kerkela R, Dallabrida SM, Zurakowski D, Nguyen L, Woulfe K, Pravda E, Cassiola F, Desai J, George S, Morgan JA, Harris DM, Ismail NS, Chen JH, Schoen FJ, Van den Abbeele AD, Demetri GD, Force T, Chen MH. Cardiotoxicity associated with tyrosine kinase inhibitor sunitinib. Lancet. 2007;370:2011–9.
114. Zhu X, Stergiopoulos K, Wu S. Risk of hypertension and renal dysfunction with an angiogenesis inhibitor sunitinib: systematic review and meta-analysis. Acta Oncol. (Stockholm, Sweden). 2009;48:9–17.
115. Wu S, Chen JJ, Kudelka A, Lu J, Zhu X. Incidence and risk of hypertension with sorafenib in patients with cancer: a systematic review and meta-analysis. Lancet Oncol. 2008;9:117–23.
116. Khakoo AY, Kassiotis CM, Tannir N, Plana JC, Halushka M, Bickford C, Trent 2nd J, Champion JC, Durand JB, Lenihan DJ. Heart failure associated with sunitinib malate: a multitargeted receptor tyrosine kinase inhibitor. Cancer. 2008;112:2500–8.
117. Ratain MJ, Eisen T, Stadler WM, Flaherty KT, Kaye SB, Rosner GL, Gore M, Desai AA, Patnaik A, Xiong HQ, Rowinsky E, Abbruzzese JL, Xia C, Simantov R, Schwartz B, O'Dwyer PJ. Phase II placebo-controlled randomized discontinuation trial of sorafenib in patients with metastatic renal cell carcinoma. J Clin Oncol. 2006;24:2505–12.
118. Chintalgattu V, Ai D, Langley RR, Zhang J, Bankson JA, Shih TL, Reddy AK, Coombes KR, Daher IN, Pati S, Patel SS, Pocius JS, Taffet GE, Buja LM, Entman ML, Khakoo AY. Cardiomyocyte PDGFR-beta signaling is an essential component of the mouse cardiac response to load-induced stress. J Clin Invest. 2010;120:472–84.
119. Shah RR, Morganroth J, Shah DR. Cardiovascular safety of tyrosine kinase inhibitors: with a special focus on cardiac repolarisation (QT interval). Drug Saf. 2013;36:295–316.
120. Telli ML, Witteles RM, Fisher GA, Srinivas S. Cardiotoxicity associated with the cancer therapeutic agent sunitinib malate. Ann Oncol. 2008;19:1613–8.
121. Escudier B, Eisen T, Stadler WM, Szczylik C, Oudard S, Siebels M, Negrier S, Chevreau C, Solska E, Desai AA, Rolland F, Demkow T, Hutson TE, Gore M, Freeman S, Schwartz B, Shan M, Simantov R, Bukowski RM. Sorafenib in advanced clear-cell renal-cell carcinoma. N Engl J Med. 2007;356:125–34.
122. Llovet JM, Ricci S, Mazzaferro V, Hilgard P, Gane E, Blanc JF, de Oliveira AC, Santoro A, Raoul JL, Forner A, Schwartz M, Porta C, Zeuzem S, Bolondi L, Greten TF, Galle PR, Seitz JF, Borbath I, Haussinger D, Giannaris T, Shan M, Moscovici M, Voliotis D, Bruix J. Sorafenib in advanced hepatocellular carcinoma. N Engl J Med. 2008;359:378–90.
123. Chen J, Tian CX, Yu M, Lv Q, Cheng NS, Wang Z, Wu X. Efficacy and safety profile of combining sorafenib with chemotherapy in patients with HER2-negative advanced breast cancer: a meta-analysis. J Breast Cancer. 2014;17:61–8.
124. Hurwitz HI, Dowlati A, Saini S, Savage S, Suttle AB, Gibson DM, Hodge JP, Merkle EM, Pandite L. Phase I trial of pazopanib in patients with advanced cancer. Clin Cancer Res. 2009;15:4220–7.
125. van der Graaf WT, Blay JY, Chawla SP, Kim DW, Bui-Nguyen B, Casali PG, Schoffski P, Aglietta M, Staddon AP, Beppu Y, Le Cesne A, Gelderblom H, Judson IR, Araki N, Ouali M, Marreaud S, Hodge R, Dewji MR, Coens C, Demetri GD, Fletcher CD, Dei Tos AP, Hohenberger P. Pazopanib for metastatic soft-tissue sarcoma (PALETTE): a randomised, double-blind, placebo-controlled phase 3 trial. Lancet. 2012;379:1879–86.
126. Heath EI, Infante J, Lewis LD, Luu T, Stephenson J, Tan AR, Kasubhai S, LoRusso P, Ma B, Suttle AB, Kleha JF, Ball HA, Dar MM. A randomized, double-blind, placebo-controlled study to evaluate the effect of repeated oral doses of pazopanib on cardiac conduction in patients with solid tumors. Cancer Chemother Pharmacol. 2013;71:565–73.
127. Rini BI, Escudier B, Tomczak P, Kaprin A, Szczylik C, Hutson TE, Michaelson MD, Gorbunova VA, Gore ME, Rusakov IG, Negrier S, Ou YC, Castellano D, Lim HY, Uemura H, Tarazi J, Cella D, Chen C, Rosbrook B, Kim S, Motzer RJ. Comparative

effectiveness of axitinib versus sorafenib in advanced renal cell carcinoma (AXIS): a randomised phase 3 trial. Lancet. 2011;378:1931–9.

128. Rini BI, Schiller JH, Fruehauf JP, Cohen EE, Tarazi JC, Rosbrook B, Bair AH, Ricart AD, Olszanski AJ, Letrent KJ, Kim S, Rixe O. Diastolic blood pressure as a biomarker of axitinib efficacy in solid tumors. Clin Cancer Res. 2011;17:3841–9.

129. Ovadia D, Esquenazi Y, Bucay M, Bachier CR. Association between takotsubo cardiomyopathy and axitinib: case report and review of the literature. J Clin Oncol. 2015;33:e1–3.

130. Abdel-Rahman O, Fouad M. Risk of cardiovascular toxicities in patients with solid tumors treated with sunitinib, axitinib, cediranib or regorafenib: an updated systematic review and comparative meta-analysis. Crit Rev Oncol Hematol. 2014;92:194–207.

131. Bachelot T, Romieu G, Campone M, Dieras V, Cropet C, Dalenc F, Jimenez M, Le Rhun E, Pierga JY, Goncalves A, Leheurteur M, Domont J, Gutierrez M, Cure H, Ferrero JM, Labbe-Devilliers C. Lapatinib plus capecitabine in patients with previously untreated brain metastases from HER2-positive metastatic breast cancer (LANDSCAPE): a single-group phase 2 study. Lancet Oncol. 2013;14:64–71.

132. Perez EA, Koehler M, Byrne J, Preston AJ, Rappold E, Ewer MS. Cardiac safety of lapatinib: pooled analysis of 3689 patients enrolled in clinical trials. Mayo Clin Proc. 2008;83:679–86.

133. Baselga J, Bradbury I, Eidtmann H, Di Cosimo S, de Azambuja E, Aura C, Gomez H, Dinh P, Fauria K, Van Dooren V, Aktan G, Goldhirsch A, Chang TW, Horvath Z, Coccia-Portugal M, Domont J, Tseng LM, Kunz G, Sohn JH, Semiglazov V, Lerzo G, Palacova M, Probachai V, Pusztai L, Untch M, Gelber RD, Piccart-Gebhart M. Lapatinib with trastuzumab for HER2-positive early breast cancer (NeoALTTO): a randomised, open-label, multicentre, phase 3 trial. Lancet. 2012;379:633–40.

134. Brunstein CG, McGlave PB. The biology and treatment of chronic myelogenous leukemia. Oncology (Williston Park). 2001;15:23–31; discussion 31–2, 35.

135. Kerkela R, Grazette L, Yacobi R, Iliescu C, Patten R, Beahm C, Walters B, Shevtsov S, Pesant S, Clubb FJ, Rosenzweig A, Salomon RN, Van Etten RA, Alroy J, Durand JB, Force T. Cardiotoxicity of the cancer therapeutic agent imatinib mesylate. Nat Med. 2006;12:908–16.

136. Atallah E, Durand JB, Kantarjian H, Cortes J. Congestive heart failure is a rare event in patients receiving imatinib therapy. Blood. 2007;110:1233–7.

137. Maharsy W, Aries A, Mansour O, Komati H, Nemer M. Ageing is a risk factor in imatinib mesylate cardiotoxicity. Eur J Heart Fail. 2014;16:367–76.

138. Verweij J, Casali PG, Kotasek D, Le Cesne A, Reichard P, Judson IR, Issels R, van Oosterom AT, Van Glabbeke M, Blay JY. Imatinib does not induce cardiac left ventricular failure in gastrointestinal stromal tumours patients: analysis of EORTC-ISG-AGITG study 62005. Eur J Cancer. 2007;43:974–8.

139. Trent JC, Patel SS, Zhang J, Araujo DM, Plana JC, Lenihan DJ, Fan D, Patel SR, Benjamin RS, Khakoo AY. Rare incidence of congestive heart failure in gastrointestinal stromal tumor and other sarcoma patients receiving imatinib mesylate. Cancer. 2010;116:184–92.

140. Saito S, Nakata K, Kajiura S, Ando T, Hosokawa A, Sugiyama T. Long-term follow-up outcome of imatinib mesylate treatment for recurrent and unresectable gastrointestinal stromal tumors. Digestion. 2013;87:47–52.

141. Apperley JF, Cortes JE, Kim DW, Roy L, Roboz GJ, Rosti G, Bullorsky EO, Abruzzese E, Hochhaus A, Heim D, de Souza CA, Larson RA, Lipton JH, Khoury HJ, Kim HJ, Sillaber C, Hughes TP, Erben P, Van Tornout J, Stone RM. Dasatinib in the treatment of chronic myeloid leukemia in accelerated phase after imatinib failure: the START a trial. J Clin Oncol. 2009;27:3472–9.

142. Bradeen HA, Eide CA, O'Hare T, Johnson KJ, Willis SG, Lee FY, Druker BJ, Deininger MW. Comparison of imatinib mesylate, dasatinib (BMS-354825), and nilotinib (AMN107) in an N-ethyl-N-nitrosourea (ENU)-based mutagenesis screen: high efficacy of drug combinations. Blood. 2006;108:2332–8.

143. Kantarjian H, Cortes J, Kim DW, Dorlhiac-Llacer P, Pasquini R, DiPersio J, Muller MC, Radich JP, Khoury HJ, Khoroshko N, Bradley-Garelik MB, Zhu C, Tallman MS. Phase 3 study of dasatinib 140 mg once daily versus 70 mg twice daily in patients with chronic myeloid leukemia in accelerated phase resistant or intolerant to imatinib: 15-month median follow-up. Blood. 2009;113:6322–9.

144. Strevel EL, Ing DJ, Siu LL. Molecularly targeted oncology therapeutics and prolongation of the QT interval. J Clin Oncol. 2007;25:3362–71.

145. Flaherty KT, Robert C, Hersey P, Nathan P, Garbe C, Milhem M, Demidov LV, Hassel JC, Rutkowski P, Mohr P, Dummer R, Trefzer U, Larkin JM, Utikal J, Dreno B, Nyakas M, Middleton MR, Becker JC, Casey M, Sherman LJ, Wu FS, Ouellet D, Martin AM, Patel K, Schadendorf D, Group MS. Improved survival with MEK inhibition in BRAF-mutated melanoma. N Engl J Med. 2012;367:107–14.

146. Wells Jr SA, Robinson BG, Gagel RF, Dralle H, Fagin JA, Santoro M, Baudin E, Elisei R, Jarzab B, Vasselli JR, Read J, Langmuir P, Ryan AJ, Schlumberger MJ. Vandetanib in patients with locally advanced or metastatic medullary thyroid cancer: a randomized, double-blind phase III trial. J Clin Oncol. 2012;30:134–41.

147. Agathocleous A, Rohatiner A, Rule S, Hunter H, Kerr JP, Neeson SM, Matthews J, Strauss S, Montoto S, Johnson P, Radford J, Lister A. Weekly versus twice weekly bortezomib given in conjunction with rituximab, in patients with recurrent follicular lymphoma, mantle cell lymphoma and Waldenstrom macroglobulinaemia. Br J Haematol. 2010;151:346–53.

148. Bringhen S, Larocca A, Rossi D, Cavalli M, Genuardi M, Ria R, Gentili S, Patriarca F, Nozzoli C, Levi A, Guglielmelli T, Benevolo G, Callea V, Rizzo V, Cangialosi C, Musto P, De Rosa L, Liberati AM, Grasso M, Falcone AP, Evangelista A, Cavo M, Gaidano G, Boccadoro M, Palumbo A. Efficacy and safety of once-weekly bortezomib in multiple myeloma patients. Blood. 2010;116:4745–53.

149. Richardson PG, Sonneveld P, Schuster MW, Irwin D, Stadtmauer EA, Facon T, Harousseau JL, Ben-Yehuda D, Lonial S, Goldschmidt H, Reece D, San-Miguel JF, Blade J, Boccadoro M, Cavenagh J, Dalton WS, Boral AL, Esseltine DL, Porter JB, Schenkein D, Anderson KC. Bortezomib or high-dose dexamethasone for relapsed multiple myeloma. N Engl J Med. 2005;352:2487–98.

150. Alsina M, Trudel S, Furman RR, Rosen PJ, O'Connor OA, Comenzo RL, Wong A, Kunkel LA, Molineaux CJ, Goy A. A phase I single-agent study of twice-weekly consecutive-day dosing of the proteasome inhibitor carfilzomib in patients with relapsed or refractory multiple myeloma or lymphoma. Clin Cancer Res. 2012;18:4830–40.

151. Kortuem KM, Stewart AK. Carfilzomib. Blood. 2013;121:893–7.

152. Siegel DS, Martin T, Wang M, Vij R, Jakubowiak AJ, Lonial S, Trudel S, Kukreti V, Bahlis N, Alsina M, Chanan-Khan A, Buadi F, Reu FJ, Somlo G, Zonder J, Song K, Stewart AK, Stadtmauer E, Kunkel L, Wear S, Wong AF, Orlowski RZ, Jagannath S. A phase 2 study of single-agent carfilzomib (PX-171-003-A1) in patients with relapsed and refractory multiple myeloma. Blood. 2012;120:2817–25.

153. Lendvai N, Hilden P, Devlin S, Landau H, Hassoun H, Lesokhin AM, Tsakos I, Redling K, Koehne G, Chung DJ, Schaffer WL, Giralt SA. A phase 2 single-center study of carfilzomib 56 mg/m2 with or without low-dose dexamethasone in relapsed multiple myeloma. Blood. 2014;124:899–906.

154. Grandin EW, Ky B, Cornell RF, Carver J, Lenihan DJ. Patterns of cardiac toxicity associated with irreversible proteasome inhibition in the treatment of multiple myeloma. J Card Fail. 2015;21:138–44.

155. Cortes JE, Kantarjian H, Shah NP, Bixby D, Mauro MJ, Flinn I, O'Hare T, Hu S, Narasimhan NI, Rivera VM, Clackson T, Turner CD, Haluska FG, Druker BJ, Deininger MW, Talpaz M. Ponatinib in refractory Philadelphia chromosome-positive leukemias. N Engl J Med. 2012;367:2075–88.

156. Cortes JE, Kim DW, Pinilla-Ibarz J, le Coutre P, Paquette R, Chuah C, Nicolini FE, Apperley JF, Khoury HJ, Talpaz M, DiPersio J, DeAngelo DJ, Abruzzese E, Rea D, Baccarani M,

Muller MC, Gambacorti-Passerini C, Wong S, Lustgarten S, Rivera VM, Clackson T, Turner CD, Haluska FG, Guilhot F, Deininger MW, Hochhaus A, Hughes T, Goldman JM, Shah NP, Kantarjian H. A phase 2 trial of ponatinib in Philadelphia chromosome-positive leukemias. N Engl J Med. 2013;369:1783–96.

157. Groarke JD, Cheng S, Moslehi J. Cancer-drug discovery and cardiovascular surveillance. N Engl J Med. 2013;369:1779–81.

158. Mross K, Frost A, Steinbild S, Hedbom S, Buchert M, Fasol U, Unger C, Kratzschmar J, Heinig R, Boix O, Christensen O. A phase I dose-escalation study of regorafenib (BAY 73-4506), an inhibitor of oncogenic, angiogenic, and stromal kinases, in patients with advanced solid tumors. Clin Cancer Res. 2012;18:2658–67.

159. Demetri GD, Reichardt P, Kang YK, Blay JY, Rutkowski P, Gelderblom H, Hohenberger P, Leahy M, von Mehren M, Joensuu H, Badalamenti G, Blackstein M, Le Cesne A, Schoffski P, Maki RG, Bauer S, Nguyen BB, Xu J, Nishida T, Chung J, Kappeler C, Kuss I, Laurent D, Casali PG and investigators Gs. Efficacy and safety of regorafenib for advanced gastrointestinal stromal tumours after failure of imatinib and sunitinib (GRID): an international, multicentre, randomised, placebo-controlled, phase 3 trial. Lancet. 2013;381:295–302.

160. Strumberg D, Scheulen ME, Schultheis B, Richly H, Frost A, Buchert M, Christensen O, Jeffers M, Heinig R, Boix O, Mross K. Regorafenib (BAY 73-4506) in advanced colorectal cancer: a phase I study. Br J Cancer. 2012;106:1722–7.

161. Grothey A, Van Cutsem E, Sobrero A, Siena S, Falcone A, Ychou M, Humblet Y, Bouche O, Mineur L, Barone C, Adenis A, Tabernero J, Yoshino T, Lenz HJ, Goldberg RM, Sargent DJ, Cihon F, Cupit L, Wagner A, Laurent D. Regorafenib monotherapy for previously treated metastatic colorectal cancer (CORRECT): an international, multicentre, randomised, placebo-controlled, phase 3 trial. Lancet. 2013;381:303–12.

162. Li J, Qin S, Xu R, Yau TC, Ma B, Pan H, Xu J, Bai Y, Chi Y, Wang L, Yeh KH, Bi F, Cheng Y, Le AT, Lin JK, Liu T, Ma D, Kappeler C, Kalmus J, Kim TW. Regorafenib plus best supportive care versus placebo plus best supportive care in Asian patients with previously treated metastatic colorectal cancer (CONCUR): a randomised, double-blind, placebo-controlled, phase 3 trial. Lancet Oncol. 2015;16:619–29.

163. Lindsay CR, MacPherson IRJ, Cassidy J. Current status of cediranib: the rapid development of a novel anti-angiogenic therapy. Future Oncol. 2009;5:421–32.

164. Hirte H, Lheureux S, Fleming GF, Sugimoto A, Morgan R, Biagi J, Wang L, McGill S, Ivy SP, Oza AM. A phase 2 study of cediranib in recurrent or persistent ovarian, peritoneal or fallopian tube cancer: A trial of the Princess Margaret, Chicago and California Phase II Consortia. Gynecol Oncol. 2015;138:55–61.

165. Spreafico A, Chi KN, Sridhar SS, Smith DC, Carducci MA, Kavsak P, Wong TS, Wang L, Ivy SP, Mukherjee SD, Kollmannsberger CK, Sukhai MA, Takebe N, Kamel-Reid S, Siu LL, Hotte SJ. A randomized phase II study of cediranib alone versus cediranib in combination with dasatinib in docetaxel resistant, castration resistant prostate cancer patients. Invest New Drugs. 2014;32:1005–16.

166. Judson I, Scurr M, Gardner K, Barquin E, Marotti M, Collins B, Young H, Jürgensmeier JM, Leahy M. Phase II study of cediranib in patients with advanced gastrointestinal stromal tumors or soft-tissue sarcoma. Clin Cancer Res. 2014;20:3603–12.

167. Matulonis UA, Berlin S, Ivy P, Tyburski K, Krasner C, Zarwan C, Berkenblit A, Campos S, Horowitz N, Cannistra SA, Lee H, Lee J, Roche M, Hill M, Whalen C, Sullivan L, Tran C, Humphreys BD, Penson RT. Cediranib, an oral inhibitor of vascular endothelial growth factor receptor kinases, is an active drug in recurrent epithelial ovarian, fallopian tube, and peritoneal cancer. J Clin Oncol. 2009;27:5601–6.

168. Van Cutsem E, Tabernero J, Lakomy R, Prenen H, Prausová J, Macarulla T, Ruff P, van Hazel GA, Moiseyenko V, Ferry D, McKendrick J, Polikoff J, Tellier A, Castan R, Allegra C. Addition of aflibercept to fluorouracil, leucovorin, and irinotecan improves survival in a phase III randomized trial in patients with metastatic colorectal cancer previously treated with an oxaliplatin-based regimen. J Clin Oncol. 2012;30:3499–506.

169. Tabernero J, Van Cutsem E, Lakomy R, Prausova J, Ruff P, van Hazel GA, Moiseyenko VM, Ferry DR, McKendrick JJ, Soussan-Lazard K, Chevalier S, Allegra CJ. Aflibercept versus placebo in combination with fluorouracil, leucovorin and irinotecan in the treatment of previously treated metastatic colorectal cancer: prespecified subgroup analyses from the VELOUR trial. Eur J Cancer (Oxford, England 1990). 2014;50:320–31.

170. Lockhart AC, Rothenberg ML, Dupont J, Cooper W, Chevalier P, Sternas L, Buzenet G, Koehler E, Sosman JA, Schwartz LH, Gultekin DH, Koutcher JA, Donnelly EF, Andal R, Dancy I, Spriggs DR, Tew WP. Phase I study of intravenous vascular endothelial growth factor trap, aflibercept, in patients with advanced solid tumors. J Clin Oncol. 2010;28:207–14.

171. Diaz-Padilla I, Siu LL, San Pedro-Salcedo M, Razak AR, Colevas AD, Shepherd FA, Leighl NB, Neal JW, Thibault A, Liu L, Lisano J, Gao B, Lawson EB, Wakelee HA. A phase I dose-escalation study of aflibercept administered in combination with pemetrexed and cisplatin in patients with advanced solid tumours. Br J Cancer. 2012;107:604–11.

172. Said R, Banchs J, Wheler J, Hess KR, Falchook G, Fu S, Naing A, Hong D, Piha-Paul S, Ye Y, Yeh E, Wolff RA, Tsimberidou AM. The prognostic significance of left ventricular ejection fraction in patients with advanced cancer treated in phase I clinical trials. Ann Oncol. 2014;25:276–82.

173. Subbiah IM, Lenihan DJ, Tsimberidou AM. Cardiovascular toxicity profiles of vascular-disrupting agents. Oncologist. 2011;16:1120–30.

Chapter 3
Screening and Monitoring for Cardiotoxicity During Cancer Treatment

Michel G. Khouri, Igor Klem, Chetan Shenoy, Jeffrey Sulpher, and Susan F. Dent

Importance of Preventing Cardiotoxicity

Mortality rates from cancer have declined over the past 30 years. More effective methods of early detection, pharmacologic treatments, and surgical approaches have resulted in significant cancer-related survival gains [1–3]. Long-term survivors with cancer are expected to increase by approximately 30 % in the next decade to an estimated 18 million by 2022 in the USA alone [4]. With prolonged survival, cancer patients are now subject to the effects of aging and to the development of other risk factors that determine their long-term risk of cardiovascular disease (CVD) [5–7]. Cardiovascular disease is already the predominant cause of mortality in breast cancer patients over 50 years of age [5, 6, 8] and a more common contributor than cancer to mortality among older survivors [9, 10].

Cancer therapies are associated with unique and varying degrees of direct (e.g., myocardial toxicity, ischemia, hypertension, arrhythmias) [11–14] as well as

Electronic supplementary material: The online version of this chapter (doi:10.1007/978-3-319-43096-6_3) contains supplementary material, which is available to authorized users.

M.G. Khouri • I. Klem
Division of Cardiology, Department of Medicine, Duke University Medical Center, Durham, NC, USA
e-mail: michel.khouri@duke.edu; igor.klem@duke.edu

C. Shenoy
Division of Cardiology, Department of Medicine, University of Minnesota Medical Center, Minneapolis, MN, USA
e-mail: cshenoy@umn.edu

J. Sulpher • S.F. Dent (✉)
Division of Medical Oncology, Department of Medicine, University of Ottawa, Ottawa, ON, Canada
e-mail: jeffrey.sulpher@bccancer.bc.ca; sdent@toh.on.ca

indirect (e.g., unfavorable lifestyle changes) insults on the cardiovascular system [11]. The most well-known direct cardiotoxic effects of cancer therapy occur with anthracycline-containing regimens (i.e., doxorubicin, epirubicin). Anthracyclines are still widely used in solid tumors (i.e., breast cancer, osteosarcoma, etc.) and hematologic malignancies (Hodgkin's/non-Hodgkin's lymphoma, acute lympho-blastic leukemia, etc.) and are well recognized to trigger dose-dependent, cumula-tive, progressive cardiac dysfunction [15, 16]. Anthracycline-associated cardiac dysfunction usually manifests as a decrease in left ventricular ejection fraction (LVEF) [17–19] and, ultimately, symptomatic heart failure (HF) in up to 5 % of patients [20]. Newer, targeted agents have dramatically improved the antitumor efficacy of therapies for various cancers but are not without adverse cardiovascular effects [13, 21–23]. Targeted therapies, particularly monoclonal antibodies and tyrosine kinase inhibitors (TKIs) targeting human epidermal growth factor receptor 2 (HER-2) (i.e., trastuzumab, pertuzumab, etc.), vascular endothelial growth factor (VEGF), VEGF receptors (VEGFRs) (i.e., bevacizumab, sunitinib, sorafenib, etc.), and Abl kinase activity (i.e., imatinib, nilotinib, dasatinib, etc.), interfere with molecular pathways crucial to cardiovascular health [23, 24]. Moreover, cardiac damage inflicted by these agents may be additive; specifically, trastuzumab (Herceptin®), a humanized monoclonal antibody used in HER-2-positive early-stage breast cancer, has demonstrated synergistic cardiotoxicity when added to anthracyclines [25, 26].

The magnitude of cardiovascular morbidity is likely to increase with the approval of newer antineoplastic agents for which the long-term cardiovascular safety profile is not yet known [27, 28]. Going forward, early detection strategies are needed to identify patients susceptible to therapy-related cardiotoxicity in order to avoid unnecessary discontinuation of essential anticancer treatment. In addition long-term cardiovascular surveillance strategies are essential for cancer survivors to prevent treatment-induced cardiovascular morbidity and mortality.

Cardiotoxicity in the Spectrum of Cancer and Heart Disease

Oncology and cardiology organizations have attempted to classify cardiotoxicity in terms of overt clinical events and subclinical injury. The National Cancer Institute (NCI) has developed a comprehensive system for cancer adverse events reporting which includes cardiotoxicity—the common terminology criteria for adverse events (CTCAE). This recognizes a broad array of important cardiac and cardio-vascular events as well as subclinical laboratory and ejection fraction changes during cytotoxic therapy. Notably, the NCI has kept the traditional criteria that define myocardial toxicity (e.g., left ventricular systolic dysfunction, HF, and LVEF decline) separate, rather than unifying these parameters under a comprehen-sive definition of cardiotoxicity [29]. The Cardiac Review and Evaluation Com-mittee (CREC) criteria were specifically developed in 2002 during an initial extensive safety review of patients treated in trastuzumab trials and defined cardiotoxicity based on physical signs, symptoms, and LVEF [30]. The American College of Cardiology/American Heart Association (ACC/AHA) have developed a staging system (stages A–D) to identify patients during the course of HF development. Asymptomatic patients who receive potential cardiotoxins (stage A) or have asymptomatic left ventricular (LV) dysfunction (stage B) are at risk to develop symptomatic HF (stages C and D) [31]. The transition from ACC/AHA stage B asymptomatic to stage C symptomatic HF has been associated with a significant decrease in 5-year survival (96 % to 75 %) equivalent to a fivefold increase in mortality risk in a community population [32].

Early detection of cardiotoxicity provides an opportunity to prevent or reverse progression to a more advanced stage; LVEF recovery and cardiac event reduction were more likely with early detection of LV dysfunction and prompt initiation of usual HF therapies in cancer patients with anthracycline-induced cardiomyopathy [33]. In this regard, the evolution of "cardio-oncology," which aims to keep pace with the rapid evolution of cancer therapies and the incidence, magnitude, and consequences of their cardiac and cardiovascular side effects, has contributed to improved recognition of the prevalence of treatment-related cardiotoxicity and the importance of early detection [34]. A common pathway for identifying patients at risk for cardiotoxicity, however, remains complicated by the nonspecific nature of treatment-related cardiac and cardiovascular damage, the unpredictability of clinical consequences (e.g., severity, timing, etc.), and, consequently, uncertainty regarding the optimal strategy for detection.

Current Approaches for Identifying Cardiotoxicity

There are currently no evidence-based guidelines for the monitoring of cancer patients receiving potentially cardiotoxic therapy [35]. Several professional societies [31, 36] provide guidance for management of heart failure, but few organizations have specifically addressed cardiovascular surveillance strategies for cancer patients during and following exposure to cardiotoxic cancer therapies [35, 37, 38].

In 2005, the American Society of Clinical Oncology (ASCO) convened an expert panel to develop guidelines for the ongoing cardiac surveillance and care of adult and pediatric survivors of cancer. The proposed guideline document was not issued by ASCO "in light of the lack of direct, high-quality evidence on the benefits and harms of screening for cardiac late effects." The document was published in 2007 as a clinical evidence review that summarized the then-current literature regarding late cardiac effects among cancer survivors [39]. The last several years has seen an exponential increase in the number of publications highlighting the potential for detrimental short- and long-term impact of cancer treatments on cardiovascular health. Nevertheless, universally accepted guidelines on surveillance strategies remain elusive. In 2011, The Heart Failure Association of the European Society of Cardiology (ESC) published recommendations on identification and surveillance strategies for those patients at risk of experiencing

Table 3.1 Surveillance strategies for cancer patients receiving potentially cardiotoxic cancer therapy

	Baseline	During cancer therapy	Following completion of cancer therapy
Heart Failure Association—European Society of Cardiology (2011) [40]	Careful cardiovascular work-up with attention to comorbidities esp. CAD and hypertension	Regular cardiovascular evaluation	Follow-up cardiac surveillance should be considered especially in those patients receiving high doses of anthracyclines
European Society of Medical Oncology (ESMO, 2012) [38]	Baseline cardiovascular evaluation (risk factors and comorbidities) Baseline 12-lead ECG and echocardiogram or MUGA Baseline biomarker (troponin, BNP) treatment of preexisting cardiopathies	Patients receiving anthracyclines +/- trastuzumab should have serial monitoring of cardiac function at 3, 6, and 9 months during treatment and then 12 and 18 months after initiation of treatment Biomarkers with each cycle	Monitoring following treatment as clinically indicated Increased vigilance for patients >60 years old Assessment of cardiac function recommended 4 and 10 years after anthracyclines in patients treated <15 years old and those >15 years old with a cumulative dose of doxorubicin >240 mg/m^2 or epirubicin >360 mg/m^2
European Association of Cardiovascular Imaging and American Society of Echocardiography (2014) [41]	Baseline cardiac assessment especially for those >65 years old and at high risk of CTRCD, LV dysfunction, or high doses of anthracyclines (>350 mg/m^2) History, physical examination, ECG, echocardiogram, and baseline global longitudinal strain (GLS), and troponin I desirable	Anthracyclines: troponin each cycle; if positive: cardiology consult. If dose >240 mg/m^2 or equivalent: recommended LVEF, GLS, and troponin prior to each additional 50 mg/m^2. Trastuzumab: LVEF, GLS, and troponin every 3 months during therapy and 6 months after treatment completed	Yearly cardiovascular assessment by a health-care provider particularly in patients not followed closely during cancer treatment imaging at the discretion of the health-care provider

cardiotoxicity during or following cancer therapy (Table 3.1). They recommended cardiovascular work-up with attention to comorbidities (especially coronary artery disease and hypertension) at baseline, regular cardiovascular evaluation during cancer therapy, and follow-up cardiac surveillance following cancer therapy especially in those patients receiving high doses of anthracyclines. Few details were provided on the recommended type and frequency of cardiac monitoring.

In 2012, the European Society of Medical Oncology (ESMO) published criteria-based recommendations of optimal screening and monitoring of cardiac function during cancer therapy based on a review of current evidence. Similar to the ESC, they recommended baseline assessment of cardiovascular risk factors and comorbidities. In addition, ESMO recommended patients receiving potentially cardiotoxic therapy have a baseline 12 lead ECG, assessment of LVEF with echocardiogram or MUGA, and measurement of biomarkers including troponin and BNP. Cardiac monitoring during cancer therapy focused on patients receiving anthracyclines +/- trastuzumab. For patients receiving anthracyclines, measurement of LVEF was recommended (in the absence of baseline troponin) every 3 months for 1 year followed by yearly assessments. In patients with normal troponin levels (during anthracycline chemotherapy), echocardiogram was recommended at 12 months and then yearly thereafter. Patients receiving trastuzumab should have LVEF assessed every 3 months during therapy and then at 12 and 18 months following initiation of treatment. Following completion of cancer therapy, cardiac assessment was recommended at 4 and 10 years in patients with higher exposure to anthracyclines (>240 mg/m^2 Adriamycin) with increased vigilance in those patients over 60 years of age. ESMO also provided stop/go rules for individuals receiving trastuzumab therapy [38]. Both ESC and ESMO reinforced that newer targeted molecular agents are associated with adverse cardiovascular events and that the early detection of cardiotoxicity needs to be an integral part of the treatment and follow-up of cancer patients [42].

In 2014, the American Society of Echocardiography and the European Association of Cardiovascular Imaging published an expert consensus on surveillance strategies for adult patients during and after cancer therapy [41] (see Table 3.1). This group recommended that echocardiography remain the cornerstone in the cardiac imaging evaluation of patients in preparation for, during, and after cancer therapy, because of its widespread availability, easy repeatability, versatility, lack of radiation exposure, and safety, particularly in patients with concomitant renal disease. Similar to ESMO, they suggested that an integrated approach combining echocardiography and biomarkers may be of utility and provide incremental value in predicting subsequent cancer therapy-related cardiac dysfunction. After the completion of therapy and particularly among patients who were not followed using a strategy aimed at early detection of subclinical LV dysfunction, the committee suggested a yearly clinical cardiovascular assessment by a health-care provider, looking for early signs and symptoms of cardiovascular disease, with further cardiac imaging ordered at the discretion of the provider. The committee highlighted that their recommendations represent a consensus of current clinical practice performed at their own respective academic institutions. Similar to other consensus statements, the group recognized the limited scientific data available and the lack of class A evidence (i.e., derived from randomized clinical trials) supporting their algorithms.

While these consensus documents provide guidance to clinicians, the impact of cardiac monitoring during and following completion of cancer therapy, on cardiovascular outcomes in cancer patients being managed in the "real-world" clinical setting, is uncertain. In addition, there is limited data in the literature on the adherence to cardiac monitoring recommendations in clinical practice. In a recent US study, 78.8 % of postmenopausal women (66 years and older) with early-stage HER2-positive breast cancer receiving trastuzumab had a baseline cardiac evaluation, while only 42.6 % had subsequent monitoring (one cardiac evaluation at least every 4 months during trastuzumab therapy). Recent year of cancer diagnosis and treatment with an anthracycline regimen was associated with higher rates of adequate cardiac monitoring [43].

Cardiovascular surveillance strategies for cancer patients have been largely limited to anthracyclines and anti-HER2 drugs such as trastuzumab. Several new classes of promising anticancer therapies have been introduced into clinical practice, several of which have unique cardiovascular toxicities (see Table 3.2). Tyrosine kinase inhibitors have demonstrated efficacy in a number of solid malignancies (renal cell carcinoma (sunitinib), hepatocellular (sorafenib), and head and neck (cetuximab)), but are associated with development of de novo or worsening hypertension. While strategies on the management and monitoring of cancer patients who develop hypertension while receiving these novel targeted drugs are emerging, there are currently no consensus or evidence-based documents to guide therapy. In the interim, patients should be managed based on current hypertension guidelines produced by organizations such as the American Society of Hypertension (www.ash-us.org), Hypertension Canada (http://guidelines.hypertension.ca), and the European Society of Hypertension (www.eshonline.org). A number of emerging cancer therapies are associated with less common cardiovascular toxicities including QTc prolongation, arrhythmias, cardiac ischemia, and thromboembolic events (see Table 3.2). Monitoring strategies for these cancer therapies should follow current evidence-based international guidelines (American (www.heart.org), Canadian (www.ccs.ca), European (www.escardio.org), UK (www.bhf.org.uk, heartuk.org.uk)).

In recognition of the increasing need for guidance, the ASCO Survivorship Guidelines Advisory Group has recently published a guideline to improve the quality of care of cancer survivors by identifying and providing guidance on prevention and monitoring of cardiac dysfunction resulting from cancer therapy; and the Canadian Cardiovascular Society has recently completed a guideline on evaluation of patients at risk for cardiovascular complications of cancer therapy [44, 45].

Table 3.2 Cardiotoxicity and cancer therapies

Anticancer therapy	Signs and symptoms of toxicity
Anthracyclines (Doxorubicin, daunorubicin, idarubicin, epirubicin, mitoxantrone)	(1) Acute toxicity: <1 %, reversible, shortly after infusion Toxicities include arrhythmias, QT prolongation +/- HF (2) Early-onset chronic progressive: 1.6–2.1 %, during treatment and up to 1 year post, not reversible, clinically resembles myocarditis, accompanying diastolic dysfunction (3) Late-onset chronic progressive: 1.6–5 %, >1 year from treatment, not reversible, clinical decompensation usually preceded by occult LVD Symptoms of mitoxantrone-induced HF are often less severe and more responsive to medical management
Cyclophosphamide	(1) Arrhythmias (2) Nonspecific ST-T abnormalities (3) Pericardial effusion (4) Hemorrhagic myopericarditis (5) Symptomatic HF (7–28 %) *Occurs within 1–14 days of dose administration and often lasts for a few days. Toxicity may resolve completely or have long-lasting consequences*
Ifosfamide	(1) Arrhythmias (2) Nonspecific ST-T changes on ECG (3) HF 17 % *Acute HF typically presents within 6–23 days of first ifosfamide dose*
Cisplatin	(1) Chest pain (2) Arrhythmias (3) ST-T changes on ECG (4) ACS (5) Thromboembolism (8.5 %)
Antimetabolites	
Fluorouracil (5-FU)	(1) Chest pain or ACS in 3–7.6 % (2) Atrial fibrillation (3) HF (4) Sudden cardiac death (rare) *Occurs during or shortly after starting treatment. Symptoms last up to 48 h, but generally resolve. ECG changes present in up to 68 % of patients treated with continuous infusion. Elevated cardiac biomarkers in up to 43 %*
Capecitabine	(1) Chest pain or ACS (3–9 %) with transient ST elevations on ECG

(continued)

Table 3.2 (continued)

Anticancer therapy	Signs and symptoms of toxicity
	Symptoms occurs 3 h–4 days after initiating therapy
	Cardiac biomarkers generally remain normal
Microtubule-targeting agents	
Paclitaxel	(1) Myocardial ischemia (1–5 %)
	(2) MI (0.5 %)
	(3) Arrhythmias and heart block
	Cardiac complications occur in up to 29 % with most being asymptomatic bradyarrhythmias. Occur during and up to 14 days after paclitaxel administration. Symptoms generally resolve with stopping therapy
Docetaxel	(1) HF 2.3–8 %
	(2) Myocardial ischemia (1.7 %)
Tyrosine kinase inhibitors	
Sunitinib	(1) Hypertension (47 %)
	(2) Asymptomatic decline in LVEF (10–21 %)
	(3) Symptomatic HF in up to 15 %
	Variable time to presentation (days–months)
Sorafenib	(1) MI (2.7–3 %)
	(2) Hypertension (17–43 %)
	(3) HF/LV dysfunction
	Less cardiac dysfunction than sunitinib
Axitinib	(1) Hypertension
Regorafenib	(1) Hypertension
Vandetanib	(1) Torsades de pointes
Imatinib	(1) LVEF reduction (0.5–1.7 %)
Dasatinib	(1) HF/LV dysfunction
Lapatinib	(1) LV dysfunction (1.6–2.2 %)
	(2) Symptomatic HF (0.2–1.4 %)
	(3) QTc prolongation
	Relatively low incidence of adverse cardiac events
Monoclonal antibodies	
Trastuzumab	(1) HF/LV dysfunction with variable rates based on definitions from clinical trials 2–7 % as monotherapy, 2–13 % with paclitaxel
	Up to 27 % with anthracyclines
Bevacizumab	(1) HTN
	(2) HF (0.8–22 %)
	(3) MI/angina (1.5 %)
	(4) ATE during treatment (median, 3 months)
Radiation therapy	(1) CAD
	(2) Valvular disease
	(3) Pericardial disease
	(4) Restrictive cardiomyopathy
	(5) Conduction system disease

CMP cardiomyopathy, *LVD* left ventricular dysfunction, *HF* heart failure, *AC* doxorubicin and cyclophosphamide, *MI* myocardial infarction, *AV* atrioventricular, *CAD* coronary artery disease, *ECG* electrocardiogram, *CVD* cardiovascular disease, *DHP* dihydropyrimidinase, *HTN* hypertension, *LVEF* left ventricular ejection fraction, *VEGF* vascular endothelial growth factor, *NO* nitric oxide, *ATE* arterial thrombotic event, *ACS* acute coronary syndrome

Defining Cardiotoxicity

Anthracycline-related symptomatic HF was first described in the 1970s [15]. In the 1970s and 1980s, multigated acquisition (MUGA) scanning, also known as resting radionuclide angiocardiography, emerged as the modality of choice for monitoring LV function in adult and pediatric patients treated with anthracyclines [46–49]. Initial guidelines were proposed by Alexander et al. grading heart failure (HF) as mild, moderate, or severe, on the basis of a progressive fall in LVEF using serial MUGA imaging [46]. These guidelines were implemented in a large single-center study over 7 years, and the use of these guidelines in conjunction with MUGA for monitoring LVEF was demonstrated to be associated with a low incidence, benign course, and reversible degree of anthracycline-related HF [49]. Accordingly, assessment of LV systolic function by resting LVEF has become routine in current practice for cardiovascular evaluation in cancer patients treated with anticancer therapy [46]. Among non-cancer populations, LVEF has been repeatedly shown to be an important and independent prognostic indicator and is used frequently in clinical decision-making [31, 50, 51]. In a cancer population, the prognosis of developing LV systolic dysfunction is presumably worse compared to the general population, given the continuous nature of the myocardial insult from cytotoxic therapy.

However, there are limitations with the current paradigm that uses resting LVEF for surveillance of changes in cardiac and cardiovascular function during and after potentially cardiotoxic anticancer therapy. First, resting LVEF provides a snapshot of cardiac performance under optimal circumstances and may not demonstrate subclinical loss of cardiac reserve from early myocyte damage [52]. Second, resting LVEF principally assesses load-dependent changes in LV cavity size. Changes in loading conditions during chemotherapy are common, and, as a result, LVEF may not reflect actual myocardial systolic function [53]. In fact, LVEF may overestimate actual LV health when intrinsic mechanisms are initially compensatory to maintain cardiac output in the face of acute myocardial injury [54]. When such compensation ultimately falters, a drop in LVEF is finally observed perhaps too late to avert irreversible cardiomyopathy and attenuate cardiac events [55, 56]. Third, cancer therapy-induced damage often extends beyond the heart and may occur in conjunction with (mal) adaptation in other organ components, which are not evaluated by resting LVEF. Many anticancer therapies cause unique and varying degrees of injury to the cardiovascular system (i.e., pulmonary-vascular/blood-skeletal muscle axis) [57]. For example, radiation and certain forms of systemic therapy (e.g., chemotherapy, molecularly targeted therapies) can cause pulmonary dysfunction, anemia, endothelial dysfunction, and pulmonary/systemic arterial stiffness as well as skeletal muscle dysfunction [11, 12, 58–60]. These direct insults occur in conjunction with "indirect" lifestyle perturbations (e.g., physical inactivity) that synergistically cause marked impairments in cardiovascular reserve capacity (CVRC) [61].

Moreover, accurate assessment of the frequency and magnitude of cardiotoxicity is challenging given differences in LVEF cut-points, monitoring frequency, and measurement modalities used in clinical trials that limit direct comparisons. There are currently no consensus criteria for cardiotoxicity [38, 41, 62]; trial-based cardiac safety end points have been heterogeneously defined as either (1) an absolute reduction of LVEF >10 % or >15 %, (2) an LVEF reduction >10 % or >15 % to a threshold of <55 % or <50 %, or (3) any LVEF decline to < 50 % [63]. Echocardiography, MUGA, or both have been used most frequently for cardiac assessments in clinical trials and practice, although LVEF measurements by these modalities are not interchangeable [64]. The validity of assumptions common to the spectrum of cardiotoxicity criteria, specifically whether an LVEF decline is always attributable to treatment-related toxicity and whether the absence of an LVEF decline can be interpreted as absence of cardiotoxicity, is also debatable [65]. Data addressing the utility of systematic follow-up LVEF assessments in adult cancer survivors with a history of cytotoxic therapy are also lacking [39]. For certain cardiotoxic agents, such as trastuzumab, serial LVEF measurements are Food and Drug Administration (FDA)-mandated in the USA [66], and stopping/holding rules (i.e., LVEF decrease of ≥ 16 % or 10–15 % below institutional lower limits of normal) that were used in the trastuzumab clinical trials [67–69] during treatment have translated to clinical monitoring practices. The most recent definition of cardiotoxicity proposed by Expert Consensus for Multimodality Imaging Evaluation of Adult Patients during and after Cancer Therapy in 2014 [41] is a decrease in the LVEF of >10 percentage points, to a value <53 %. Moving forward it will be imperative that a common definition of cardiotoxicity be adopted in order to gain a better understanding of cardiac dysfunction in cancer patients exposed to anticancer agents.

Available Modalities for Screening and Monitoring for Cardiotoxicity

Conventional Imaging Modalities

In current practice, multigated acquisition (MUGA) scanning and two-dimensional echocardiography (2DE) are most frequently used to evaluate resting LVEF.

MUGA uses 99mTc-labeled erythrocytes to visualize the cardiac blood pool with gated acquisition using a gamma camera. A series of planar images at each stage of the cardiac cycle are acquired for the quantification of left ventricular volumes and LVEF (Fig. 3.1). Following the findings of Schwartz et al. [49], MUGA soon became popular as the technique of choice for monitoring cardiotoxicity, and detection of an asymptomatic decline in LVEF by MUGA was preferred over surveillance for the development of CHF symptoms. Serial MUGA imaging also allowed the administration of high cumulative doses of

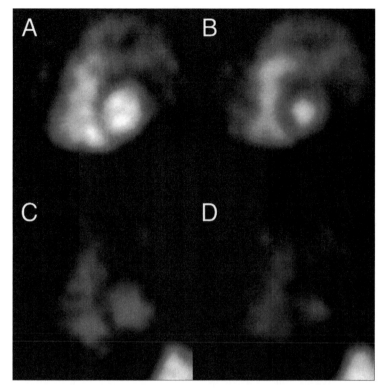

Fig. 3.1 Example MUGA images from cancer patients. (**a**) and (**b**) are end-diastolic and end-systolic MUGA images, respectively, from a 61-year-old male whose LVEF was analyzed to be abnormal at 47.0 %; (**c**) and (**d**) are end-diastolic and end-systolic MUGA images, respectively, from a 61-year-old female whose LVEF was analyzed to be normal at 69.2 %

anthracyclines and the use of anthracyclines when the baseline LVEF was abnormal. MUGA was also demonstrated to have high reproducibility and low variability, making it well suited for serial use [48, 70]. On the basis of this body of evidence, MUGA came to be widely used in oncology clinical trials and in clinical practice. This practice still continues within the oncology community, while the cardiology community has largely moved away from MUGA in favor of echocardiography and cardiac magnetic resonance (CMR) imaging for the evaluation of LV systolic function. Cardiologists favor echocardiography and CMR because these modalities provide additional clinically valuable information not provided by MUGA such as assessment of diastolic function, right ventricular size and function, atrial size and function, valvular disease, pericardial disease, intracardiac thrombus, and extra-cardiac pathology [71]. A recently published study of 2203 breast cancer patients from the SEER-Medicare cohort who received adjuvant trastuzumab showed that 42 % were monitored by echocardiogram, 28 % were monitored by MUGA, and 23 % had imaging alternating between the two modalities [72].

Advantages of MUGA imaging include the ability to image almost all patients without limitations due to body size or obesity, poor acoustic windows, or the presence of cardiac devices such as pacemakers or defibrillators. MUGA is also widely available [71]. Limitations of MUGA include the potential of lower hematocrit and commonly used drugs such as digoxin, heparin, prazosin, and hydralazine to adversely affect the efficiency of erythrocyte labeling [73]. Medications that decrease erythrocyte labeling will reduce the target-to-background ratio and lead to error. Due to the need for cardiac gating, the accuracy of LVEF assessments is limited by arrhythmias such as atrial fibrillation [73]. MUGA is also associated with an average typical effective ionizing radiation dose of 8 mSv [74, 75]. Thus, in a hypothetical breast cancer patient receiving adjuvant trastuzumab who is recommended to have LVEF assessment before starting treatment, every 3 months during, upon completion of treatment, and every 6 months for at least 2 years following completion of treatment [76], the use of MUGA would result in a cumulative effective dose of 72 mSv. Based on published estimates of the radiation-related secondary cancer risk from technetium-99 m myocardial perfusion studies [77], a hypothetical 50-year-old female who undergoes nine MUGAs would be estimated to have a lifetime risk of 0.64 % for a radiation-related secondary cancer. This is not an insignificant risk when considered in light of the excellent survival rates for patients diagnosed with breast cancer today—a 5-year relative survival rate of 89 % and a 10-year relative survival rate of 82 % [78]. Finally, the high reproducibility of LVEF measurements reported in the 1970s and 1980s may not apply to current gamma cameras. Those early MUGA studies were performed using small-field-of-view, single-headed gamma cameras that allowed optimal positioning of the patient and good separation between the left and the right ventricles. Current gamma cameras are primarily large-field-of-view, dual-headed systems that do not permit this degree of patient positioning [71].

Two-dimensional echocardiography has emerged as the primary cardiac imaging modality in patients who are preparing for, are receiving, or have completed anticancer therapy. Accurate measurement of LVEF by 2DE requires sufficient visualization of the LV endocardial border to enable manual tracing of the end-systolic and end-diastolic volumes from which LVEF is calculated. Visual LVEF assessments by 2DE are also common in echocardiography laboratories in clinical practice [79] and prior studies suggest visual LVEF assessments correlate with quantitative methods [79, 80]. Echocardiography has well-described disadvantages, including reliance on adequate acoustic windows and assumptions of LV geometry (for 2DE). These limitations diminish the reproducibility and accuracy for assessment of LV volumes and LVEF by 2DE and reduce sensitivity among serial measurements for detection of small changes in LV function; on occasion, measurement variability of LVEF by 2DE may be higher than thresholds used to define cardiotoxicity [81]. However, 2DE has many significant advantages as well, including wide availability, portability, ease of use, and safety given its lack of exposure to radiation and to potentially nephrotoxic contrast agents. Finally, 2DE without contrast does not require intravenous access.

Novel Imaging Modalities

Transthoracic Echocardiography

Three-dimensional echocardiography (3DE) preserves many of the advantages of echocardiography while mitigating some of the limitations that exist with 2DE. In adjuvant breast cancer, 3DE was superior to 2DE in terms of accuracy and reproducibility, and had similar accuracy to MUGA [with cardiac magnetic resonance (CMR) imaging as the gold standard] for LVEF in early breast cancer [82]. Similarly, 3DE may provide more reliable detection of LVEF changes, which is clinically important given the threshold magnitude of LVEF decline (10 %) used to adjudicate subclinical cancer therapy-related cardiac dysfunction by existing criteria [62]. In a prospective comparison of 2DE and 3DE in 56 breast cancer patients, Thavendiranathan et al. [81] found that the temporal variability of LVEF by 3DE was 5–6 % compared with 10–13 % by 2DE. In the same study, non-contrast 3DE measurement of LVEF had the best intra- and interobserver as well as test-retest variability, compared with 2DE. Despite its superiority for LVEF assessments, 3DE requires greater expertise and is less available than 2DE, limiting its use in standard monitoring at most centers.

While evaluation of contractile function with echocardiography has traditionally been limited to volume-based assessment of LVEF and assessment of regional wall motion or visual estimation of regional thickening, there has been interest in the past few years in techniques that provide more objective and reproducible measures of contractile function through imaging of myocardial deformation. Deformation imaging, in the broadest sense, allows for direct assessment of myocardial muscle shortening and lengthening throughout the cardiac cycle. There are several indices available to assess myocardial deformation, including strain, strain rate, and torsion. Current echocardiographic assessments of myocardial deformation are based on tissue Doppler imaging (TDI) or speckle-based tracking (STE), the two-dimensional tracking of unique speckle patterns created by the constructive and destructive interference of ultrasound beams within tissue, which has technical advantages compared to TDI. These speckles are tracked on a frame-by-frame basis and the accuracy of speckle tracking has been validated against sonomicrometry and tagged CMR imaging [83]. Strain reflects the global deformation of ventricular myocardium during the cardiac cycle, is typically measured at peak systole (i.e., at aortic valve closure), and can be determined in the longitudinal (GLS), radial (GRS), and circumferential (GCS) planes [83]. Beyond measuring linear deformations, peak systolic LV torsion by STE can also measure myocardial rotational deformation due to helical orientation of the myocardial fibers, by calculating the maximum instantaneous difference between peak systolic apical rotation relative to basal rotation [84].

These parameters have emerged as more sensitive measures of subclinical LV dysfunction and may be useful approaches for the early detection of cancer therapy-induced cardiotoxicity and for following patients longitudinally [85]. Reduced TDI

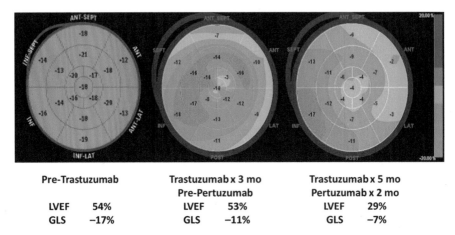

	Pre-Trastuzumab		Trastuzumab x 3 mo Pre-Pertuzumab		Trastuzumab x 5 mo Pertuzumab x 2 mo	
LVEF	54%		LVEF	53%	LVEF	29%
GLS	−17%		GLS	−11%	GLS	−7%

Fig. 3.2 Echocardiographic strain imaging for early detection of cardiotoxicity. In many disease states, measurements of global longitudinal strain (GLS) by two-dimensional echocardiographic speckle tracking are more sensitive for detecting impaired myocardial systolic performance than left ventricular ejection fraction (LVEF) and less susceptible to alterations in loading conditions. In toxin-induced myocardial damage, both in the preclinical and clinical setting, reduced strain and strain rate have revealed impaired myocardial function prior to LVEF decline and heart failure symptoms

strain and strain rate revealed impaired myocardial function prior to LVEF decline [86–88] and HF symptoms [89] in patients treated with anthracycline-containing therapy although the predictive value of these parameters was not evaluated. Global longitudinal strain by STE detects subclinical LV systolic dysfunction among cancer patients with preserved LVEF, including early-stage breast cancer patients undergoing anthracycline-trastuzumab therapy [85, 90] and adult survivors of pediatric malignancies treated with anthracyclines and/or chest radiation [91]. In separate small studies, Sawaya et al. [90, 92] found that impaired absolute GLS (> −19 %) at 3 months and Negishi et al. [93] found that relative GLS decline (≥11 %) from baseline to 6 months predicted LVEF decline in breast cancer patients treated with trastuzumab with or without anthracyclines (Fig. 3.2). GLS also appears to provide superior prognostic information to LVEF in non-cancer populations; a recent meta-analysis showed that GLS independently predicted mortality better than LVEF in 5721 patients with diverse cardiac conditions including HF, acute myocardial infarction, valvular heart disease, and cardiac amyloidosis [51]. Impairments in torsion and torsion velocities in the absence of LVEF changes have been observed 1 month after anthracycline therapy in 25 leukemia/lymphoma patients [94] and after 7 years in 35 anthracycline-treated childhood cancer survivors [95]. Finally, three-dimensional (3D) STE is a novel modality that can comprehensively assess LV myocardial mechanics, tracking linear myocardial deformation in multiple dimensions simultaneously as well as torsion and mechanical dyssynchrony, and has demonstrated early promise in this context, with sensitive detection of altered LV mechanics in childhood cancer survivors treated with anthracyclines [96].

Despite their potential, echocardiographic myocardial deformation indices have important considerations currently limiting their widespread use in cardio-oncology. The optimal timing for assessments in relation to chemotherapy completion and cutoff values for positive tests remain undetermined. Strain echocardiography is dependent on high-quality images, has variability related to different vendor acquisition and analysis platforms, and has uncertainty regarding the optimal parameter of myocardial deformation and interinstitutional reproducibility [41]. However, longitudinal strain has been demonstrated to be more reproducible [97] and the emerging evidence suggests myocardial deformation indices have a potential role for early detection of therapy-related cardiotoxicity that merits further investigation and validation in large cohort studies.

Cardiac Magnetic Resonance

Cardiac magnetic resonance (CMR) imaging became a routine clinical test only about a decade ago. This was made possible by dramatic advances in technology, which changed this modality from providing mostly static, tomographic images of organ morphology to high-resolution, dynamic images allowing the assessment of cardiac function with excellent resolution and contrast. Moreover, advances in tissue characterization techniques, have made CMR the gold standard for assessment of myocardial viability, fibrosis, infiltrative, and inflammatory diseases [98, 99]. In this section we will discuss established and routinely available CMR techniques for cardiotoxicity screening during cancer treatment, which at present relies primarily on imaging left ventricular systolic function. Furthermore, we will discuss which additional information can be obtained in the same routine CMR exam for monitoring cardio-oncology patients, namely, early detection of myocardial tissue damage, impaired myocardial blood flow, tumor involvement of the heart and pericardium, and thrombus formation. We will also address promising, new technological developments, which are being explored for use in this patient population.

CMR for Evaluation of Ventricular Function and Volumes

CMR is widely accepted in the cardiac imaging community as the gold standard for assessment of cardiac volumes, left ventricular mass, and function [100] and endorsed by the American College of Cardiology/American Heart Association as a method to screen for chemotherapy-related cardiotoxicity [101]. From a conceptual standpoint, the key parameter for being able to detect changes in ventricular function on serial imaging is the inter-study reproducibility of the imaging modality used for LVEF measurements. This is determined by the standard deviation (SD) of the mean difference between repeat imaging studies. With wider margins in variability (usually expressed as ±2 SD), the ability to detect these subclinical, often small, changes in LVEF decreases. As a consequence, patients may develop HF symptoms without detecting a significant reduction in LVEF in serial imaging. Conversely, important treatment may be held due to a "measurement error," without a true decline in LVEF. Some information of the relative reproducibility of modalities can be gleaned from prior studies where both image acquisitions and LVEF measurements were repeated in the same patients. Grothues et al. studied 60 patients twice with 2D echocardiography and CMR and found superior reproducibility of LVEF measurements with CMR compared with 2D echocardiography with a mean difference and SD of −0.5±1.7 and 0.5±5.6, respectively [102]. Similar direct comparisons of LVEF measurements of MUGA vs. CMR are not available; however, the reported mean differences for repeated MUGA LVEF measurements are 1.8 %, with SD ranging between 4.4 and 6.9 % [103, 104]. To illustrate, a 5 % SD of the mean difference means that in repeat assessments, notably without any true change in LVEF, this imaging modality will produce LVEF results that are within 20 % of each other (i.e., ±2 SD). With that in mind, it may not be surprising that Swain et al. found in their analysis of 630 patients receiving doxorubicin that 66 % of patients who developed HF had no significant LVEF reduction noticed on serial MUGA scans and many patients had similar EF changes without HF occurrence [16]. The authors concluded that LVEF measurements [with MUGA] are not an accurate predictor of HF in patients who receive doxorubicin. The question though is whether the reproducibility of the modality rather than the physiologic concept of LVEF monitoring is flawed, knowing that occurrence of HF symptoms in the context of cardiotoxicity is uniformly associated with a significant drop in LVEF.

Current guideline cutoffs for detecting cardiotoxicity are based on studies using MUGA showing LVEF variability of 5.4 ± 4.4 % in normal patients and 2.1 ± 2.0 % in abnormal patients [47]. Since the variability of CMR is lower, using CMR we may be able to reliably detect smaller changes and diagnose cardiotoxicity earlier, before there is a large (>10 %) drop in LVEF. Therefore, further research is needed on using CMR LVEFs to detect cardiotoxicity, and based on this research, guidelines may need to be refined. One study supporting this thought is by Drafts et al. [105] who found smaller changes in LVEF of <10 % (58 ± 1 % to 53 ± 1 %), whereas other features such as strain, pulse wave velocity, and biomarkers confirmed that these patients did have cardiotoxicity even though they technically did not meet the current guideline cutoffs for change in LVEF.

Although CMR has been used in cardiotoxicity screening with substantial improvements in diagnosis of cardiomyopathy after cancer treatment [106], at present its use in oncology practice is limited. Arguments raised against its use are primarily concerns regarding availability and cost [62]. Concerning the latter, a closer look at 2014 Medicare National Coverage Determinations Manual demonstrates however a de facto lower cost for the pertinent CMR procedure compared to MUGA and echocardiography procedures (CPT 75557 "cardiac magnetic resonance imaging for morphology and function without contrast material" at $ 294.78 vs. CPT 78473 "cardiac blood pool imaging, gated equilibrium wall motion

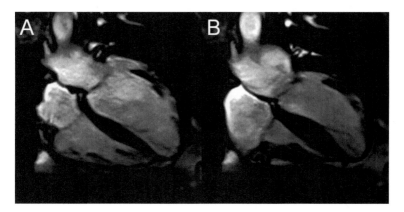

Fig. 3.3 Example CMR images demonstrating cardiomyopathy. A 47-year-old patient with breast cancer treated with anthracyclines, demonstrating cardiomyopathy. Panel A shows a diastolic frame and Panel B shows a systolic frame. The LVEF was quantified at 42 %

with ejection fraction" at $ 397.32 vs. CPT 93306 "echocardiography, transthoracic" at $ 427.00) [107, 108]. Second, the USA has a high availability of MRI scanners with a total of about 12,000 scanners or 38 MRI scanners per million population, and the basic functionality for LVEF measurements can easily be implemented on a clinical scanner and performed with little additional cost and training.

Thus, the main practical limitations to performing MRI for screening in cancer arise in patients with pathologic claustrophobia, which in most patients is mild and can be overcome with conscious sedation, and with implantable devices such as older non-MRI compatible pacemakers and implantable cardioverter-defibrillators. Some breast tissue expanders have magnetic ports, such as the Contour Profile Tissue Expander (Mentor, Santa Barbara, CA), and are not considered safe for an MRI examination. Using current state-of-the-art CMR technology, LVEF measurements can be accomplished within a 15 min examination, which does not require intravenous access or contrast administration. Off-line image analysis of the 3D data set can be accomplished on commercially available workstations within 5 min (Figs. 3.3 and 3.4). Importantly, there are no limitations to visualizing the heart due to acoustic window (which may be obscured by breast expanders such as saline or silicone implants, bone or lung tissue), and radiation doses typically in the order of 7 mSv for each serial MUGA scan can be avoided in these patients with already high radiation exposure due to the need for cancer staging [109].

Delayed Enhancement CMR for Myocardial fibrosis

Cardiac fibrosis can occur without a decrease in LVEF [110, 111] and is a highly sensitive marker of structural heart disease. Cardiac fibrosis occurs in two forms—reactive and replacement. In reactive fibrosis, collagen accumulates diffusely in

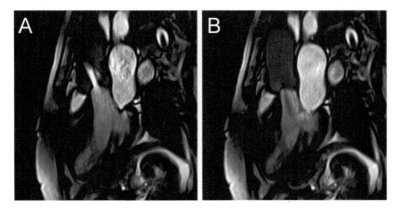

Fig. 3.4 Example CMR images demonstrating valvular disease. A 61-year-old patient with lymphoma treated with chemotherapy and radiation, demonstrating aortic stenosis (**a**) and aortic regurgitation (**b**)

perivascular and interstitial tissues without cardiomyocyte loss, while replacement fibrosis involves loss of cardiomyocytes. Cardiac fibrosis plays an important role in the development and progression of systolic and diastolic heart failure [112, 113]. Increasing cardiac fibrosis results in progressive deterioration of cardiac function, with more extensive cardiac fibrosis identified in patients with advanced heart failure, regardless of the etiology of cardiomyopathy [114, 115]. The presence and extent of cardiac fibrosis has been associated with heart failure [114] and death [115, 116], even in subjects without known cardiac disease [110, 117, 119]. In recent years, cardiac fibrosis has been demonstrated to have an adverse prognostic impact in various forms of heart disease such as ischemic heart disease [120], nonischemic dilated cardiomyopathy [121], hypertrophic cardiomyopathy [122], cardiac sarcoidosis [123], cardiac amyloidosis [124], myocarditis [125], and aortic stenosis [126]. Thus, cardiac fibrosis is not only a highly sensitive but also a prognostically important marker of structural heart disease. Importantly, imaging techniques that are used routinely for assessment of LVEF in cancer patients—echocardiography and MUGA scanning [72]—cannot assess cardiac fibrosis. CMR allows accurate detection and quantification of both reactive and replacement fibrosis [98, 127–129]—reactive fibrosis by T1 mapping and replacement fibrosis by delayed enhancement CMR (DE-CMR).

Two retrospective and one prospective studies from the group at the University of Manitoba described the presence of subepicardial delayed enhancement with a prevalence of 94–100 % in the context of cardiomyopathy in patients with breast cancer during [130, 131] and at the end of treatment [132] with anthracyclines and trastuzumab. However, subsequent studies from other groups [105, 133] have demonstrated that chemotherapy-related cardiotoxicity is not typically associated with any delayed enhancement during or early after treatment. In our collective experience, we have also observed no delayed enhancement in patients with cardiotoxicity during or soon after chemotherapy with either anthracyclines or trastuzumab.

Some patients with chronic cardiomyopathy from cardiotoxicity may develop delayed enhancement that is basal mid-myocardial or at the right ventricular insertion points [133]. The prevalence of these patterns is low [133–135]. These patterns are nonspecific and shared by chronic cardiomyopathies of any etiology. A study of 62 childhood cancer survivors treated with anthracyclines and imaged 7.8 years later described no delayed enhancement [136]. Thus, there is no pattern of delayed enhancement or replacement fibrosis that is unique to chemotherapy-related cardiotoxicity.

Since chemotherapy-related cardiotoxicity is not typically associated with replacement fibrosis, fibrosis seen on CMR with delayed enhancement imaging in the setting of a low LVEF could point to an alternative explanation for the cardiomyopathy, such as an ischemic cardiomyopathy or myocarditis [99]. Thus, delayed enhancement imaging is nevertheless useful in the evaluation of presumed chemotherapy-related cardiotoxicity to confirm the etiology of the cardiomyopathy and to rule out other diagnoses with important implications, such as ischemic heart disease.

CMR for Assessment of Concomitant Cardiac Disease in Cancer Patients

With the increasing number of older patients newly diagnosed with breast and other cancers [137], and as a result thereof the increasing prevalence of co-existing cardiovascular disease, timely diagnosis and initiation of treatment of these is essential prior to exposure to potentially cardiotoxic drug regimens. This is particularly important since preexisting cardiac conditions such as coronary artery disease or cardiomyopathy are known risk factors for both anthracycline-[55, 138] and trastuzumab-related [139] cardiac complications.

A CMR study is modular allowing the expansion of the basic CMR test protocol for LVEF assessment to include evaluation for ischemic heart disease and/or cardiomyopathy as indicated based on patients' history of risk factors and symptoms. For the assessment of myocardial ischemia, there are few additional steps required, including intravenous access and contrast administration. Most elderly and cancer patients have limited exercise tolerance; therefore, pharmacological stress with vasodilators such as adenosine or regadenoson will be more practical in most cases. This "ischemia" protocol, which is typically combined with assessment of myocardial viability/scar with the delayed enhancement technique discussed above, adds approximately 20 min to the baseline exam without contrast. The diagnostic performance of stress CMR for detection of CAD in a recent meta-analysis was reported having a sensitivity of 91 % and specificity of 81 % [140]. Moreover, CMR was shown to be useful in women, who pose in general challenges for noninvasive CAD diagnosis due to smaller heart size, more frequent intermediate severity, and limited extent of CAD, with a sensitivity and specificity of 84 and 88 %, respectively [141].

The pericardium may be affected in cancer patients as the primary affected organ such as in pericardial mesothelioma, but this is rarely diagnosed clinically [142]. However, autopsy studies show that 19–40 % of patients dying of lung cancer, and 10–28 % dying of breast cancer have pericardial involvement, which is typically from direct spread of the primary chest tumor [143]. A sequela of pericardial tumor involvement is pericardial effusion, which can result in tamponade. Pericardial effusion can also be the cardiotoxic sequela of various anticancer agents [12]. Pericardial morphology and the presence of an effusion can be assessed by the same image data set obtained for LVEF assessment. These dynamic images also provide information on the hemodynamic relevance, if collapse of the right atrium and ventricle is present and if the inferior vena cava is dilated [144]. On delayed enhancement images obtained for myocardial tissue characterization, pericardial enhancement indicates the presence of inflammation. Pericardial thickening and typical findings of increased ventricular interdependence on dynamic cine imaging during respiration are hallmarks of constrictive pericarditis [145].

Strain Imaging by CMR

To better characterize the complex deformation and shortening of the helical myocardial layers during contraction, and to differentiate passive tethering of dysfunctional myocardial regions from active contraction, strain imaging was introduced [146, 147]. Strain is a measurement of the percent change in the fiber length and can be obtained in radial, circumferential, and longitudinal direction. A widely validated and reproducible tool for this purpose is tagged CMR, whereby noninvasive markers (e.g., tags) are placed in a grid-like format by locally induced perturbations of magnetization with selective radiofrequency saturation. Several motion quantification techniques are available; the most commonly used is harmonic phase (HARP) analysis [148]. Normal values for maximal longitudinal strain (%; mean $\pm$ SD) depend on age and gender and are highest at the apex and smallest at the base, ranging from -0.13 ± 0.04 to -0.15 ± 0.03 at the base to -0.18 ± 0.05 to -0.19 ± 0.04 at the apex [149]. One study assessed myocardial strain by speckle tracking echocardiography and CMR in childhood cancer survivors exposed to anthracycline therapy with normal systolic function. The authors found that both circumferential and longitudinal myocardial strains were reduced in these individuals compared to normal controls [average mid-peak circumferential strain magnitude -14.9 ± 1.4 versus -19.5 ± 2.1 ($P < 0.001$) and peak longitudinal strain magnitude -13.5 ± 1.9 versus -17.3 ± 1.4 ($P < 0.001$) by CMR] [150]. The added benefit of strain imaging is expected to be the detection of subclinical cardiotoxicity in patients receiving potentially cardiotoxic chemotherapies. To investigate changes in circumferential strain over the course of anthracycline therapy, Drafts et al. performed serial CMR imaging before and 1, 3, and 6 months after therapy in 53 patients. The authors found deterioration in circumferential strain (-17.7 ± 0.4 to -15.1 ± 0.4; $p = 0.0003$); interestingly this was accompanied by a likewise small but significant change in LVEF ($58 \pm 1\%$ to $53 \pm 1\%$; $p = 0.0002$) [105]. This small study raises a question needing further investigation about how much additional diagnostic information is gained by both imaging (strain, etc.) and non-imaging (troponin, etc.) tests over small changes in LVEF that can be detected by CMR as an indication for cardiotoxicity.

T1 and T2 Mapping by CMR to Characterize the Myocardium

T1 and T2 myocardial mapping are promising newer CMR techniques that offer a quantitative assessment of the myocardium (by using T1 and T2 relaxation times) in the evaluation of diffuse myocardial disease (fibrosis and edema).

Reactive fibrosis is most often assessed by CMR using the T1 mapping technique and is expressed using "native" T1 values when performed without contrast and as extracellular volume fraction (ECV) when performed with contrast. The longitudinal relaxation time T1 of a tissue indicates how rapidly protons recover after a radiofrequency pulse. Pre-contrast (or "native") T1 varies with water content and may increase due to diffuse myocardial fibrosis, but it reflects a composite signal from both myocardial cells and the interstitium, and it varies with the measurement technique and CMR field strength. After gadolinium-based contrast administration, T1 times are shortened. The T1 times are a primary reflection of and are inversely proportional to the concentration of gadolinium in the interstitium. Thus, measuring T1 after contrast administration gives a better measure of the interstitial space. However, post-contrast T1 also varies with gadolinium dose, clearance rate, time after contrast administration, body composition, hematocrit, and the heart rate. If the change in T1 after contrast administration is measured in both the myocardium and blood after equilibration of the contrast distribution, the partition coefficient can be calculated. By correcting for the hematocrit level, the myocardial ECV is derived. The ECV is largely independent of the measurement technique and CMR field strength and is an inherent measure of the individual's myocardial interstitial space.

T1 mapping has great potential for the evaluation of chemotherapy-related cardiotoxicity because the predominant type of fibrosis seen in cardiotoxicity is reactive fibrosis and not replacement fibrosis. Diffuse reactive fibrosis is, in fact, a hallmark of the condition. Animal studies of chronic anthracycline cardiotoxicity have shown higher native T1 values compared to controls [151, 152]. ECV has been shown to correlate with anthracycline dose, functional capacity, LV dysfunction, and markers of adverse LV remodeling in pediatric [153] and adult [154] patients after completion of anthracycline-based chemotherapy. Similarly, CMR measures of contrast-enhanced T1-weighted signal intensity were higher 3 months after initiating potentially cardiotoxic chemotherapy in a study of 65 cancer patients [155]. Thus, diffuse reactive fibrosis assessed by CMR has an important role in the pathophysiology and likely the prognosis of chemotherapy-related cardiotoxicity.

T2-weighted CMR is useful in distinguishing acute from chronic myocardial infarction according to the presence or absence of edema. However, T2-weighted sequences have a number of disadvantages including their susceptibility to artifacts and relatively lower differences in signal intensity between edematous and normal myocardium, making the image interpretation difficult. Also, similar to DE-CMR, T2-weighted imaging is based on identification of focally increased signal intensity compared to "normal remote" myocardium. Such a technique would not be useful to identify the presence of diffuse edema in the entire myocardium, as would be expected with chemotherapy-related cardiotoxicity. It is in this regard that T2 mapping would provide an objective and quantitative measure of diffuse myocardial edema.

In an animal study of early anthracycline cardiotoxicity, T2 values were increased in explanted hearts of anthracycline-treated rats in comparison to controls, even in the absence of LV dysfunction or histopathologic evidence of cardiac fibrosis or necrosis [156]. However, another rat study of anthracycline cardiotoxicity did not show any significant changes in T2 values in explanted hearts of anthracycline-treated rats [151]. In a human study of 65 cancer patients treated with anthracyclines who had CMRs before and 3 months after initiation of chemotherapy and had small but significant LVEF declines, there was no significant increase in myocardial relative enhancement (quantified as the ratio of myocardial to skeletal muscle signal intensity) on T2-weighted images [155]. There are three main explanations for the negative finding: one, there may be absence of significant edema with cardiotoxicity; two, this study only noted small declines in LVEF and edema may be seen in those with larger declines in LVEF; or three, imaging at 3 months may not be the right timing to detect edema from cardiotoxicity. Therefore, further research is warranted to investigate whether T2 mapping could be used for the early detection of cardiotoxicity.

Targeted Nuclear Imaging by CMR

Cell death by apoptosis is believed to be an important mechanism in ischemic and nonischemic cardiomyopathies [157]. An early event in apoptosis is translocation of phosphatidylserine on the extracellular surface of the cell membrane, where annexin V, a commercially available soluble protein, can bind. This protein has been recently conjugated to superparamagnetic iron oxide (SPIO), which is a negative MRI contrast agent that can be visualized using a T2*-weighted MRI pulse sequence. Dash et al. have tested this technique to detect apoptosis in a mouse model of doxorubicin cardiotoxicity. They found a good correlation between CMR T2* signal loss and number of apoptotic cells in tissue samples. In vivo, they were able to detect apoptotic activity up to 10 days after doxorubicin exposure and moreover demonstrated that apoptosis is a reversible and treatable process with alpha-1-adrenergic receptor agonists [158].

Detection of Vascular Injury by CMR

In addition to HF from myocardial toxicity, damage to the endothelium and increased risk for vascular disease have been demonstrated after anthracyclines [59], hormone therapy [159], and therapies targeting the vascular endothelial growth factor (VGEF) pathway with bevacizumab [160] and sorafenib [161]. Using the phase-contrast velocity flow mapping technique, which allows the measurement of blood flow and the generation of flow velocity time curves, Chaosuwannakit et al. were able to demonstrate an increase in aortic stiffness after anthracycline therapy. They studied aortic blood flow in 40 patients before and after anthracycline treatment and demonstrated an increase in pulse wave velocities and decrease in aortic distensibility in treated patients but not in controls [59]. Endothelial function can be assessed noninvasively by flow-mediated arterial dilatation (FMAD) [162] and could be used in studies investigating vascular effects of chemotherapies.

Nuclear Cardiology Techniques

New radiopharmaceuticals and technical advances in scintigraphy have contributed to an evolution in nuclear cardiac imaging for cancer patients starting from MUGA, used to quantitate LVEF, to higher-order functional techniques capable of visualizing pathophysiologic and neurophysiologic processes at the cardiac tissue level. Molecular imaging techniques including ^{111}In-antimyosin (marker specific for myocardial cell necrosis) and ^{123}I-metaiodobenzylguanidine (imaging the efferent sympathetic nervous innervation) have demonstrated potential as early predictors of chemotherapy-induced cardiotoxicity in anthracycline-treated patients. In one study, ^{111}In-antimyosin uptake was more intense in patients with low LVEF and correlated with LVEF values [163] while increased uptake at intermediate cumulative doses identified patients at risk for cardiotoxicity before LVEF deterioration [164]. The same group showed that patients with more intense ^{111}In-antimyosin uptake at intermediate doses tended to have more severe cardiac functional impairment at maximal cumulative doses [165]. Another small prospective study found that at low doxorubicin and epirubicin dose levels, ^{111}In-antimyosin uptake occurred in the absence of LV systolic and diastolic dysfunction suggesting that ^{111}In-antimyosin is very sensitive in detecting myocyte damage that precedes LV dysfunction [166]. Declines in ^{123}I-metaiodobenzylguanidine uptake have also demonstrated correlation with higher cumulative anthracycline doses and preceded changes in LVEF [165, 167]. Nevertheless, despite promising results, these techniques, which were investigated more than a decade ago, still have not been integrated into standard clinical practice.

Blood-Based Cardiac Biomarkers

Blood-based cardiac biomarkers, specifically troponins, have emerged as potentially useful noninvasive markers of cardiotoxicity in cancer based on the findings of numerous small studies. Cardiac troponins (troponins I, T, etc.) are released into the serum as a result of cardiac myocyte death and are the established gold standard for detecting cardiomyocyte necrosis from any cause. A transient rise in cardiac troponin I has been demonstrated to predict the occurrence [168, 169] as well as the magnitude of LVEF decline [169–169] in patients with hematologic and solid malignancies receiving high-dose anthracyclines (Table 3.3). In women receiving anthracycline-trastuzumab-containing therapy, detectable troponin I levels (>0.08 ng/ml) were associated with a 23-fold increased risk of "cardiotoxicity" (LVEF decline >10 % to <50 %) and a ~3-fold increased risk of LVEF irreversibility following drug discontinuation [56]. Early changes in highly and ultrasensitive troponin I have shown incremental prognostic power, particularly in combination with STE, to predict HF in early breast cancer patients treated with anthracycline-trastuzumab therapy [90, 92]. However, as reported by Sawaya et al. [90], the sensitivity and specificity of ultrasensitive troponin I for predicting anthracycline-trastuzumab cardiotoxicity are not high at 48 % (95 % CI, 27 %–69 %) and 73 % (95 % CI, 59 %–84 %), respectively, and the clinical utility of troponin measurements is not as well established for non-anthracycline-based chemotherapeutic regimens [172]. The family of natriuretic peptides (e.g., brain natriuretic peptide (BNP), N-terminal pro-BNP, and N-terminal pro-atrial natriuretic peptide) which measure myocardial stress/stretch and are prognostic in general HF populations appears to be less reliable than troponins in predicting LVEF decline in the oncology setting [174, 175].

Overall, the studies of troponins and natriuretic peptides do have notable limitations. The predictive role of these biomarkers has been investigated in small studies with heterogeneous cancer populations receiving a variety of cytotoxic and targeted therapies [175]. Moreover, standardization of timing of assessments, measurement assays, and cutoff points remain undetermined, currently limiting translation into clinical practice.

Stress-Related Functional Testing

Cancer therapy is associated with reduced cardiovascular reserve attributed to either the direct effects of therapy or the indirect effects of therapy-associated lifestyle changes [11, 176]. Application of "system stress" (via pharmacology or exercise) is an established method to detect subclinical impairments in myocardial function, and determination of contractile reserve is an independent predictor of prognosis beyond LVEF in patients with coronary artery disease (CAD), although these methods have received limited attention in cancer therapy-related cardiotoxicity [61]. Using exercise stress echocardiography in 57 asymptomatic

Table 3.3 Troponin for early detection and prediction of cancer therapy-related cardiotoxicity

Reference	Patient population	Treatment	N	Detection	Cutoff	% BM+	LVEF modality	Mean ↓LVEF BM+	Mean ↓LVEF BM−	Incidence of ↓LVEF >10% or LVEF <50% BM+	Incidence of ↓LVEF >10% or LVEF <50% BM−	Incidence of HF symptoms BM+	Incidence of HF symptoms BM−	BM predicted (P sig) ↓LVEF	BM predicted (P sig) HF
Sawaya [92]	Breast	ANT, H	43	hsTnI	0.015 µg/L	28 %	Echo	–	–	50 %	10 %	–	–	Yes	–
Sawaya [90]	Breast	ANT, H	81	usTnI	30 pg/mL	14 %	Echo	–	–	42 %	27 %	8 %	5 %	Yes	–
Fallah-Rad [132]	Breast	FEC, H AC, H	42	cTnT	0.01 ng/mL	0 %	Echo	–	~4 %	–	24 %	–	24 %	No	No
Cardinale [168]	Multiple diagnoses	HDC	204	cTnI	0.4 ng/ml	32 %	Echo	>10 %	~0 %	29 %	0 %	5 %	0 %	Yes	Yes[a]
Cardinale [169]	Multiple diagnoses	HDC	703	cTnI	0.08 ng/ml	30 %	Echo	–	–	71 %	2 %	22 %	0.2 %	Yes	Yes[b]
Cardinale [170]	Breast	HDC	211	cTnI	0.5 ng/ml	33 %	Echo	>15 %	~0 %	–	–	14 %	0 %	Yes	–
Sandri [171]	Multiple diagnoses	HDC	179	cTnI	0.08 µg/ml	32 %	Echo	18 %	3 %	–	–	–	–	Yes	–
Cardinale [56]	Breast	H	251	cTnI	0.08 ng/ml	14 %	Echo	–	–	72 %	7 %	19 %	0 %	Yes	Yes[b]
Morris [172]	Breast	ddAC → THL	95	cTnI	0.04–0.06 ng/ml	67 %	RNA	–	–	5 %	19 %	2 %	7 %	No	No

↓ = decline or impairment; Δ = change

Table adapted from Khouri et al. [173]

AC doxorubicin and cyclophosphamide; ANT anthracyclines; BM biomarker; cTnI cardiac troponin I; cTnT cardiac troponin T; dd dose-dense; FEC fluorouracil, epirubicin, cyclophosphamide; H trastuzumab; HDC high-dose chemotherapy; HF heart failure; hsTnI high-sensitivity troponin I; L lapatinib; LVEF left ventricular ejection fraction; RNA radionuclide angiography; T paclitaxel; usTnI ultrasensitive troponin I

[a]All patients (n = 3) developing HF during study were cTnI+

[b]Elevated cTnI predicted composite cardiac events, including heart failure

early-stage breast cancer survivors with resting LVEF $\geq$ 50 %, Khouri et al. found that change in LV stroke volume and cardiac index (from rest) were significantly reduced by 12 and 24 %, respectively, compared to controls, suggesting that patients have impaired LV contractile reserve (LVCR) [177]. McKillop et al. [178] examined radionuclide-determined LVEF at rest and during graded exercise testing in 37 patients receiving doxorubicin; exercise LVEF improved the sensitivity for detection of cardiotoxicity from 58 to 100 %. Civelli et al. [179] measured LVCR (defined as the difference between peak and resting LVEF) with low-dose dobutamine during and after high-dose chemotherapy in women with advanced breast cancer; an asymptomatic decline in LVCR of $\geq$5 units from baseline predicted LVEF decline to <50 %. By comparison, multiple exercise and pharmacologic stress studies have been performed in anthracycline-treated adult survivors of pediatric malignancies with mixed results regarding the incremental sensitivity of exercise [180–183] or pharmacologic [184, 185] stress echocardiography to detect subclinical therapy-induced cardiotoxicity over resting echocardiography alone.

Cancer therapy-related cardiac damage also occurs in conjunction with (mal) adaptation in other organ components [11, 61, 105, 153]. Thus, tools with the ability to evaluate integrated cross talk between cardiovascular organ components, like VO_{2peak}, may provide a more comprehensive measure of therapy-related global cardiovascular effects in the setting of cancer [61]. As a measure of global cardiovascular function and reserve capacity, VO_{2peak} is also inversely correlated with cardiovascular and all-cause mortality in a broad range of adult populations, including lung cancer [186–189]. In breast cancer, Jones et al. [190] found that despite preserved resting LVEF $\geq$ 50 %, 130 patients, on average 3 years following the completion of adjuvant therapy, had VO_{2peak} that was 22 % below that of sedentary age-matched women without a history of breast cancer. Studies investigating the predictive value of VO_{2peak} for acute and late-occurring cardiac dysfunction and other cardiovascular events in cancer patients are warranted.

Genetic Risk Profiling

Future strategies to treat and prevent anticancer therapy-induced cardiotoxicity are likely to include personalized approaches that tailor patients to specific therapies using geneomic(s)-based approaches [191]. Gene polymorphisms may explain, in part, observed heterogeneity in the incidence rates of cardiotoxicity and may contribute to myocardial injury from trastuzumab [192] and anthracyclines [193–195]. Homozygosis for the G allele in carbonyl reductase 3 (CBR3) contributed to increased cardiomyopathy risk among childhood cancer survivors treated with low-to moderate-dose anthracyclines [193], whereas breast cancer susceptibility gene 2 (BRCA2) deficiency was demonstrated to increase anthracycline-induced DNA damage, apoptosis, and risk of cardiac failure in mouse models [194]. Furthermore, analyses of single nucleotide polymorphisms (SNPs) among anthracycline-treated children found that using patients' genetic information in combination with clinical risk factors improved discrimination of risk for anthracycline-induced cardiotoxicity beyond clinical risk factors alone [195]. Although preliminary, these studies support the potential for genetic testing to enhance surveillance and prediction of cardiotoxicity, and further study is required.

Conclusions

Cardiovascular disease and cancer lead to significant morbidity and mortality in the North American population. Improvements in cancer therapies have led to increased survivorship; however, these treatments may contribute to cardiac morbidity and mortality. Guidance on how to best monitor cancer patients during and following these treatments is lacking. Current imaging modalities used to detect cardiotoxicity, such as resting LVEF, are insensitive. Many alternative techniques have been proposed including advanced cardiac imaging modalities, functional capacity testing, blood-based biomarkers, and genetic testing, but no best approach or combination of approaches has yet to clearly emerge. Research evaluating the role of biomarkers, alternate imaging strategies, and the optimal timing and frequency of these detection techniques is needed. Large prospective, multi-institutional studies will determine whether these techniques can be used practically to improve not only detection of cardiotoxicity but also prediction of cardiovascular and overall survival, thereby facilitating early interventions that may reduce risk of downstream cardiovascular morbidity without compromising the efficacy of anti-cancer therapy.

References

1. Jemal A, Ward E, Hao Y, Thun M. Trends in the leading causes of death in the United States, 1970–2002. JAMA. 2005;294(10):1255–9.
2. Jemal A, Ward E, Thun M. Declining death rates reflect progress against cancer. PLoS One. 2010;5(3):e9584.
3. Howlader N, Ries LA, Mariotto AB, Reichman ME, Ruhl J, Cronin KA. Improved estimates of cancer-specific survival rates from population-based data. J Natl Cancer Inst. 2010;102 (20):1584–98.
4. Siegel R, DeSantis C, Virgo K, Stein K, Mariotto A, Smith T, et al. Cancer treatment and survivorship statistics, 2012. CA Cancer J Clin. 2012;62(4):220–41.
5. Chapman JA, Meng D, Shepherd L, Parulekar W, Ingle JN, Muss HB, et al. Competing causes of death from a randomized trial of extended adjuvant endocrine therapy for breast cancer. J Natl Cancer Inst. 2008;100(4):252–60.
6. Hanrahan EO, Gonzalez-Angulo AM, Giordano SH, Rouzier R, Broglio KR, Hortobagyi GN, et al. Overall survival and cause-specific mortality of patients with stage T1a, bN0M0 breast carcinoma. J Clin Oncol. 2007;25(31):4952–60.
7. Lloyd-Jones DM, Leip EP, Larson MG, D'Agostino RB, Beiser A, Wilson PW, et al. Prediction of lifetime risk for cardiovascular disease by risk factor burden at 50 years of age. Circulation. 2006;113(6):791–8.

8. Schairer C, Mink PJ, Carroll L, Devesa SS. Probabilities of death from breast cancer and other causes among female breast cancer patients. J Natl Cancer Inst. 2004;96(17):1311–21.
9. Patnaik JL, Byers T, Diguiseppi C, Dabelea D, Denberg TD. Cardiovascular disease competes with breast cancer as the leading cause of death for older females diagnosed with breast cancer: a retrospective cohort study. Breast Cancer Res. 2011;13(3):R64.
10. Colzani E, Liljegren A, Johansson AL, Adolfsson J, Hellborg H, Hall PF, et al. Prognosis of patients with breast cancer: causes of death and effects of time since diagnosis, age, and tumor characteristics. J Clin Oncol. 2011;29(30):4014–21.
11. Jones LW, Haykowsky MJ, Swartz JJ, Douglas PS, Mackey JR. Early breast cancer therapy and cardiovascular injury. J Am Coll Cardiol. 2007;50(15):1435–41.
12. Yeh ET, Bickford CL. Cardiovascular complications of cancer therapy: incidence, pathogenesis, diagnosis, and management. J Am Coll Cardiol. 2009;53(24):2231–47.
13. Chu TF, Rupnick MA, Kerkela R, Dallabrida SM, Zurakowski D, Nguyen L, et al. Cardiotoxicity associated with tyrosine kinase inhibitor sunitinib. Lancet. 2007;370(9604):2011–9.
14. Hall PS, Harshman LC, Srinivas S, Witteles RM. The frequency and severity of cardiovascular toxicity from targeted therapy in advanced renal cell carcinoma patients. JACC Heart Fail. 2013;1(1):72–8.
15. Von Hoff DD, Layard MW, Basa P, Davis Jr HL, Von Hoff AL, Rozencweig M, et al. Risk factors for doxorubicin-induced congestive heart failure. Ann Intern Med. 1979;91(5):710–7.
16. Swain SM, Whaley FS, Ewer MS. Congestive heart failure in patients treated with doxorubicin: a retrospective analysis of three trials. Cancer. 2003;97(11):2869–79.
17. Perez EA, Suman VJ, Davidson NE, Kaufman PA, Martino S, Dakhil SR, et al. Effect of doxorubicin plus cyclophosphamide on left ventricular ejection fraction in patients with breast cancer in the North Central Cancer Treatment Group N9831 Intergroup Adjuvant Trial. J Clin Oncol. 2004;22(18):3700–4.
18. Meinardi MT, van Veldhuisen DJ, Gietema JA, Dolsma WV, Boomsma F, van den Berg MP, et al. Prospective evaluation of early cardiac damage induced by epirubicin-containing adjuvant chemotherapy and locoregional radiotherapy in breast cancer patients. J Clin Oncol. 2001;19(10):2746–53.
19. Mackey JR, Martin M, Pienkowski T, Rolski J, Guastalla JP, Sami A, et al. Adjuvant docetaxel, doxorubicin, and cyclophosphamide in node-positive breast cancer: 10-year follow-up of the phase 3 randomised BCIRG 001 trial. Lancet Oncol. 2013;14(1):72–80.
20. Wouters KA, Kremer LC, Miller TL, Herman EH, Lipshultz SE. Protecting against anthracycline-induced myocardial damage: a review of the most promising strategies. Br J Haematol. 2005;131(5):561–78.
21. Schmidinger M, Zielinski CC, Vogl UM, Bojic A, Bojic M, Schukro C, et al. Cardiac toxicity of sunitinib and sorafenib in patients with metastatic renal cell carcinoma. J Clin Oncol. 2008;26(32):5204–12.
22. Tocchetti CG, Ragone G, Coppola C, Rea D, Piscopo G, Scala S, et al. Detection, monitoring, and management of trastuzumab-induced left ventricular dysfunction: an actual challenge. Eur J Heart Fail. 2012;14(2):130–7.
23. Force T, Kolaja KL. Cardiotoxicity of kinase inhibitors: the prediction and translation of preclinical models to clinical outcomes. Nat Rev Drug Discov. 2011;10(2):111–26.
24. Ky B, Vejpongsa P, Yeh ET, Force T, Moslehi JJ. Emerging paradigms in cardiomyopathies associated with cancer therapies. Circ Res. 2013;113(6):754–64.
25. Tan-Chiu E, Yothers G, Romond E, Geyer Jr CE, Ewer M, Keefe D, et al. Assessment of cardiac dysfunction in a randomized trial comparing doxorubicin and cyclophosphamide followed by paclitaxel, with or without trastuzumab as adjuvant therapy in node-positive, human epidermal growth factor receptor 2-overexpressing breast cancer: NSABP B-31. J Clin Oncol. 2005;23(31):7811–9.
26. Perez EA, Rodeheffer R. Clinical cardiac tolerability of trastuzumab. J Clin Oncol. 2004;22(2):322–9.

27. Cheng H, Force T. Molecular mechanisms of cardiovascular toxicity of targeted cancer therapeutics. Circ Res. 2010;106(1):21–34.

28. Telli ML, Hunt SA, Carlson RW, Guardino AE. Trastuzumab-related cardiotoxicity: calling into question the concept of reversibility. J Clin Oncol. 2007;25(23):3525–33.

29. Common Terminology Criteria for Adverse Events v4.03 (CTCAE). http://evs.nci.nih.gov/ftp1/CTCAE. Publish date: June 14 DaN, 2011.

30. Seidman A, Hudis C, Pierri MK, Shak S, Paton V, Ashby M, et al. Cardiac dysfunction in the trastuzumab clinical trials experience. J Clin Oncol. 2002;20(5):1215–21.

31. Yancy CW, Jessup M, Bozkurt B, Butler J, Casey Jr DE, Drazner MH, et al. 2013 ACCF/AHA guideline for the management of heart failure: a report of the American College of Cardiology Foundation/American Heart Association Task Force on Practice Guidelines. J Am Coll Cardiol. 2013;62(16):e147–239.

32. Ammar KA, Jacobsen SJ, Mahoney DW, Kors JA, Redfield MM, Burnett Jr JC, et al. Prevalence and prognostic significance of heart failure stages: application of the American College of Cardiology/American Heart Association heart failure staging criteria in the community. Circulation. 2007;115(12):1563–70.

33. Cardinale D, Colombo A, Lamantia G, Colombo N, Civelli M, De Giacomi G, et al. Anthracycline-induced cardiomyopathy: clinical relevance and response to pharmacologic therapy. J Am Coll Cardiol. 2010;55(3):213–20.

34. Lenihan DJ, Sawyer DB. Heart disease in cancer patients: a burgeoning field where optimizing patient care is requiring interdisciplinary collaborations. Heart Fail Clin. 2011;7(3):xxi–xxiii.

35. Schmitz KH, Prosnitz RG, Schwartz AL, Carver JR. Prospective surveillance and management of cardiac toxicity and health in breast cancer survivors. Cancer. 2012;118 (8 Suppl):2270–6.

36. Arnold JM, Howlett JG, Dorian P, Ducharme A, Giannetti N, Haddad H, et al. Canadian Cardiovascular Society Consensus Conference recommendations on heart failure update 2007: Prevention, management during intercurrent illness or acute decompensation, and use of biomarkers. Can J Cardiol. 2007;23(1):21–45.

37. Davis M, Witteles RM. Cardiac testing to manage cardiovascular risk in cancer patients. Semin Oncol. 2013;40(2):147–55.

38. Curigliano G, Cardinale D, Suter T, Plataniotis G, de Azambuja E, Sandri MT, et al. Cardiovascular toxicity induced by chemotherapy, targeted agents and radiotherapy: ESMO Clinical Practice Guidelines. Ann Oncol. 2012;23 Suppl 7:vii155–66.

39. Carver JR, Shapiro CL, Ng A, Jacobs L, Schwartz C, Virgo KS, et al. American Society of Clinical Oncology clinical evidence review on the ongoing care of adult cancer survivors: cardiac and pulmonary late effects. J Clin Oncol. 2007;25(25):3991–4008.

40. McDonagh TA, Blue L, Clark AL, Dahlström U, Ekman I, Lainscak M, et al. European Society of Cardiology Heart Failure Association Standards for delivering heart failure care. Eur J Heart Fail. 2011;13(3):235–41.

41. Plana JC, Galderisi M, Barac A, Ewer MS, Ky B, Scherrer-Crosbie M, et al. Expert consensus for multimodality imaging evaluation of adult patients during and after cancer therapy: a report from the American Society of Echocardiography and the European Association of Cardiovascular Imaging. J Am Soc Echocardiogr. 2014;27(9):911–39.

42. Carver JR, Szalda D, Ky B. Asymptomatic cardiac toxicity in long-term cancer survivors: defining the population and recommendations for surveillance. Semin Oncol. 2013;40 (2):229–38.

43. Chavez-MacGregor M, Niu J, Zhang N, Elting LS, Smith BD, Banchs J, et al. Cardiac monitoring during adjuvant trastuzumab-based chemotherapy among older patients with breast cancer. J Clin Oncol. 2015:JCO. 2014.58. 9465.

44. Armenian SH, et al. Prevention and monitoring of cardiac dysfunction in survivors of adult cancers: American society of clinical oncology clinical practice guideline. J Clin Oncol. 2016 (Epub ahead of print).

45. Virani SA, et al. Canadian cardiovascular society guidelines for evaluation and management of cardiovascular complications of cancer therapy. Can J Cardiol. 2016;32:831–41.

46. Alexander J, Dainiak N, Berger HJ, Goldman L, Johnstone D, Reduto L, et al. Serial assessment of doxorubicin cardiotoxicity with quantitative radionuclide angiocardiography. N Engl J Med. 1979;300(6):278–83.
47. Wackers FJ, Berger HJ, Johnstone DE, Goldman L, Reduto LA, Langou RA, et al. Multiple gated cardiac blood pool imaging for left ventricular ejection fraction: validation of the technique and assessment of variability. Am J Cardiol. 1979;43(6):1159–66.
48. Upton MT, Rerych SK, Newman GE, Bounous Jr EP, Jones RH. The reproducibility of radionuclide angiographic measurements of left ventricular function in normal subjects at rest and during exercise. Circulation. 1980;62(1):126–32.
49. Schwartz RG, McKenzie WB, Alexander J, Sager P, D'Souza A, Manatunga A, et al. Congestive heart failure and left ventricular dysfunction complicating doxorubicin therapy. Seven-year experience using serial radionuclide angiocardiography. Am J Med. 1987;82 (6):1109–18.
50. McMurray JJ, Adamopoulos S, Anker SD, Auricchio A, Bohm M, Dickstein K, et al. ESC Guidelines for the diagnosis and treatment of acute and chronic heart failure 2012: The Task Force for the Diagnosis and Treatment of Acute and Chronic Heart Failure 2012 of the European Society of Cardiology. Developed in collaboration with the Heart Failure Association (HFA) of the ESC. Eur Heart J. 2012;33(14):1787–847.
51. Kalam K, Otahal P, Marwick TH. Prognostic implications of global LV dysfunction: a systematic review and meta-analysis of global longitudinal strain and ejection fraction. Heart. 2014;100(21):1673–80.
52. Ewer MS, Ali MK, Mackay B, Wallace S, Valdivieso M, Legha SS, et al. A comparison of cardiac biopsy grades and ejection fraction estimations in patients receiving Adriamycin. J Clin Oncol. 1984;2(2):112–7.
53. Delgado V, Mollema SA, Ypenburg C, Tops LF, van der Wall EE, Schalij MJ, et al. Relation between global left ventricular longitudinal strain assessed with novel automated function imaging and biplane left ventricular ejection fraction in patients with coronary artery disease. J Am Soc Echocardiogr. 2008;21(11):1244–50.
54. Mann DL, Bristow MR. Mechanisms and models in heart failure: the biomechanical model and beyond. Circulation. 2005;111(21):2837–49.
55. Doyle JJ, Neugut AI, Jacobson JS, Grann VR, Hershman DL. Chemotherapy and cardiotoxicity in older breast cancer patients: a population-based study. J Clin Oncol. 2005;23(34):8597–605.
56. Cardinale D, Colombo A, Torrisi R, Sandri MT, Civelli M, Salvatici M, et al. Trastuzumab-induced cardiotoxicity: clinical and prognostic implications of troponin I evaluation. J Clin Oncol. 2010;28(25):3910–6.
57. Jones LW, Eves ND, Haykowsky M, Freedland SJ, Mackey JR. Exercise intolerance in cancer and the role of exercise therapy to reverse dysfunction. Lancet Oncol. 2009;10 (6):598–605.
58. Lakoski SG, Eves ND, Douglas PS, Jones LW. Exercise rehabilitation in patients with cancer. Nat Rev Clin Oncol. 2012;9(5):288–96.
59. Chaosuwannakit N, D'Agostino Jr R, Hamilton CA, Lane KS, Ntim WO, Lawrence J, et al. Aortic stiffness increases upon receipt of anthracycline chemotherapy. J Clin Oncol. 2010;28 (1):166–72.
60. Beckman JA, Thakore A, Kalinowski BH, Harris JR, Creager MA. Radiation therapy impairs endothelium-dependent vasodilation in humans. J Am Coll Cardiol. 2001;37(3):761–5.
61. Koelwyn GJ, Khouri M, Mackey JR, Douglas PS, Jones LW. Running on empty: cardiovascular reserve capacity and late effects of therapy in cancer survivorship. J Clin Oncol. 2012;30(36):4458–61.
62. Khouri MG, Douglas PS, Mackey JR, Martin M, Scott JM, Scherrer-Crosbie M, et al. Cancer therapy-induced cardiac toxicity in early breast cancer: addressing the unresolved issues. Circulation. 2012;126(23):2749–63.

63. Verma S, Ewer MS. Is cardiotoxicity being adequately assessed in current trials of cytotoxic and targeted agents in breast cancer? Ann Oncol. 2011;22(5):1011–8.

64. Bellenger NG, Burgess MI, Ray SG, Lahiri A, Coats AJ, Cleland JG, et al. Comparison of left ventricular ejection fraction and volumes in heart failure by echocardiography, radionuclide ventriculography and cardiovascular magnetic resonance; are they interchangeable? Eur Heart J. 2000;21(16):1387–96.

65. Ewer MS, Lenihan DJ. Left ventricular ejection fraction and cardiotoxicity: is our ear really to the ground? J Clin Oncol. 2008;26(8):1201–3.

66. Trastuzumab (Herceptin). Package Insert. San Francisco CG, Inc.

67. Romond EH, Jeong JH, Rastogi P, Swain SM, Geyer Jr CE, Ewer MS, et al. Seven-year follow-up assessment of cardiac function in NSABP B-31, a randomized trial comparing doxorubicin and cyclophosphamide followed by paclitaxel (ACP) with ACP plus trastuzumab as adjuvant therapy for patients with node-positive, human epidermal growth factor receptor 2-positive breast cancer. J Clin Oncol. 2012;30(31):3792–9.

68. Romond EH, Perez EA, Bryant J, Suman VJ, Geyer Jr CE, Davidson NE, et al. Trastuzumab plus adjuvant chemotherapy for operable HER2-positive breast cancer. N Engl J Med. 2005;353(16):1673–84.

69. Slamon D, Eiermann W, Robert N, Pienkowski T, Martin M, Press M, et al. Adjuvant trastuzumab in HER2-positive breast cancer. N Engl J Med. 2011;365(14):1273–83.

70. van Royen N, Jaffe CC, Krumholz HM, Johnson KM, Lynch PJ, Natale D, et al. Comparison and reproducibility of visual echocardiographic and quantitative radionuclide left ventricular ejection fractions. Am J Cardiol. 1996;77(10):843–50.

71. Plana JC, Galderisi M, Barac A, Ewer MS, Ky B, Scherrer-Crosbie M, et al. Expert consensus for multimodality imaging evaluation of adult patients during and after cancer therapy: a report from the American Society of Echocardiography and the European Association of Cardiovascular Imaging. Eur Heart J Cardiovasc Imaging. 2014;15(10):1063–93.

72. Chavez-MacGregor M, Niu J, Zhang N, Elting LS, Smith BD, Banchs J, et al. Cardiac monitoring during adjuvant trastuzumab-based chemotherapy among older patients with breast cancer. J Clin Oncol. 2015;33(19):2176–83.

73. Corbett JR, Akinboboye OO, Bacharach SL, Borer JS, Botvinick EH, DePuey EG, et al. Equilibrium radionuclide angiocardiography. J Nucl Cardiol. 2006;13(6):e56–79.

74. Einstein AJ, Berman DS, Min JK, Hendel RC, Gerber TC, Carr JJ, et al. Patient-centered imaging: shared decision making for cardiac imaging procedures with exposure to ionizing radiation. J Am Coll Cardiol. 2014;63(15):1480–9.

75. Chen J, Einstein AJ, Fazel R, Krumholz HM, Wang Y, Ross JS, et al. Cumulative exposure to ionizing radiation from diagnostic and therapeutic cardiac imaging procedures: a population-based analysis. J Am Coll Cardiol. 2010;56(9):702–11.

76. Herceptin (Trastuzumab) Prescribing Information. Available online at http://wwwgenecom/download/pdf/herceptin_prescribing.pdf. Date checked 30 Aug 2015.

77. Berrington de Gonzalez A, Kim KP, Smith-Bindman R, McAreavey D. Myocardial perfusion scans: projected population cancer risks from current levels of use in the United States. Circulation. 2010;122(23):2403–10.

78. DeSantis CE, Lin CC, Mariotto AB, Siegel RL, Stein KD, Kramer JL, et al. Cancer treatment and survivorship statistics, 2014. CA Cancer J Clin. 2014;64(4):252–71.

79. Shih T, Lichtenberg R, Jacobs W. Ejection fraction: subjective visual echocardiographic estimation versus radionuclide angiography. Echocardiography. 2003;20(3):225–30.

80. Jensen-Urstad K, Bouvier F, Hojer J, Ruiz H, Hulting J, Samad B, et al. Comparison of different echocardiographic methods with radionuclide imaging for measuring left ventricular ejection fraction during acute myocardial infarction treated by thrombolytic therapy. Am J Cardiol. 1998;81(5):538–44.

81. Thavendiranathan P, Grant AD, Negishi T, Plana JC, Popovic ZB, Marwick TH. Reproducibility of echocardiographic techniques for sequential assessment of left

ventricular ejection fraction and volumes: application to patients undergoing cancer chemotherapy. J Am Coll Cardiol. 2013;61(1):77–84.

82. Walker J, Bhullar N, Fallah-Rad N, Lytwyn M, Golian M, Fang T, et al. Role of three-dimensional echocardiography in breast cancer: comparison with two-dimensional echocardiography, multiple-gated acquisition scans, and cardiac magnetic resonance imaging. J Clin Oncol. 2010;28(21):3429–36.

83. Gorcsan 3rd J, Tanaka H. Echocardiographic assessment of myocardial strain. J Am Coll Cardiol. 2011;58(14):1401–13.

84. Sengupta PP, Tajik AJ, Chandrasekaran K, Khandheria BK. Twist mechanics of the left ventricle: principles and application. JACC Cardiovasc Imaging. 2008;1(3):366–76.

85. Thavendiranathan P, Poulin F, Lim KD, Plana JC, Woo A, Marwick TH. Use of myocardial strain imaging by echocardiography for the early detection of cardiotoxicity in patients during and after cancer chemotherapy: a systematic review. J Am Coll Cardiol. 2014;63 (25 Pt A):2751–68.

86. Ganame J, Claus P, Uyttebroeck A, Renard M, D'Hooge J, Bijnens B, et al. Myocardial dysfunction late after low-dose anthracycline treatment in asymptomatic pediatric patients. J Am Soc Echocardiogr. 2007;20(12):1351–8.

87. Jurcut R, Wildiers H, Ganame J, D'Hooge J, De Backer J, Denys H, et al. Strain rate imaging detects early cardiac effects of pegylated liposomal Doxorubicin as adjuvant therapy in elderly patients with breast cancer. J Am Soc Echocardiogr. 2008;21(12):1283–9.

88. Hare JL, Brown JK, Leano R, Jenkins C, Woodward N, Marwick TH. Use of myocardial deformation imaging to detect preclinical myocardial dysfunction before conventional measures in patients undergoing breast cancer treatment with trastuzumab. Am Heart J. 2009;158 (2):294–301.

89. Mercuro G, Cadeddu C, Piras A, Dessi M, Madeddu C, Deidda M, et al. Early epirubicin-induced myocardial dysfunction revealed by serial tissue Doppler echocardiography: correlation with inflammatory and oxidative stress markers. Oncologist. 2007;12(9):1124–33.

90. Sawaya H, Sebag IA, Plana JC, Januzzi JL, Ky B, Tan TC, et al. Assessment of echocardiography and biomarkers for the extended prediction of cardiotoxicity in patients treated with anthracyclines, taxanes, and trastuzumab. Circ Cardiovasc Imaging. 2012;5(5):596–603.

91. Armstrong GT, Joshi VM, Ness KK, Marwick TH, Zhang N, Srivastava D, et al. Comprehensive echocardiographic detection of treatment-related cardiac dysfunction in adult survivors of childhood cancer: results from the St. Jude Lifetime Cohort Study. J Am Coll Cardiol. 2015;65(23):2511–22.

92. Sawaya H, Sebag IA, Plana JC, Januzzi JL, Ky B, Cohen V, et al. Early detection and prediction of cardiotoxicity in chemotherapy-treated patients. Am J Cardiol. 2011;107 (9):1375–80.

93. Negishi K, Negishi T, Hare JL, Haluska BA, Plana JC, Marwick TH. Independent and incremental value of deformation indices for prediction of trastuzumab-induced cardiotoxicity. J Am Soc Echocardiogr. 2013;26(5):493–8.

94. Motoki H, Koyama J, Nakazawa H, Aizawa K, Kasai H, Izawa A, et al. Torsion analysis in the early detection of anthracycline-mediated cardiomyopathy. Eur Heart J Cardiovasc Imaging. 2012;13(1):95–103.

95. Cheung YF, Li SN, Chan GC, Wong SJ, Ha SY. Left ventricular twisting and untwisting motion in childhood cancer survivors. Echocardiography. 2011;28(7):738–45.

96. Yu HK, Yu W, Cheuk DK, Wong SJ, Chan GC, Cheung YF. New three-dimensional speckle-tracking echocardiography identifies global impairment of left ventricular mechanics with a high sensitivity in childhood cancer survivors. J Am Soc Echocardiogr. 2013;26(8):846–52.

97. Risum N, Ali S, Olsen NT, Jons C, Khouri MG, Lauridsen TK, et al. Variability of global left ventricular deformation analysis using vendor dependent and independent two-dimensional speckle-tracking software in adults. J Am Soc Echocardiogr. 2012;25(11):1195–203.

98. Kim RJ, Fieno DS, Parrish TB, Harris K, Chen EL, Simonetti O, et al. Relationship of MRI delayed contrast enhancement to irreversible injury, infarct age, and contractile function. Circulation. 1999;100(19):1992–2002.

99. Senthilkumar A, Majmudar MD, Shenoy C, Kim HW, Kim RJ. Identifying the etiology: a systematic approach using delayed-enhancement cardiovascular magnetic resonance. Heart Fail Clin. 2009;5(3):349–67. vi.

100. Pennell DJ, Sechtem UP, Higgins CB, Manning WJ, Pohost GM, Rademakers FE, et al. Clinical indications for cardiovascular magnetic resonance (CMR): Consensus Panel report. Eur Heart J. 2004;25(21):1940–65.

101. Hendel RC, Patel MR, Kramer CM, Poon M, Hendel RC, Carr JC, et al. ACCF/ACR/SCCT/ SCMR/ASNC/NASCI/SCAI/SIR 2006 appropriateness criteria for cardiac computed tomography and cardiac magnetic resonance imaging: a report of the American College of Cardiology Foundation Quality Strategic Directions Committee Appropriateness Criteria Working Group, American College of Radiology, Society of Cardiovascular Computed Tomography, Society for Cardiovascular Magnetic Resonance, American Society of Nuclear Cardiology, North American Society for Cardiac Imaging, Society for Cardiovascular Angiography and Interventions, and Society of Interventional Radiology. J Am Coll Cardiol. 2006;48 (7):1475–97.

102. Grothues F, Smith GC, Moon JC, Bellenger NG, Collins P, Klein HU, et al. Comparison of interstudy reproducibility of cardiovascular magnetic resonance with two-dimensional echocardiography in normal subjects and in patients with heart failure or left ventricular hypertrophy. Am J Cardiol. 2002;90(1):29–34.

103. Hoilund-Carlsen PF, Lauritzen SL, Marving J, Rasmussen S, Hesse B, Folke K, et al. The reliability of measuring left ventricular ejection fraction by radionuclide cardiography: evaluation by the method of variance components. Br Heart J. 1988;59(6):653–62.

104. Dymond DS, Elliott A, Stone D, Hendrix G, Spurrell R. Factors that affect the reproducibility of measurements of left ventricular function from first-pass radionuclide ventriculograms. Circulation. 1982;65(2):311–22.

105. Drafts BC, Twomley KM, D'Agostino Jr R, Lawrence J, Avis N, Ellis LR, et al. Low to moderate dose anthracycline-based chemotherapy is associated with early noninvasive imaging evidence of subclinical cardiovascular disease. JACC Cardiovasc Imaging. 2013;6 (8):877–85.

106. Armstrong GT, Plana JC, Zhang N, Srivastava D, Green DM, Ness KK, et al. Screening adult survivors of childhood cancer for cardiomyopathy: comparison of echocardiography and cardiac magnetic resonance imaging. J Clin Oncol. 2012;30(23):2876–84.

107. CMS. CMS Website HOPPS CY2014 Final Rule.

108. ASE. [Available from: http://asecho.org/wordpress/wp-content/uploads/2014/06/2014-reim bursement-newsletter-.pdf.

109. Thomas G. Dehn M, FACR, Chief Medical Officer, National Imaging Associates. Ionizing Radiation Exposure from Radiologic Imaging: The Issue and What We Can Do [Available from: http://www1.radmd.com/media/126106/n-o100rev2-radsafety-provider-edu.pdf.

110. Kim HW, Klem I, Shah DJ, Wu E, Meyers SN, Parker MA, et al. Unrecognized non-Q-wave myocardial infarction: prevalence and prognostic significance in patients with suspected coronary disease. PLoS Med. 2009;6(4):e1000057.

111. Su MY, Lin LY, Tseng YH, Chang CC, Wu CK, Lin JL, et al. CMR-verified diffuse myocardial fibrosis is associated with diastolic dysfunction in HFpEF. JACC Cardiovasc Imaging. 2014;7(10):991–7.

112. Paulus WJ, Tschope C. A novel paradigm for heart failure with preserved ejection fraction: comorbidities drive myocardial dysfunction and remodeling through coronary microvascular endothelial inflammation. J Am Coll Cardiol. 2013;62(4):263–71.

113. Schelbert EB, Fonarow GC, Bonow RO, Butler J, Gheorghiade M. Therapeutic targets in heart failure: refocusing on the myocardial interstitium. J Am Coll Cardiol. 2014;63 (21):2188–98.

114. Sun Y, Weber KT. Cardiac remodelling by fibrous tissue: role of local factors and circulating hormones. Ann Med. 1998;30 Suppl 1:3–8.

115. Heling A, Zimmermann R, Kostin S, Maeno Y, Hein S, Devaux B, et al. Increased expression of cytoskeletal, linkage, and extracellular proteins in failing human myocardium. Circ Res. 2000;86(8):846–53.

116. Wong TC, Piehler KM, Zareba KM, Lin K, Phrampus A, Patel A, et al. Myocardial damage detected by late gadolinium enhancement cardiovascular magnetic resonance is associated with subsequent hospitalization for heart failure. J Am Heart Assoc. 2013;2(6):e000416.

117. Schelbert EB, Cao JJ, Sigurdsson S, Aspelund T, Kellman P, Aletras AH, et al. Prevalence and prognosis of unrecognized myocardial infarction determined by cardiac magnetic resonance in older adults. JAMA. 2012;308(9):890–6.

118. Wong TC, Piehler K, Meier CG, Testa SM, Klock AM, Aneizi AA, et al. Association between extracellular matrix expansion quantified by cardiovascular magnetic resonance and short-term mortality. Circulation. 2012;126(10):1206–16.

119. Kwong RY, Chan AK, Brown KA, Chan CW, Reynolds HG, Tsang S, et al. Impact of unrecognized myocardial scar detected by cardiac magnetic resonance imaging on event-free survival in patients presenting with signs or symptoms of coronary artery disease. Circulation. 2006;113(23):2733–43.

120. Gerber BL, Rousseau MF, Ahn SA, le Polain de Waroux JB, Pouleur AC, Phlips T, et al. Prognostic value of myocardial viability by delayed-enhanced magnetic resonance in patients with coronary artery disease and low ejection fraction: impact of revascularization therapy. J Am Coll Cardiol. 2012;59(9):825–35.

121. Gulati A, Jabbour A, Ismail TF, Guha K, Khwaja J, Raza S, et al. Association of fibrosis with mortality and sudden cardiac death in patients with nonischemic dilated cardiomyopathy. JAMA. 2013;309(9):896–908.

122. Chan RH, Maron BJ, Olivotto I, Pencina MJ, Assenza GE, Haas T, et al. Prognostic value of quantitative contrast-enhanced cardiovascular magnetic resonance for the evaluation of sudden death risk in patients with hypertrophic cardiomyopathy. Circulation. 2014;130 (6):484–95.

123. Greulich S, Deluigi CC, Gloekler S, Wahl A, Zurn C, Kramer U, et al. CMR imaging predicts death and other adverse events in suspected cardiac sarcoidosis. JACC Cardiovasc Imaging. 2013;6(4):501–11.

124. Austin BA, Tang WH, Rodriguez ER, Tan C, Flamm SD, Taylor DO, et al. Delayed hyper-enhancement magnetic resonance imaging provides incremental diagnostic and prognostic utility in suspected cardiac amyloidosis. JACC Cardiovasc Imaging. 2009;2(12):1369–77.

125. Grun S, Schumm J, Greulich S, Wagner A, Schneider S, Bruder O, et al. Long-term follow-up of biopsy-proven viral myocarditis: predictors of mortality and incomplete recovery. J Am Coll Cardiol. 2012;59(18):1604–15.

126. Barone-Rochette G, Pierard S, De Meester de Ravenstein C, Seldrum S, Melchior J, Maes F, et al. Prognostic significance of LGE by CMR in aortic stenosis patients undergoing valve replacement. J Am Coll Cardiol. 2014;64(2):144–54.

127. Mewton N, Liu CY, Croisille P, Bluemke D, Lima JA. Assessment of myocardial fibrosis with cardiovascular magnetic resonance. J Am Coll Cardiol. 2011;57(8):891–903.

128. Jerosch-Herold M, Kwong RY. Cardiac T(1) imaging. Top Magn Reson Imaging. 2014;23 (1):3–11.

129. Iles LM, Ellims AH, Llewellyn H, Hare JL, Kaye DM, McLean CA, et al. Histological validation of cardiac magnetic resonance analysis of regional and diffuse interstitial myocardial fibrosis. Eur Heart J Cardiovasc Imaging. 2015;16(1):14–22.

130. Wadhwa D, Fallah-Rad N, Grenier D, Krahn M, Fang T, Ahmadie R, et al. Trastuzumab mediated cardiotoxicity in the setting of adjuvant chemotherapy for breast cancer: a retrospective study. Breast Cancer Res Treat. 2009;117(2):357–64.

131. Fallah-Rad N, Lytwyn M, Fang T, Kirkpatrick I, Jassal DS. Delayed contrast enhancement cardiac magnetic resonance imaging in trastuzumab induced cardiomyopathy. J Cardiovasc Magn Reson. 2008;10:5.

132. Fallah-Rad N, Walker JR, Wassef A, Lytwyn M, Bohonis S, Fang T, et al. The utility of cardiac biomarkers, tissue velocity and strain imaging, and cardiac magnetic resonance imaging in predicting early left ventricular dysfunction in patients with human epidermal growth factor receptor II-positive breast cancer treated with adjuvant trastuzumab therapy. J Am Coll Cardiol. 2011;57(22):2263–70.

133. Neilan TG, Coelho-Filho OR, Pena-Herrera D, Shah RV, Jerosch-Herold M, Francis SA, et al. Left ventricular mass in patients with a cardiomyopathy after treatment with anthracyclines. Am J Cardiol. 2012;110(11):1679–86.

134. Lunning MA, Kutty S, Rome ET, Li L, Padiyath A, Loberiza F, et al. Cardiac magnetic resonance imaging for the assessment of the myocardium after doxorubicin-based chemotherapy. Am J Clin Oncol. 2013;38(4):377–81.

135. Lawley C, Wainwright C, Segelov E, Lynch J, Beith J, McCrohon J. Pilot study evaluating the role of cardiac magnetic resonance imaging in monitoring adjuvant trastuzumab therapy for breast cancer. Asia Pac J Clin Oncol. 2012;8(1):95–100.

136. Ylanen K, Poutanen T, Savikurki-Heikkila P, Rinta-Kiikka I, Eerola A, Vettenranta K. Cardiac magnetic resonance imaging in the evaluation of the late effects of anthracyclines among long-term survivors of childhood cancer. J Am Coll Cardiol. 2013;61(14):1539–47.

137. Yancik R, Ries LA. Aging and cancer in America. Demographic and epidemiologic perspectives. Hematol Oncol Clin North Am. 2000;14(1):17–23.

138. Pinder MC, Duan Z, Goodwin JS, Hortobagyi GN, Giordano SH. Congestive heart failure in older women treated with adjuvant anthracycline chemotherapy for breast cancer. J Clin Oncol. 2007;25(25):3808–15.

139. Perez EA, Suman VJ, Davidson NE, Sledge GW, Kaufman PA, Hudis CA, et al. Cardiac safety analysis of doxorubicin and cyclophosphamide followed by paclitaxel with or without trastuzumab in the North Central Cancer Treatment Group N9831 adjuvant breast cancer trial. J Clin Oncol. 2008;26(8):1231–8.

140. Nandalur KR, Dwamena BA, Choudhri AF, Nandalur MR, Carlos RC. Diagnostic performance of stress cardiac magnetic resonance imaging in the detection of coronary artery disease: a meta-analysis. J Am Coll Cardiol. 2007;50(14):1343–53.

141. Klem I, Greulich S, Heitner JF, Kim H, Vogelsberg H, Kispert EM, et al. Value of cardiovascular magnetic resonance stress perfusion testing for the detection of coronary artery disease in women. JACC Cardiovasc Imaging. 2008;1(4):436–45.

142. Vavalle J, Bashore TM, Klem I. Surprising finding of a primary pericardial mesothelioma. Int J Cardiovasc Imaging. 2010;26(6):625–7.

143. Lestuzzi C. Neoplastic pericardial disease: old and current strategies for diagnosis and management. World J Cardiol. 2010;2(9):270–9.

144. Grizzard JD, Ang GB. Magnetic resonance imaging of pericardial disease and cardiac masses. Cardiol Clin. 2007;25(1):111–40. vi.

145. Francone M, Dymarkowski S, Kalantzi M, Bogaert J. Real-time cine MRI of ventricular septal motion: a novel approach to assess ventricular coupling. J Magn Reson Imaging. 2005;21(3):305–9.

146. Edvardsen T, Gerber BL, Garot J, Bluemke DA, Lima JA, Smiseth OA. Quantitative assessment of intrinsic regional myocardial deformation by Doppler strain rate echocardiography in humans: validation against three-dimensional tagged magnetic resonance imaging. Circulation. 2002;106(1):50–6.

147. Shehata ML, Cheng S, Osman NF, Bluemke DA, Lima JA. Myocardial tissue tagging with cardiovascular magnetic resonance. J Cardiovasc Magn Reson. 2009;11:55.

148. Osman NF, Kerwin WS, McVeigh ER, Prince JL. Cardiac motion tracking using CINE harmonic phase (HARP) magnetic resonance imaging. Magn Reson Med. 1999;42 (6):1048–60.

149. Kawel-Boehm N, Maceira A, Valsangiacomo-Buechel ER, Vogel-Claussen J, Turkbey EB, Williams R, et al. Normal values for cardiovascular magnetic resonance in adults and children. J Cardiovasc Magn Reson. 2015;17:29.

150. Toro-Salazar OH, Gillan E, O'Loughlin MT, Burke GS, Ferranti J, Stainsby J, et al. Occult cardiotoxicity in childhood cancer survivors exposed to anthracycline therapy. Circ Cardiovasc Imaging. 2013;6(6):873–80.

151. Thompson RC, Canby RC, Lojeski EW, Ratner AV, Fallon JT, Pohost GM. Adriamycin cardiotoxicity and proton nuclear magnetic resonance relaxation properties. Am Heart J. 1987;113(6):1444–9.

152. Lightfoot JC, D'Agostino Jr RB, Hamilton CA, Jordan J, Torti FM, Kock ND, et al. Novel approach to early detection of doxorubicin cardiotoxicity by gadolinium-enhanced cardio-vascular magnetic resonance imaging in an experimental model. Circ Cardiovasc Imaging. 2010;3(5):550–8.

153. Tham EB, Haykowsky MJ, Chow K, Spavor M, Kaneko S, Khoo NS, et al. Diffuse myocardial fibrosis by T1-mapping in children with subclinical anthracycline cardiotoxicity: relationship to exercise capacity, cumulative dose and remodeling. J Cardiovasc Magn Reson. 2013;15:48.

154. Neilan TG, Coelho-Filho OR, Shah RV, Feng JH, Pena-Herrera D, Mandry D, et al. Myo-cardial extracellular volume by cardiac magnetic resonance imaging in patients treated with anthracycline-based chemotherapy. Am J Cardiol. 2013;111(5):717–22.

155. Jordan JH, D'Agostino Jr RB, Hamilton CA, Vasu S, Hall ME, Kitzman DW, et al. Longi-tudinal assessment of concurrent changes in left ventricular ejection fraction and left ven-tricular myocardial tissue characteristics after administration of cardiotoxic chemotherapies using T1-weighted and T2-weighted cardiovascular magnetic resonance. Circ Cardiovasc Imaging. 2014;7(6):872–9.

156. Cottin Y, Ribuot C, Maupoil V, Godin D, Arnould L, Brunotte F, et al. Early incidence of adriamycin treatment on cardiac parameters in the rat. Can J Physiol Pharmacol. 1994;72 (2):140–5.

157. Garg S, Narula J, Chandrashekhar Y. Apoptosis and heart failure: clinical relevance and therapeutic target. J Mol Cell Cardiol. 2005;38(1):73–9.

158. Dash R, Chung J, Chan T, Yamada M, Barral J, Nishimura D, et al. A molecular MRI probe to detect treatment of cardiac apoptosis in vivo. Magn Reson Med. 2011;66(4):1152–62.

159. Hu JC, Williams SB, O'Malley AJ, Smith MR, Nguyen PL, Keating NL. Androgen-deprivation therapy for nonmetastatic prostate cancer is associated with an increased risk of peripheral arterial disease and venous thromboembolism. Eur Urol. 2012;61(6):1119–28.

160. Miller K, Wang M, Gralow J, Dickler M, Cobleigh M, Perez EA, et al. Paclitaxel plus bevacizumab versus paclitaxel alone for metastatic breast cancer. N Engl J Med. 2007;357 (26):2666–76.

161. Escudier B, Eisen T, Stadler WM, Szczylik C, Oudard S, Staehler M, et al. Sorafenib for treatment of renal cell carcinoma: Final efficacy and safety results of the phase III treatment approaches in renal cancer global evaluation trial. J Clin Oncol. 2009;27(20):3312–8.

162. Lee JM, Shirodaria C, Jackson CE, Robson MD, Antoniades C, Francis JM, et al. Multi-modal magnetic resonance imaging quantifies atherosclerosis and vascular dysfunction in patients with type 2 diabetes mellitus. Diab Vasc Dis Res. 2007;4(1):44–8.

163. Estorch M, Carrio I, Berna L, Martinez-Duncker C, Alonso C, Germa JR, et al. Indium-111-antimyosin scintigraphy after doxorubicin therapy in patients with advanced breast cancer. J Nucl Med. 1990;31(12):1965–9.

164. Carrio I, Lopez-Pousa A, Estorch M, Duncker D, Berna L, Torres G, et al. Detection of doxorubicin cardiotoxicity in patients with sarcomas by indium-111-antimyosin monoclonal antibody studies. J Nucl Med. 1993;34(9):1503–7.

165. Carrio I, Estorch M, Berna L, Lopez-Pousa J, Tabernero J, Torres G. Indium-111-antimyosin and iodine-123-MIBG studies in early assessment of doxorubicin cardiotoxicity. J Nucl Med. 1995;36(11):2044–9.

166. Valdes Olmos RA, Carrio I, Hoefnagel CA, Estorch M, ten Bokkel Huinink WW, Lopez-Pousa J, et al. High sensitivity of radiolabelled antimyosin scintigraphy in assessing

anthracycline related early myocyte damage preceding cardiac dysfunction. Nucl Med Commun. 2002;23(9):871–7.

167. Valdes Olmos RA, ten Bokkel Huinink WW, ten Hoeve RF, van Tinteren H, Bruning PF, van Vlies B, et al. Assessment of anthracycline-related myocardial adrenergic derangement by [123I]metaiodobenzylguanidine scintigraphy. Eur J Cancer. 1995;31A(1):26–31.

168. Cardinale D, Sandri MT, Martinoni A, Tricca A, Civelli M, Lamantia G, et al. Left ventricular dysfunction predicted by early troponin I release after high-dose chemotherapy. J Am Coll Cardiol. 2000;36(2):517–22.

169. Cardinale D, Sandri MT, Colombo A, Colombo N, Boeri M, Lamantia G, et al. Prognostic value of troponin I in cardiac risk stratification of cancer patients undergoing high-dose chemotherapy. Circulation. 2004;109(22):2749–54.

170. Cardinale D, Sandri MT, Martinoni A, Borghini E, Civelli M, Lamantia G, et al. Myocardial injury revealed by plasma troponin I in breast cancer treated with high-dose chemotherapy. Ann Oncol. 2002;13(5):710–5.

171. Sandri MT, Cardinale D, Zorzino L, Passerini R, Lentati P, Martinoni A, et al. Minor increases in plasma troponin I predict decreased left ventricular ejection fraction after high-dose chemotherapy. Clin Chem. 2003;49(2):248–52.

172. Morris PG, Chen C, Steingart R, Fleisher M, Lin N, Moy B, et al. Troponin I and C-reactive protein are commonly detected in patients with breast cancer treated with dose-dense chemotherapy incorporating trastuzumab and lapatinib. Clin Cancer Res. 2011;17(10):3490–9.

173. Khouri MG, Klein MR, Velazquez EJ, Jones LW. Current and emerging modalities for detection of cardiotoxicity in cardio-oncology. Future Cardiol. 2015;11(4):471–84.

174. Ky B, Putt M, Sawaya H, French B, Januzzi Jr JL, Sebag IA, et al. Early increases in multiple biomarkers predict subsequent cardiotoxicity in patients with breast cancer treated with doxorubicin, taxanes, and trastuzumab. J Am Coll Cardiol. 2014;63(8):809–16.

175. Cardinale D, Sandri MT. Role of biomarkers in chemotherapy-induced cardiotoxicity. Prog Cardiovasc Dis. 2010;53(2):121–9.

176. Lakoski SG, Barlow CE, Koelwyn GJ, Hornsby WE, Hernandez J, Defina LF, et al. The influence of adjuvant therapy on cardiorespiratory fitness in early-stage breast cancer seven years after diagnosis: the Cooper Center Longitudinal Study. Breast Cancer Res Treat. 2013;138(3):909–16.

177. Khouri MG, Hornsby WE, Risum N, Velazquez EJ, Thomas S, Lane A, et al. Utility of 3-dimensional echocardiography, global longitudinal strain, and exercise stress echocardiography to detect cardiac dysfunction in breast cancer patients treated with doxorubicin-containing adjuvant therapy. Breast Cancer Res Treat. 2014;143(3):531–9.

178. McKillop JH, Bristow MR, Goris ML, Billingham ME, Bockemuehl K. Sensitivity and specificity of radionuclide ejection fractions in doxorubicin cardiotoxicity. Am Heart J. 1983;106(5 Pt 1):1048–56.

179. Civelli M, Cardinale D, Martinoni A, Lamantia G, Colombo N, Colombo A, et al. Early reduction in left ventricular contractile reserve detected by dobutamine stress echo predicts high-dose chemotherapy-induced cardiac toxicity. Int J Cardiol. 2006;111(1):120–6.

180. Smibert E, Carlin JB, Vidmar S, Wilkinson LC, Newton M, Weintraub RG. Exercise echocardiography reflects cumulative anthracycline exposure during childhood. Pediatr Blood Cancer. 2004;42(7):556–62.

181. De Souza AM, Potts JE, Potts MT, De Souza ES, Rowland TW, Pritchard SL, et al. A stress echocardiography study of cardiac function during progressive exercise in pediatric oncology patients treated with anthracyclines. Pediatr Blood Cancer. 2007;49(1):56–64.

182. Guimaraes-Filho FV, Tan DM, Braga JC, Rodrigues A, Waib PH, Matsubara BB. Ventricular systolic reserve in asymptomatic children previously treated with low doses of anthracyclines: a longitudinal, prospective exercise echocardiography study. Pediatr Blood Cancer. 2012;59(3):548–52.

183. Sieswerda E, Kremer LC, Vidmar S, De Bruin ML, Smibert E, Sjoberg G, et al. Exercise echocardiography in asymptomatic survivors of childhood cancer treated with anthracyclines: a prospective follow-up study. Pediatr Blood Cancer. 2010;54(4):579–84.
184. Klewer SE, Goldberg SJ, Donnerstein RL, Berg RA, Hutter Jr JJ. Dobutamine stress echocardiography: a sensitive indicator of diminished myocardial function in asymptomatic doxorubicin-treated long-term survivors of childhood cancer. J Am Coll Cardiol. 1992;19 (2):394–401.
185. Lanzarini L, Bossi G, Laudisa ML, Klersy C, Arico M. Lack of clinically significant cardiac dysfunction during intermediate dobutamine doses in long-term childhood cancer survivors exposed to anthracyclines. Am Heart J. 2000;140(2):315–23.
186. Gupta S, Rohatgi A, Ayers CR, Willis BL, Haskell WL, Khera A, et al. Cardiorespiratory fitness and classification of risk of cardiovascular disease mortality. Circulation. 2011;123 (13):1377–83.
187. Gulati M, Pandey DK, Arnsdorf MF, Lauderdale DS, Thisted RA, Wicklund RH, et al. Exercise capacity and the risk of death in women: the St James Women Take Heart Project. Circulation. 2003;108(13):1554–9.
188. Jones LW, Watson D, Herndon 2nd JE, Eves ND, Haithcock BE, Loewen G, et al. Peak oxygen consumption and long-term all-cause mortality in nonsmall cell lung cancer. Cancer. 2010;116(20):4825–32.
189. Jones LW, Hornsby WE, Goetzinger A, Forbes LM, Sherrard EL, Quist M, et al. Prognostic significance of functional capacity and exercise behavior in patients with metastatic non-small cell lung cancer. Lung Cancer. 2012;76(2):248–52.
190. Jones LW, Courneya KS, Mackey JR, Muss HB, Pituskin EN, Scott JM, et al. Cardiopulmonary function and age-related decline across the breast cancer survivorship continuum. J Clin Oncol. 2012;30(20):2530–7.
191. Ginsburg GS, Seo D, Frazier C. Microarrays coming of age in cardiovascular medicine: standards, predictions, and biology. J Am Coll Cardiol. 2006;48(8):1618–20.
192. Beauclair S, Formento P, Fischel JL, Lescaut W, Largillier R, Chamorey E, et al. Role of the HER2 [Ile655Val] genetic polymorphism in tumorogenesis and in the risk of trastuzumab-related cardiotoxicity. Ann Oncol. 2007;18(8):1335–41.
193. Blanco JG, Sun CL, Landier W, Chen L, Esparza-Duran D, Leisenring W, et al. Anthracycline-related cardiomyopathy after childhood cancer: role of polymorphisms in carbonyl reductase genes--a report from the Children's Oncology Group. J Clin Oncol. 2012;30(13):1415–21.
194. Singh KK, Shukla PC, Quan A, Desjardins JF, Lovren F, Pan Y, et al. BRCA2 protein deficiency exaggerates doxorubicin-induced cardiomyocyte apoptosis and cardiac failure. J Biol Chem. 2012;287(9):6604–14.
195. Visscher H, Ross CJ, Rassekh SR, Barhdadi A, Dube MP, Al-Saloos H, et al. Pharmacogenomic prediction of anthracycline-induced cardiotoxicity in children. J Clin Oncol. 2012;30(13):1422–8.

Chapter 4
Management of Chemotherapy-Associated Cardiomyopathy

Lauren Gilstrap, Mike Harrison, Gretchen G. Kimmick, and Anju Nohria

Introduction

Cardiovascular complications of cancer therapies are not uncommon, especially in the setting of preexisting heart disease. The frequency of cardiovascular complications of cancer therapies has increased with the introduction of novel combinations and with new targeted biologic therapies [1]. There are many well-documented, long-term cardiovascular complications of chemotherapy including cardiomyopathy, myocardial infarction, and arrhythmia [2]. This chapter will focus on the management of cancer treatment-induced cardiomyopathy.

Over the past two decades, the survival rate for most cancers has improved substantially, due to better screening and treatment modalities. However, as patients survive longer, we are increasingly aware of side effects and toxicities associated with cancer therapies. Cardiotoxicity, in particular, is of clinical

---

Electronic supplementary material: The online version of this chapter (doi:10.1007/978-3-319-43096-6_4) contains supplementary material, which is available to authorized users.

L. Gilstrap (✉)
Newton-Wesley Hospital, Newton, MA, USA

Cardiovascular Medicine, Brigham and Women's Hospital, Boston, MA, USA
e-mail: lgilstrap@partners.org

M. Harrison
Duke Cancer Institute, Duke University Medical Center, Durham, NC, USA
e-mail: michael.harrison@duke.edu

G.G. Kimmick
Department of Medicine, Duke University Medical Center, Durham, NC, USA
e-mail: Gretchen.kimmick@duke.edu

A. Nohria
Brigham and Womens Hospital, Brigham and Womens Cardiology, 70 Francis St, Boston, MA 02115, USA
e-mail: anohria@partners.org

© Springer International Publishing Switzerland 2017
G.G. Kimmick et al. (eds.), *Cardio-Oncology*, DOI 10.1007/978-3-319-43096-6_4

significance for two reasons. First, its development may limit or preclude potentially lifesaving chemotherapy options. Second, among patients who survive their cancer, the cardiotoxicity associated with chemotherapy exposure can cause significant clinical symptoms and limit life expectancy, independent of the patient's oncologic prognosis [3].

Chemotherapies Most Commonly Associated with Cardiomyopathy

The chemotherapy agents most commonly associated with the development of cardiomyopathy are anthracyclines and human epidermal growth factor receptor-2 (HER-2)-targeted agents. Other agents that have been associated with cardiomyopathy are shown in Table 4.1. The majority of data on the management of chemotherapy-induced cardiomyopathy is derived from patients treated with anthracyclines and trastuzumab. Therefore, these will be discussed in detail, in addition to the general management of all chemotherapy-induced cardiomyopathies.

Table 4.1 Chemotherapy agents associated with cardiomyopathy

Class of chemotherapy	Examples
Anthracycline	Daunorubicin
	Doxorubicin
	Epirubicin
	Mitoxantrone
Alkylating agents	Cyclophosphamide
	Cisplatin
Microtubule-targeting agents	Paclitaxel
	Docetaxel
Topoisomerase II inhibitors	Etoposide
Biologic response modifiers	Interferon
	Interleukin-2
Antimetabolites	Fluorouracil
Antibodies	Trastuzumab
	Pertuzumab
	T-DM1
	Bevacizumab
	Alemtuzumab
Tyrosine kinase inhibitors	Sunitinib
	Sorafenib
	Imatinib
	Lapatinib
	Trametinib
Proteasome inhibitors	Carfilzomib

Anthracyclines

As early as 1967, there were reports of congestive heart failure (CHF) in children treated with daunomycin for leukemia [4]. Anthracyclines, such as doxorubicin, daunorubicin, epirubicin, and idarubicin, exert their antitumor effects by (1) intercalation between base pairs of the DNA/RNA strands to inhibit DNA and RNA synthesis [5]; (2) inhibition of topoisomerase II, thereby blocking DNA transcription and replication [6]; (3) iron-mediated generation of oxygen free radicals [7]; and (4) induction of histone eviction from chromatin that deregulates the DNA damage response [8].

The exact mechanism of anthracycline-mediated cardiotoxicity remains unclear. Proposed mechanisms include [9] (1) increased myocardial oxidative stress via redox cycling of the quinone moiety of anthracyclines and through the formation of anthracycline-iron complexes, (2) disruption of cellular and mitochondrial calcium homeostasis, (3) disruption of mitochondrial energetics, (4) degradation of ultrastructural proteins including titin and dystrophin, (5) direct DNA damage via inhibition of topoisomerase 2β [10], (6) inhibition of pro-survival pathways such as neuregulin-1 and ErbB, and (7) direct cytotoxic effects on cardiac progenitor cells diminishing repair potential after myocardial injury [11].

Clinical Presentation

Anthracycline cardiotoxicity can present as either acute, early-onset chronic progressive, or late-onset chronic progressive cardiotoxicity [12]. Acute cardiotoxicity often presents within the first week of anthracycline exposure and usually recovers with withdrawal of the offending agent. Recent prospective observational data in 2625 adults treated with anthracyclines suggests that the majority (98 %) of anthracycline cardiotoxicity presents early within the first year of therapy [13]. This can progress to chronic cardiomyopathy, with a predominantly dilated phenotype in adults and a restrictive phenotype in pediatric patients [14]. Anthracyclines can also cause a more subtle, chronic cardiomyopathy which presents years to decades after anthracycline treatment [15]. This form of anthracycline-associated cardiomyopathy often results in ventricular dysfunction [15] with the subsequent development of clinical heart failure and arrhythmias [16].

Risk Factors

There are no reported risk factors for the development of acute cardiotoxicity related to anthracycline administration. Risk factors for early- and late-onset anthracycline cardiotoxicity include cumulative anthracycline dose, concurrent mediastinal radiation, extremes of age, female gender, and cardiac risk factors or preexisting heart disease [14]. A formula for estimating the likelihood of developing cardiomyopathy from anthracycline exposure is shown below:

$$Y = (X)^2/a$$

where Y = the likelihood of developing cardiomyopathy, X = the number of cycles of anthracycline therapy, and $a = a$ correction constant determined by the cycle dose and the duration between cycles [3].

Recommended Monitoring

Asymptomatic cardiomyopathy can progress to symptomatic heart failure and carries an adverse prognosis. Since the physical exam alone may miss over 50 % of early and potentially reversible cases of anthracycline-induced cardiomyopathy [17], serial and post-therapy monitoring with electrocardiograms (ECGs), echocardiograms, and biomarkers, such as troponin I, may be beneficial in high-risk patients and has been recommended by some groups [18]. However, this strategy is not universally agreed upon and is an active area of guideline development.

Traditionally, multi-gated blood pool imaging (MUGA) was used to assess serial left ventricular ejection fractions (LVEF) during chemotherapy. Due to concerns related to the radiation exposure associated with MUGA, two-dimensional echocardiography has become the accepted modality for assessing serial LVEF in patients treated with anthracyclines. Based on data using MUGA, a baseline evaluation of LVEF is recommended prior to starting anthracyclines. If the baseline LVEF is >50 %, serial measurement is recommended after a cumulative anthracycline dose of 250–300 mg/m^2, then after 450 mg/m^2, and after each subsequent cycle at doses >450 mg/m^2. Anthracycline therapy should be discontinued if the LVEF declines ≥10 % from baseline to ≤50 % [19]. For patients with preexisting LV dysfunction (baseline LVEF <50 %), anthracycline therapy is not recommended for LVEF <30 %. Patients with an LVEF 30–50 % can receive anthracyclines, but their LVEF should be carefully monitored before each subsequent dose, and anthracyclines should be discontinued if the EF falls ≥10 % from baseline to <30 % [19].

A recent consensus statement released by the American Society of Echocardiography and the European Association of Cardiovascular Imaging updated these recommendations to suggest that in patients receiving ≤240 mg/m^2 of anthracyclines, echocardiograms should be performed at baseline, at completion, and 6 months after the completion of anthracycline therapy [18]. In patients receiving >240 mg/m^2, additional imaging is recommended before each additional 50 mg/m^2. Newer echocardiographic techniques such as strain rate imaging, a marker of myocardial deformation, may predict early cardiotoxicity prior to the development of overt LV dysfunction [20]. Measurement of global longitudinal strain along with LVEF has also been recommended to identify at-risk patients who may benefit from early intervention [20]. None of these screening recommendations have been incorporated into guidelines or uniformly accepted in clinical practice.

Biomarkers, such as B-type natriuretic peptide (BNP) and troponins, have been used in research settings to stratify patients into baseline risk categories prior to anthracycline administration. There is data to suggest that the presence of an elevated troponin at any time during anthracycline administration increases the risk of cardiotoxicity [21]. The likelihood of toxicity is even greater among patients with a persistently elevated troponin, even after discontinuation of anthracycline therapy [22]. An elevated troponin, at any time during anthracycline administration, has been used as a marker to identify high-risk patients who might benefit from early initiation of cardiac therapy [23].

Prevention of Anthracycline-Induced Cardiomyopathy

The American Heart Association and American College of Cardiology define four stages of heart failure that reflect progressive disease and can be used to guide heart failure therapy (Table 4.2). Patients receiving potentially cardiotoxic chemotherapies are defined as having Stage A heart failure or are deemed to be "at risk" for the development of heart failure. As such, several strategies have been examined to reduce the risk of anthracycline cardiotoxicity.

Dose limitation and continuous, rather than bolus, infusions to limit peak serum concentrations appear to decrease cardiotoxicity [24]. There have been modifications of doxorubicin which may reduce the overall cardiotoxic effects; liposomal preparations, epirubicin, and mitoxantrone all appear to be associated with a lower

Table 4.2 American Heart Association/American College of Cardiology Stages of Heart Failure

	At risk for HF		Heart failure	
	Stage A	Stage B	Stage C	Stage D
Symptoms	Hypertension	Prior MI	Structural disease	HF symptoms at rest despite maximal medical therapy
	Atherosclerosis, Diabetes, Obesity	LV hypertrophy	*AND*	
	Metabolic syndrome	Decreased EF	Dyspnea	
	OR	Valve disease (asymptomatic)	Fatigue	
	Prior cardiotoxin use (including chemotherapy)		Decreased exercise tolerance	
	Familial cardiomyopathy			

(continued)

Table 4.2 (continued)

	At risk for HF		Heart failure	
	Stage A	Stage B	Stage C	Stage D
Goals of therapy	Risk factor management including:	Risk factor management including:	Risk factor management including:	Risk factor management including:
	Treat hypertension	Treat hypertension	Treat hypertension	Treat hypertension
	Smoking cessation	Smoking cessation	Smoking cessation	Smoking cessation
	Lipid management	Lipid management	Lipid management	Lipid management
	Regular exercise	Regular exercise	Regular exercise	Regular exercise
	Decrease/eliminate alcohol	Decrease/eliminate alcohol	Decrease/eliminate alcohol	Decrease/eliminate alcohol
	Eliminate illicit drug use	Eliminate illicit drug use	Eliminate illicit drug use	Eliminate illicit drug use
	Control metabolic syndrome	Control metabolic syndrome	Control metabolic syndrome	Control metabolic syndrome
			Dietary salt restriction	Dietary salt restriction
				Address goals of care and appropriate level of care
Standard drug therapy	ACEi/ARBs for patients with diabetes and/or known vascular disease	ACEi/ARBs for patients with diabetes and/or known vascular disease	ACEi	ACEi
		Beta-blockers for patients with prior MI, decreased EF or valve disease (when appropriate)	Beta-blockers	Beta-blockers
			Diuretics	Diuretics
Drug therapy to consider in selected patients			Aldosterone antagonist	Aldosterone antagonist
			ARB's	ARB's
			Digitalis	Digitalis
			Hydralazine/nitrates	Hydralazine/nitrates

(continued)

Table 4.2 (continued)

	At risk for HF		Heart failure	
	Stage A	Stage B	Stage C	Stage D
Additional therapies to consider in selected patients			Biventricular pacing	Biventricular pacing
			Defibrillator	Defibrillator
				Heart transplant
				Chronic inotropes
				Permanent mechanical support
				Experimental drugs and/or surgeries
				Compassionate care/Hospice Care

Adapted from ACC/AHA 2005 Guideline Update for the Diagnosis and Management of Chronic Heart Failure in the Adult—Summary Article A Report of the American College of Cardiology/ American Heart Association Task Force on Practice Guidelines (Writing Committee to Update the 2001 Guidelines for the Evaluation and Management of Heart Failure): Developed in Collaboration With the American College of Chest Physicians and the International Society for Heart and Lung Transplantation: Endorsed by the Heart Rhythm Society. (Circulation 2005;112:1825–52.)
ACEi Angiotensin converting enzyme inhibitors, *ARB* Angiotensin receptor blockers, *EF* Ejection fraction, *HF* Heart failure, *LV* Left ventricle, *MI* Myocardial infarction

risk of heart failure than doxorubicin [25]. However, the data comparing these agents are not robust except for liposomal-encapsulated doxorubicin which is associated with a significantly lower rate of both asymptomatic and symptomatic heart failure than conventional doxorubicin [26]. Dexrazoxane is an iron chelator that binds free iron and prevents the formation of anthracycline-iron complexes that contribute to oxygen free radical formation. Dexrazoxane has proven to be effective in reducing anthracycline-mediated cardiotoxicity when doxorubicin has been administered at doses ≥ 300 mg/m^2, without compromising the efficacy of cancer treatment [27]. Unfortunately, dexrazoxane treatment in children has been associated with an increased risk of myelodysplastic syndrome and acute myelogenous leukemia when given in combination with other drugs known to be associated with secondary leukemias [28]. While there is considerable debate that this increase in late hematologic malignancies may be related to other chemotherapies administered to children rather than dexrazoxane, this observation has led the US Food and Drug Administration and the European Medicines Agency to restrict the use of dexrazoxane to adult patients with advanced or metastatic breast cancer who have already received a certain amount of the anthracyclines: doxorubicin (300 mg/m^2)

or epirubicin (540 mg/m^2). Novel agents such as engineered bivalent neuregulin-1β have been shown to reduce the double-stranded DNA breaks associated with anthracycline exposure and attenuate LV dysfunction in animal models of anthracycline-induced cardiomyopathy [29]. However, neuregulin analogs may have pro-neoplastic effects, and further translational studies are needed to evaluate their utility as cardioprotective agents.

Prophylactic use of angiotensin converting enzyme inhibitors (ACEi) has also been proposed. In a randomized open-label trial, 125 lymphoma patients who had received doxorubicin were assigned 1:1:1 to enalapril, metoprolol, or no therapy. There was no significant difference in left ventricular ejection fraction (LVEF) or heart failure between the three groups over a median follow-up period of 31 months [30]. In another study of 473 patients, troponin I levels were measured following each cycle of anthracyclines. The 114 patients with a positive troponin were randomized to receive enalapril or placebo starting one month after the final cycle. None of the patients in the enalapril-treated group developed subsequent cardiomyopathy ($>10\%$ reduction in LVEF from baseline to $<50\%$) compared to 43% in the placebo group [23].

Beta-blockers have also been evaluated for the prevention of heart failure related to anthracyclines. Carvedilol has been shown in a small, randomized study of 50 patients to prevent LV dysfunction in patients being treated with high-dose (mean >500 mg/m^2) anthracyclines [31]. By 6 months, patients treated with carvedilol 12.5 mg once daily had no change in their LVEF compared to a mean reduction in LVEF from 69% to 52% in the placebo-treated group [31]. Similar findings were noted in a trial of 45 patients being treated with anthracyclines randomized to nebivolol vs. placebo [32].

The OVERCOME (preventiOn of left Ventricular dysfunction with Enalapril and caRvedilol in patients submitted to intensive ChemOtherapy for the treatment of Malignant hEmopathies) trial randomized 90 patients with hematologic malignancies undergoing high-dose chemotherapy, followed by autologous hematopoietic stem cell transplantation, to either placebo or a combination of enalapril (mean daily dose 8.6 mg) and carvedilol (mean daily dose 23.8 mg) [33]. Patients treated with enalapril and carvedilol had no significant change in LVEF, compared to an absolute 3% reduction in LVEF in the placebo group as estimated both with echocardiography and cardiac MRI at baseline and six months. There was also a significant reduction in the composite end point of death, heart failure, or LVEF $<45\%$ in the treatment group by 6 months (6.7 vs. 24.4%, $p = 0.02$) [33]. The recently completed PRADA (PRevention of cArdiac Dysfunction during Adjuvant breast cancer therapy) trial evaluated the effect of prophylactic candesartan and metoprolol in 120 patients with early breast cancer treated with anthracyclines $\pm$ trastuzumab and radiation [34]. In this study, patients were randomized in a 2×2 factorial design to candesartan (8–32 mg daily), metoprolol (25–100 mg daily), or placebo prior to initiating anthracyclines and were evaluated for change in LVEF by cardiac MRI from baseline to the end of adjuvant chemotherapy. LVEF declined less in candesartan-treated patients relative to placebo (0.6 vs. 2.6%, $p = 0.021$). However, there was no difference in LVEF between metoprolol- and placebo-treated patients [34]. Thus, in totality, while there is data supporting the prophylactic use of ACEi, angiotensin receptor blockers, and certain beta-blockers to prevent anthracycline-induced cardiomyopathy, the small size of these clinical trials, limited follow-up, and the large number of patients that would need to be placed on these medications have prevented the routine use of these medications in clinical practice.

Incidental use of statins has also been associated with a lower rate of heart failure in a small propensity score-matched retrospective study [35]. However, at this point there is insufficient data to recommend initiation of statin therapy in patients without a preexisting indication.

Trastuzumab and HER-2-Targeted Agents

Trastuzumab is a monoclonal antibody that targets HER-2. The HER-2 gene is amplified in 20–30 % of early-stage breast cancers [36, 37]. The HER-2 gene encodes a transmembrane tyrosine kinase receptor that belongs to the epidermal growth factor family. This family has four members that function by stimulating pathways such as PI3kinase-AKT-mTOR pathway. Activation of these pathways occurs via ligand-mediated hetero- or homo-dimerization. Overexpression of HER-2 leads to constitutive activation of these signaling pathways, enabling rapid proliferation of cancer cells [38]. Trastuzumab binds to domain IV of the extracellular segment of the HER2-neu receptor, thereby blocking this pathway [39]. This results in cellular arrest during the G1 phase of the cell cycle and a reduction in cellular proliferation. Members of this family (ErbB2 and ErbB4) are receptor tyrosine kinases that are also expressed in cardiac myocytes [40]. - Neuregulin-1 binds to ErbB4 which, along with its coreceptor ErbB2, appears to be involved in growth and survival signaling pathways and is inhibited by trastuzumab [40]. The neuregulin-1 signaling pathway is also altered by anthracyclines, which may explain the synergistic cardiotoxicity of anthracyclines and trastuzumab [41].

Clinical Presentation

Trastuzumab-induced cardiomyopathy most often presents as an asymptomatic decrease in LVEF and less commonly as overt heart failure during trastuzumab treatment. In contrast to anthracyclines, trastuzumab-induced cardiac dysfunction does not appear to be dose dependent, and the cardiotoxicity is often reversible with discontinuation of therapy.

In a phase III trial of chemotherapy with or without trastuzumab for metastatic breast cancer, 33 patients continued therapy with trastuzumab for an additional 6–7 months despite developing a cardiac event (most often an asymptomatic decline in

LVEF). After stopping trastuzumab therapy, the LVEF was stable or improved for 85 % of patients, and heart failure symptoms were completely reversible for 75 % of patients treated with standard heart failure therapy [42].

In the pivotal trial by Slamon et al., the incidence of cardiotoxicity in patients with metastatic breast cancer treated with trastuzumab alone was 3–7 % [43]. The incidence of cardiotoxicity in patients treated with trastuzumab, anthracyclines, and cyclophosphamide was as high as 27 % [44]. In 2012, a meta-analysis of 8 trials and almost 12,000 patients with HER-2-positive breast cancer demonstrated a significantly increased risk of asymptomatic cardiomyopathy (relative risk 1.83) and "severe" heart failure (relative risk 5.11) in patients treated with trastuzumab versus non-trastuzumab chemotherapy. The rate of severe heart failure among those treated with non-trastuzumab regimens was 0.4 % compared to 2.5 % among those treated with trastuzumab-based chemotherapies [45].

Risk Factors

Age greater than 50 years and previous or concurrent anthracycline use are the primary risk factors for the development of trastuzumab-induced cardiomyopathy [46]. Patients who receive concurrent anthracyclines, especially when the anthracycline is doxorubicin and the cumulative dose exceeds 300 mg/m^2, are at the highest risk of developing trastuzumab-induced cardiomyopathy [47–49]. Other cardiovascular risk factors such as hypertension, obesity, and a prior diagnosis of heart disease increase the risk of trastuzumab-induced cardiomyopathy [46, 50]. There is limited data to suggest that in elderly women, the risk of cardiotoxicity is higher among those with diabetes [51].

Recommended Monitoring

LVEF should be assessed prior to the initiation of trastuzumab therapy. When trastuzumab therapy follows anthracycline treatment, LVEF should be assessed after the completion of anthracycline therapy and prior to the initiation of the trastuzumab [52]. Patients with a normal baseline LVEF can begin trastuzumab therapy. Patients with a mildly reduced LVEF 40–50 % should have the risks and benefits carefully weighed before initiating trastuzumab and may benefit from pretreatment cardiology consultation.

There are no established guidelines for LVEF monitoring during trastuzumab therapy. In the adjuvant setting, echocardiography is recommended at baseline and every 3 months during trastuzumab therapy [18, 52]. In the metastatic setting, most recommend LVEF monitoring at baseline and thereafter as clinically indicated. If the LVEF declines more than 15 % from baseline or 10 % from baseline to below 50 %, trastuzumab should be held for a month before the LVEF is reassessed. If the

LVEF remains low or there is evidence of symptomatic heart failure, trastuzumab should be discontinued [53].

Given that an elevation in troponin predicts cardiotoxicity with anthracyclines, studies have examined the utility of baseline and post-trastuzumab troponin monitoring. In a multivariable analysis of over 250 patients, an elevated troponin at baseline was a significant predictor of trastuzumab-induced decline in LVEF [54]. Older patients, those with a positive troponin, those with a marked reduction in LVEF, or those who develop cardiotoxicity early in the course of trastuzumab treatment are less likely to recover left ventricular function to baseline values [54].

Prevention of Trastuzumab-Induced Cardiotoxicity

Like anthracyclines, patients receiving HER-2-targeted therapies are believed to have Stage A heart failure. Data supporting the use of prophylactic beta-blockers in patients treated with trastuzumab are derived from a retrospective, propensity-matched cohort study. This study found that breast cancer patients on incident beta-blockers were less likely to develop trastuzumab-induced heart failure, compared to those who were not treated with a beta-blocker [55]. The recent MANTI-CORE (Multidisciplinary Approach to Novel Therapies In Cardiology Oncology REsearch) trial evaluated the cardioprotective effects of prophylactic perindopril (target daily dose 8 mg) or bisoprolol (target daily dose 10 mg) in 94 patients with HER-2-positive breast cancer treated with trastuzumab [56]. Neither drug prevented trastuzumab-induced LV remodeling which was the primary end point of the study. However, in a secondary analysis, both perindopril (3 %) and bisoprolol (1 %) resulted in a smaller decline in LVEF from baseline to 12 months, compared to placebo (5 %). Furthermore, both perindopril (1/33) and bisoprolol (1/31) resulted in fewer trastuzumab interruptions compared to placebo (8/30) [56]. Several randomized clinical trials are currently underway to assess whether prophylactic ACEi and/or beta-blockers reduce the risk of trastuzumab-induced cardiotoxicity.

General Principles of Heart Failure Management

There is very little data that specifically addresses the management of chemotherapy-induced cardiomyopathies. As a result, much of the management of chemotherapy-induced cardiomyopathy is based on the recommended guidelines for the management of heart failure with reduced ejection fraction (HFrEF) due to other etiologies (Table 4.2) [54, 57–59]. It is therefore worth reviewing the central tenets of HFrEF management and any data specific to the post-chemotherapy setting.

Guideline Review of Chemotherapy-Induced Cardiomyopathy

The 2013 American College of Cardiology Foundation/American Heart Association Task Force guidelines and the 2006 Canadian Cardiovascular Society guidelines do not specifically mention chemotherapy-induced cardiomyopathy [57, 58]. The 2010 Heart Failure Society of America guidelines recommend that in patients with established heart failure who are undergoing treatment with potential cardiotoxic chemotherapy, repeat measurements of LVEF should be considered as long as there is no clinical evidence of deterioration [54]. The 2012 European Society of Cardiology guidelines contain a paragraph about cardiomyopathy in the setting of concurrent cancer. These guidelines name anthracyclines and trastuzumab specifically as the "best recognized" chemotherapy agents associated with left ventricular systolic dysfunction. The guidelines state that dexrazoxane may confer some cardioprotection. Finally, the European guidelines recommend at least pre- and post-anthracycline LVEF assessment. Furthermore, they recommend that patients who develop systolic dysfunction should have their anthracyclines stopped and should undergo "standard" treatment for HFrEF [59].

Pharmacologic Management Principles

Pharmacologic therapy in heart failure is intended to reverse or prevent progressive adverse left ventricular remodeling, improve clinical symptoms, and reduce morbidity and mortality.

Angiotensin Converting Enzyme Inhibitors (ACEi)

ACEi are one of the most important classes of drugs in the management of HFrEF. ACEi have been shown to improve survival in both asymptomatic (Stage B) and symptomatic (Stage C) patients with LVEF ≤40 [60–62]. Notably, similarly positive results have been seen with angiotensin receptor blockers (ARBs) in patients who are unable to tolerate ACEi [63].

Serial imaging as per the recommended consensus statements permits the detection of left ventricular dysfunction prior to the development of symptomatic heart failure (Stage B). According to published cardiology guidelines, all patients with Stage B heart failure should receive an ACEi or ARB to promote recovery/stabilization of left ventricular function and prevent the development of symptoms. In a prospective study of 2625 anthracycline-treated patients followed by serial echocardiography, 9 % developed cardiomyopathy (defined as a >10 % decline in LVEF from baseline to <50 %) over a median follow-up of 5.2 years. Most of these patients (81 %) had none or minimal heart failure symptoms, and early initiation of

ACEi and beta-blocker therapy resulted in either full (11 %) or partial recovery (71 %) of LV function in majority of patients [54]. Similarly, in a cohort of 251 breast cancer patients treated with trastuzumab and followed by serial echocardiography, 17 % developed cardiotoxicity. Interruption of trastuzumab and initiation of ACEi and beta-blockers facilitated recovery of LVEF to >50 % in 60 % of patients [54]. In contrast, the effectiveness of ACEi in childhood cancer survivors with anthracycline cardiotoxicity remains unclear [64].

When initiating an ACEi, it is prudent to start at a low dose (i.e., short-acting captopril 6.25 mg three times daily or long-acting lisinopril 5 mg daily) to minimize the risk of hypotension and renal insufficiency [65]. A 10–20 % increase in creatinine is expected within the first 2 weeks after starting ACEi therapy. If the creatinine increases >30 %, the ACEi should be stopped. In patients with baseline renal insufficiency (creatinine >1.4 mg/dL), creatinine and potassium levels must both be monitored 1 week after initiating ACEi and periodically thereafter. There is evidence that ACEi decrease the progression of renal disease in most patients with baseline renal insufficiency. Therefore, under careful surveillance, an ACEi should be continued, even in a patient with renal insufficiency, unless the creatinine increases >30 % from baseline [66].

Once patients are able to tolerate low doses of ACEi (based on blood pressure, creatinine, and potassium), the dose should be increased every 1–2 days (in an inpatient setting) or 1–2 weeks (in an outpatient setting) to a target of short-acting captopril 50 mg three times daily or long-acting lisinopril 40 mg daily (Table 4.3). Attempts should be made to achieve the target doses used in clinical trials. However, in patients who cannot tolerate target doses, the maximum dose tolerated should be continued [67].

The most common reasons ACEi cannot be tolerated or uptitrated include cough, hypotension, renal insufficiency, and allergic reaction. Patients with cough should be switched to an ARB. Blood pressure and routine laboratory studies including electrolytes and renal function should be checked 1–2 weeks after changing or starting an ACEi. Given the risk of hyperkalemia, anytime there is an abrupt change in renal function on routine laboratory evaluation; electrolytes should be checked in patients on ACEi therapy.

Beta-Blockers

There have been numerous clinical trials demonstrating the mortality benefit of beta-blocker therapy in both asymptomatic (Stage B) and symptomatic patients (Stage C) with HFrEF [68]. Beta-blocker pharmacology varies greatly between agents, and therefore the guidelines recommend one of the three beta-blockers proven to be efficacious in randomized clinical trials. These include carvedilol, metoprolol, and bisoprolol.

Carvedilol has the most balanced profile of β-1 and β-2 receptor antagonism, whereas metoprolol and bisoprolol are more selective β-1 receptor blockers.

Table 4.3 Drug dosages for the management of heart failure with reduced ejection fraction

Drug class	Starting dose	Target dose
ACE inhibitors (ACEi)		
Captopril	6.25–12.5 mg TID	25–50 mg TID
Lisinopril	2.5–5 mg QD	20–40 mg QD
Enalapril	1.25–2.5 mg BID	10–20 mg BID
Ramipril	1.25–2.5 mg QD	10 mg QD
Angiotensin receptor blockers (ARBs)		
Candesartan	4 mg QD	32 mg QD
Valsartan	40 mg BID	160 mg BID
Losartan	12.5 mg QD	150 mg QD
Beta-blockers		
Carvedilol	3.125 mg BID	25 mg BID
Metoprolol succinate	12.5–25 mg QD	200 mg QD
Bisoprolol	1.25 mg QD	10 mg QD
Aldosterone antagonists		
Spironolactone	12.5 mg QD	50 mg QD
Eplerenone	25 mg QD	50 mg QD
Vasodilators		
Hydralazine	10 mg TID	75 mg TID
Isosorbide dinitrate	10 mg TID	40 mg TID
Isosorbide mononitrate	30 mg QD	120 mg QD

Carvedilol is also the only agent with clinically relevant α-1 receptor antagonism. Of these agents, carvedilol has the greatest blood pressure-lowering effect due to its α-1 blocking properties and has been associated with decreased insulin resistance. Metoprolol succinate and bisoprolol offer once daily dosing and are associated with less bronchospasm and hypotension. There is limited data about the efficacy of commonly prescribed beta-blockers, such as atenolol, in HFrEF, and when possible, patients with an LVEF <40% should be switched to carvedilol, metoprolol, or bisoprolol.

In general, beta-blockers should not be initiated when a patient has acute decompensated heart failure. In compensated patients, beta-blockers should be started at relatively low doses and increased as tolerated by heart rate and blood pressure. Carvedilol is dosed twice a day, with a starting dose of 3.125 mg twice daily and a maximum target dose of 25 mg twice daily. Metoprolol comes in short- and long- acting formulations. Metoprolol tartrate is the short-acting form and can be started as low as 12.5 mg twice daily. Metoprolol succinate (the extended release version) can be dosed daily or twice daily for patient with HFrEF [69]. The target dose of metoprolol tartrate is 50–100 mg twice daily, while the target dose for metoprolol succinate is 200 mg daily. The starting dose of bisoprolol is 1.25 mg daily and the target dose for HFrEF is 5–10 mg daily (Table 4.3).

Common side effects of beta-blockers include bradycardia, hypotension, lethargy, and impotence. Depression may also be exacerbated in susceptible patients.

The dose of beta-blockers may need to be decreased in patients with these symptoms. Beta-blockers can also exacerbate bronchospasm in patients with concomitant lung disease, and therefore agents that are more β-1 selective, such as bisoprolol or metoprolol, should be preferentially used in these patients. Similar to ACEi, the maximum benefit is seen at the higher doses used in clinical trials, but even lower doses are felt to be beneficial [70].

Other Heart Failure Drugs

There is no data specific to cancer patients as to the efficacy of additional heart failure treatments such as aldosterone antagonists, hydralazine/nitrates, and diuretics. Aldosterone antagonists, such as spironolactone or eplerenone, have a mortality benefit in symptomatic (Stage C) patients with an LVEF <35 % [71, 72]. Therefore, in chemotherapy-induced HFrEF patients with symptomatic heart failure and LVEF <35 % (Stage C), it is reasonable to consider aldosterone antagonist therapy. The initial dose of spironolactone can be as low as 12.5 mg daily and the target dose is 50 mg daily (Table 4.3). As this medication causes an increase in potassium levels, electrolytes should be followed at 3 days, 1 week, and monthly for the first 3 months after the initiation of therapy. Careful consideration should be given to patients with borderline renal function or who are receiving nephrotoxic chemotherapies.

Hydralazine with or without nitrate therapy is clinically used to reduce cardiac afterload in patients unable to tolerate ACEi/ARB therapy (typically secondary to renal dysfunction). The combination has a proven mortality benefit compared to placebo in patients with symptomatic (Stage C) heart failure [73], but is less effective than ACEi therapy [74]. Interestingly, the addition of hydralazine and nitrates to standard heart failure treatment has been shown to improve outcomes in African American patients [64]. Therefore, current guidelines recommend the addition of hydralazine and nitrate therapy for African American patients with symptomatic HFrEF, but do not recommend the routine use of hydralazine and nitrates for non-African American patients who are already tolerating an ACEi/ARB (Table 4.3) [58].

Digoxin is one of the oldest heart failure drugs, commonly used to control heart failure symptoms and provide rate control in patients with atrial fibrillation. Notably, while digoxin has been shown to reduce heart failure hospitalizations, it has no mortality benefit in HFrEF [75]. The 2013 ACC/AHA guidelines recommend starting digoxin in patients with LVEF <40 % who continue to have heart failure symptoms, despite maximal medical therapy with ACEi, beta-blocker, and aldosterone antagonists [58]. The typical starting dose of digoxin is 0.125 mg daily. In patients with impaired renal function, the drug can be started at 0.0625 mg daily or every other day. After several doses, a serum digoxin level should be checked and the recommended level is 0.5–0.8 ng/mL. Anytime there is an abrupt change in renal function, a digoxin level should be rechecked [76].

Diuretics are used to control symptoms of volume overload in HFrEF. This must be balanced against the stress that aggressive diuretic therapy places on the kidneys. The most commonly used diuretic is furosemide. Starting doses in heart failure are often 20–40 mg daily and can be increased to 200 mg twice daily. In patients with significant volume overload or recurrent heart failure hospitalizations, other diuretics with greater bioavailability such as torsemide and bumetanide should be considered.

Implantable cardioverter-defibrillator (ICD) therapy to reduce the risk of sudden cardiac death should be considered in symptomatic patients with an LVEF < 35 % who have a life expectancy greater than 1 year [57, 59]. Cardiac resynchronization therapy (CRT) should be considered in appropriate patients with symptomatic heart failure, LVEF < 35 %, and left bundle branch block to reduce heart failure morbidity and mortality [57, 59].

Chemotherapy-Induced Cardiomyopathy and Advanced Therapies

Approximately 2–4 % of patients with chemotherapy-induced cardiomyopathy progress to end-stage heart failure (Stage D) and may require consideration of advanced therapies including cardiac transplantation and mechanical circulatory support [11]. Among patients with nonischemic cardiomyopathy undergoing cardiac transplantation, approximately 2.5 % have chemotherapy-induced heart failure [77]. The posttransplant survival rates in these patients are 86 % at 1 year and 71 % at 5 years, which are similar to those in patients undergoing transplantation for non-chemotherapy-related etiologies of heart failure [78]. Similarly, the overall survival rates after mechanical circulatory support in patients with chemotherapy-induced heart failure are 73 % at 1 year and 63 % at 2 years, which are also not significantly different from other patient populations [78]. Therefore, while end-stage heart failure due to chemotherapy is not a contraindication to transplantation or mechanical circulatory support, certain factors specific to this patient population must be considered.

A history of active malignancy within the past 5 years is considered an absolute contraindication to cardiac transplantation. This is largely driven by the potential risk of recurrent malignant disease and shortened posttransplant survival in a resource-constrained environment. While recurrent malignancies are uncommon, the rates of novel malignancies are higher in patients with chemotherapy-induced cardiomyopathy compared to other etiologies (5 % vs. 2 %) [77]. Despite this, posttreatment malignancy-related death rates at 1 and 5 years do not differ significantly between patients with chemotherapy-related heart failure and heart failure due to other causes [77].

Patients with restrictive cardiomyopathy, either due to chest irradiation or childhood anthracycline exposure, have a significantly worse prognosis compared to other patients transplanted for restrictive cardiomyopathies. They have a 1.8-fold greater risk of mortality, with a 1-, 5-, and 10-year survival of only 71 %, 47 %, and 32 %, respectively [79]. Most of this risk is attributable to the multiple cardiovascular and pulmonary complications of chest irradiation therapy. In addition to myocardial dysfunction, radiation therapy can affect the coronary arteries, valves, and pericardium. Thus, many patients undergoing cardiac transplantation may have had prior cardiac surgery. Furthermore, radiation-induced scarring of the chest wall, lungs, and intrathoracic vessels further complicates cardiac surgery leading to greater ischemic times and worse outcomes. In addition, there is an increase in early mortality due to impaired sternal wound healing and a higher rate of postsurgical respiratory complications, postoperative RV dysfunction, and postoperative bleeding [80]. These patients also have an increased risk of secondary malignancies, limiting long-term posttransplant survival [81]. Thus, while patients with restrictive cardiomyopathies related to cancer treatment should be considered for advanced therapies, careful consideration should be given to other treatment-related comorbidities.

Patients with chemotherapy-induced heart failure are more likely to undergo mechanical circulatory support as durable, life-prolonging destination therapy rather than as a bridge to cardiac transplantation [78]. This is either due to the presence of recent or active malignancy or due to comorbidities that are often related to their cancer treatment. Furthermore, patients with chemotherapy-induced cardiomyopathy are more likely to require biventricular support, which carries a higher risk than isolated left ventricular support. In a retrospective analysis of 3812 patients enrolled in the Interagency Registry for Mechanically Assisted Circulatory Support, 19 % of patients with chemotherapy-induced cardiomyopathy undergoing mechanical circulatory support required right ventricular support, compared to 11 % with other nonischemic etiologies and 6 % with ischemic cardiomyopathy [78]. At present, biventricular assist devices are approved only as a bridge to transplantation, and therefore transplant-ineligible patients who require biventricular support cannot receive mechanical circulatory support. However, these patients can still be considered for home inotropes as palliative therapy. Additionally, chemotherapy-induced cardiomyopathy is associated with a greater risk of postoperative bleeding after ventricular assist device implantation, but there is no increase in the rate of neurologic complications, device malfunction, or infection compared to patients with non-chemotherapy-induced cardiomyopathy [78].

Progress in cancer treatment has increased cancer survivorship and the realization of long-term toxicities related to cancer therapy. Chemotherapeutic agents such as anthracyclines and HER-2-targeted therapies have been associated with cardiomyopathy. Serial monitoring for early markers of left ventricular dysfunction or asymptomatic disease allows initiation of cardiac therapies that may prevent the development of progressive heart failure. Further work is needed to identify the optimal screening tools and medication regimens that would allow successful delivery of cancer treatment while minimizing long-term cardiac toxicity.

Summary of Recommendations

- Patients undergoing treatment with potentially cardiotoxic chemotherapies are at risk for developing heart failure (Stage A) and measures should be taken to minimize cardiotoxicity.
- Limiting the cumulative anthracycline dose, using less cardiotoxic alternatives, and concomitant use of agents such as dexrazoxane should be considered to minimize cardiotoxicity.
- Limited data suggests that prophylactic use of ACEi and/or beta-blockers may be cardioprotective in patients undergoing potentially cardiotoxic chemotherapy.
- Serial monitoring of LVEF by echocardiography can help identify asymptomatic left ventricular dysfunction (Stage B).
- Initiation of ACEi and beta-blockers ± interruption/discontinuation of cardiotoxic chemotherapy can help reverse/prevent further progression of heart failure in patients with Stage B disease.
- The general principles of the management of heart failure with reduced ejection fraction apply to chemotherapy-induced cardiomyopathy.
- All patients with symptomatic heart failure (Stage C) should receive guideline-based therapy with ACEi/ARB, beta-blockers, and aldosterone antagonists as tolerated.
- Diuretics should be used as needed for symptom relief.
- Hydralazine plus nitrates and digoxin should be considered in certain patient populations.
- Patients with end-stage heart failure (Stage D) can be considered for advanced therapies (home inotropes, mechanical circulatory support, and cardiac transplantation).
- Patients with end-stage heart failure (Stage D) who are cancer-free for ≥5 years can be considered for cardiac transplantation.
- Careful consideration should be given to comorbidities that might worsen surgical outcomes, especially in patients with prior thoracic irradiation.
- Patients undergoing mechanical circulatory support should be carefully evaluated for right ventricular dysfunction to guide appropriate device selection.
- In patients who are ineligible for transplant or mechanical circulatory support, home inotropes can be considered for palliation.
- Patients with a history of cancer who require advanced cardiac therapy consideration should be referred to a tertiary center with experience dealing with this unique patient population.

References

1. Monsuez JJ, Charniot JC, Vignat N, Artigou JY. Cardiac side-effects of cancer chemotherapy. Int J Cardiol. 2010;144:3–15.
2. Floyd JD, Nguyen DT, Lobins RL, Bashir Q, Doll DC, Perry MC. Cardiotoxicity of cancer therapy. J Clin Oncol. 2005;23:7685–96.
3. Shakir DK, Rasul KI. Chemotherapy induced cardiomyopathy: pathogenesis, monitoring and management. J Clin Med Res. 2009;1:8–12.
4. Tan C, Tasaka H, Yu KP, Murphy ML, Karnofsky DA. Daunomycin, an antitumor antibiotic, in the treatment of neoplastic disease. Clinical evaluation with special reference to childhood leukemia. Cancer. 1967;20:333–53.
5. Minotti G, Menna P, Salvatorelli E, Cairo G, Gianni L. Anthracyclines: molecular advances and pharmacologic developments in antitumor activity and cardiotoxicity. Pharmacol Rev. 2004;56:185–229.
6. Jensen PB, Sorensen BS, Sehested M, Demant EJ, Kjeldsen E, Friche E, Hansen HH. Different modes of anthracycline interaction with topoisomerase II. Separate structures critical for DNA-cleavage, and for overcoming topoisomerase II-related drug resistance. Biochem Pharmacol. 1993;45:2025–35.
7. Xu X, Persson HL, Richardson DR. Molecular pharmacology of the interaction of anthracyclines with iron. Mol Pharmacol. 2005;68:261–71.
8. Pang B, Qiao X, Janssen L, Velds A, Groothuis T, Kerkhoven R, Nieuwland M, Ovaa H, Rottenberg S, van Tellingen O, Janssen J, Huijgens P, Zwart W, Neefjes J. Drug-induced histone eviction from open chromatin contributes to the chemotherapeutic effects of doxorubicin. Nat Commun. 2013;4:1908.
9. Hahn VS, Lenihan DJ, Ky B. Cancer therapy-induced cardiotoxicity: basic mechanisms and potential cardioprotective therapies. J Am Heart Assoc. 2014;3, e000665.
10. Lyu YL, Kerrigan JE, Lin CP, Azarova AM, Tsai YC, Ban Y, Liu LF. Topoisomerase II-beta mediated DNA double-strand breaks: implications in doxorubicin cardiotoxicity and prevention by dexrazoxane. Cancer Res. 2007;67:8839–46.
11. Yeh ET, Bickford CL. Cardiovascular complications of cancer therapy: incidence, pathogenesis, diagnosis, and management. J Am Coll Cardiol. 2009;53:2231–47.
12. Shan K, Lincoff AM, Young JB. Anthracycline-induced cardiotoxicity. Ann Intern Med. 1996;125:47–58.
13. Cardinale D, Colombo A, Bacchiani G, Tedeschi I, Meroni CA, Veglia F, Civelli M, Lamantia G, Colombo N, Curigliano G, Fiorentini C, Cipolla CM. Early detection of anthracycline cardiotoxicity and improvement with heart failure therapy. Circulation. 2015;131:1981–8.
14. Von Hoff DD, Rozencweig M, Layard M, Slavik M, Muggia FM. Daunomycin-induced cardiotoxicity in children and adults. A review of 110 cases. Am J Med. 1977;62:200–8.
15. Haq MM, Legha SS, Choksi J, Hortobagyi GN, Benjamin RS, Ewer M, Ali M. Doxorubicin-induced congestive heart failure in adults. Cancer. 1985;56:1361–5.
16. Steinherz LJ, Steinherz PG, Tan C. Cardiac failure and dysrhythmias 6-19 years after anthracycline therapy: a series of 15 patients. Med Pediatr Oncol. 1995;24:352–61.
17. Dresdale A, Bonow RO, Wesley R, Palmeri ST, Barr L, Mathison D, D'Angelo T, Rosenberg SA. Prospective evaluation of doxorubicin-induced cardiomyopathy resulting from postsurgical adjuvant treatment of patients with soft tissue sarcomas. Cancer. 1983;52:51–60.
18. Plana JC, Galderisi M, Barac A, Ewer MS, Ky B, Scherrer-Crosbie M, Ganame J, Sebag IA, Agler DA, Badano LP, Banchs J, Cardinale D, Carver J, Cerqueira M, DeCara JM, Edvardsen T, Flamm SD, Force T, Griffin BP, Jerusalem G, Liu JE, Magalhaes A, Marwick T, Sanchez LY, Sicari R, Villarraga HR, Lancellotti P. Expert consensus for multimodality imaging evaluation of adult patients during and after cancer therapy: a report from the american society of echocardiography and the european association of cardiovascular imaging. J Am Soc Echocardiogr. 2014;27:911–39.

19. Schwartz RG, McKenzie WB, Alexander J, Sager P, D'Souza A, Manatunga A, Schwartz PE, Berger HJ, Setaro J, Surkin L, et al. Congestive heart failure and left ventricular dysfunction complicating doxorubicin therapy. Seven-year experience using serial radionuclide angiocardiography. Am J Med. 1987;82:1109–18.
20. Sawaya H, Sebag IA, Plana JC, Januzzi JL, Ky B, Cohen V, Gosavi S, Carver JR, Wiegers SE, Martin RP, Picard MH, Gerszten RE, Halpern EF, Passeri J, Kuter I, Scherrer-Crosbie M. Early detection and prediction of cardiotoxicity in chemotherapy-treated patients. Am J Cardiol. 2011;107:1375–80.
21. Cardinale D, Sandri MT, Colombo A, Colombo N, Boeri M, Lamantia G, Civelli M, Peccatori F, Martinelli G, Fiorentini C, Cipolla CM. Prognostic value of troponin I in cardiac risk stratification of cancer patients undergoing high-dose chemotherapy. Circulation. 2004;109:2749–54.
22. Lipshultz SE, Rifai N, Dalton VM, Levy DE, Silverman LB, Lipsitz SR, Colan SD, Asselin BL, Barr RD, Clavell LA, Hurwitz CA, Moghrabi A, Samson Y, Schorin MA, Gelber RD, Sallan SE. The effect of dexrazoxane on myocardial injury in doxorubicin-treated children with acute lymphoblastic leukemia. N Engl J Med. 2004;351:145–53.
23. Cardinale D, Colombo A, Sandri MT, Lamantia G, Colombo N, Civelli M, Martinelli G, Veglia F, Fiorentini C, Cipolla CM. Prevention of high-dose chemotherapy-induced cardiotoxicity in high-risk patients by angiotensin-converting enzyme inhibition. Circulation. 2006;114:2474–81.
24. Legha SS, Benjamin RS, Mackay B, Ewer M, Wallace S, Valdivieso M, Rasmussen SL, Blumenschein GR, Freireich EJ. Reduction of doxorubicin cardiotoxicity by prolonged continuous intravenous infusion. Ann Intern Med. 1982;96:133–9.
25. Smith LA, Cornelius VR, Plummer CJ, Levitt G, Verrill M, Canney P, Jones A. Cardiotoxicity of anthracycline agents for the treatment of cancer: systematic review and meta-analysis of randomised controlled trials. BMC Cancer. 2010;10:337.
26. van Dalen EC, Michiels EM, Caron HN, Kremer LC. Different anthracycline derivates for reducing cardiotoxicity in cancer patients. Cochrane Datab Syst Rev. 2010:CD005006.
27. Swain SM, Whaley FS, Gerber MC, Weisberg S, York M, Spicer D, Jones SE, Wadler S, Desai A, Vogel C, Speyer J, Mittelman A, Reddy S, Pendergrass K, Velez-Garcia E, Ewer MS, Bianchine JR, Gams RA. Cardioprotection with dexrazoxane for doxorubicin-containing therapy in advanced breast cancer. J Clin Oncol. 1997;15:1318–32.
28. Tebbi CK, London WB, Friedman D, Villaluna D, De Alarcon PA, Constine LS, Mendenhall NP, Sposto R, Chauvenet A, Schwartz CL. Dexrazoxane-associated risk for acute myeloid leukemia/myelodysplastic syndrome and other secondary malignancies in pediatric Hodgkin's disease. J Clin Oncol. 2007;25:493–500.
29. Jay SM, Murthy AC, Hawkins JF, Wortzel JR, Steinhauser ML, Alvarez LM, Gannon J, Macrae CA, Griffith LG, Lee RT. An engineered bivalent neuregulin protects against doxorubicin-induced cardiotoxicity with reduced proneoplastic potential. Circulation. 2013;128:152–61.
30. Georgakopoulos P, Roussou P, Matsakas E, Karavidas A, Anagnostopoulos N, Marinakis T, Galanopoulos A, Georgiakodis F, Zimeras S, Kyriakidis M, Ahimastos A. Cardioprotective effect of metoprolol and enalapril in doxorubicin-treated lymphoma patients: a prospective, parallel-group, randomized, controlled study with 36-month follow-up. Am J Hematol. 2010;85:894–6.
31. Kalay N, Basar E, Ozdogru I, Er O, Cetinkaya Y, Dogan A, Inanc T, Oguzhan A, Eryol NK, Topsakal R, Ergin A. Protective effects of carvedilol against anthracycline-induced cardiomyopathy. J Am Coll Cardiol. 2006;48:2258–62.
32. Kaya MG, Ozkan M, Gunebakmaz O, Akkaya H, Kaya EG, Akpek M, Kalay N, Dikilitas M, Yarlioglues M, Karaca H, Berk V, Ardic I, Ergin A, Lam YY. Protective effects of nebivolol against anthracycline-induced cardiomyopathy: a randomized control study. Int J Cardiol. 2013;167:2306–10.

33. Bosch X, Rovira M, Sitges M, Domenech A, Ortiz-Perez JT, de Caralt TM, Morales-Ruiz M, Perea RJ, Monzo M, Esteve J. Enalapril and carvedilol for preventing chemotherapy-induced left ventricular systolic dysfunction in patients with malignant hemopathies: The OVER-COME trial (preventiOn of left Ventricular dysfunction with Enalapril and caRvedilol in patients submitted to intensive ChemOtherapy for the treatment of Malignant hEmopathies). J Am Coll Cardiol. 2013;61:2355–62.
34. Gulati G, Heck SL, Hoffman P, et al. Prevention of cardiac dysfunction during adjuvant breast cancer therapy (PRADA): primary results of a randomized, 2×2 factorial, placebo-controlled, double-blind clinical trial. 2015.
35. Seicean S, Seicean A, Plana JC, Budd GT, Marwick TH. Effect of statin therapy on the risk for incident heart failure in patients with breast cancer receiving anthracycline chemotherapy: an observational clinical cohort study. J Am Coll Cardiol. 2012;60:2384–90.
36. Bange J, Zwick E, Ullrich A. Molecular targets for breast cancer therapy and prevention. Nat Med. 2001;7:548–52.
37. Wolff AC, Hammond ME, Hicks DG, Dowsett M, McShane LM, Allison KH, Allred DC, Bartlett JM, Bilous M, Fitzgibbons P, Hanna W, Jenkins RB, Mangu PB, Paik S, Perez EA, Press MF, Spears PA, Vance GH, Viale G, Hayes DF, American Society of Clinical O, College of American P. Recommendations for human epidermal growth factor receptor 2 testing in breast cancer: American society of clinical oncology/college of american pathologists clinical practice guideline update. J Clin Oncol. 2013;31:3997–4013.
38. Feldman AM, Koch WJ, Force TL. Developing strategies to link basic cardiovascular sciences with clinical drug development: another opportunity for translational sciences. Clin Pharmacol Ther. 2007;81:887–92.
39. Calabro P, Yeh ET. Multitasking of the 3-hydroxy-3-methylglutaryl coenzyme a reductase inhibitor: Beyond cardiovascular diseases. Curr Atheroscler Rep. 2004;6:36–41.
40. Chen MH, Kerkela R, Force T. Mechanisms of cardiac dysfunction associated with tyrosine kinase inhibitor cancer therapeutics. Circulation. 2008;118:84–95.
41. Sawyer DB, Zuppinger C, Miller TA, Eppenberger HM, Suter TM. Modulation of anthracycline-induced myofibrillar disarray in rat ventricular myocytes by neuregulin-1beta and anti-erbb2: potential mechanism for trastuzumab-induced cardiotoxicity. Circulation. 2002;105:1551–4.
42. Tripathy D, Seidman A, Keefe D, Hudis C, Paton V, Lieberman G. Effect of cardiac dysfunction on treatment outcomes in women receiving trastuzumab for her2-overexpressing metastatic breast cancer. Clin Breast Cancer. 2004;5:293–8.
43. Slamon DJ, Leyland-Jones B, Shak S, Fuchs H, Paton V, Bajamonde A, Fleming T, Eiermann W, Wolter J, Pegram M, Baselga J, Norton L. Use of chemotherapy plus a monoclonal antibody against her2 for metastatic breast cancer that overexpresses her2. N Engl J Med. 2001;344:783–92.
44. Seidman A, Hudis C, Pierri MK, Shak S, Paton V, Ashby M, Murphy M, Stewart SJ, Keefe D. Cardiac dysfunction in the trastuzumab clinical trials experience. J Clin Oncol. 2002;20:1215–21.
45. Moja L, Tagliabue L, Balduzzi S, Parmelli E, Pistotti V, Guarneri V, D'Amico R. Trastuzumab containing regimens for early breast cancer. Cochrane Database Syst Rev. 2012;4, CD006243.
46. Ewer SM, Ewer MS. Cardiotoxicity profile of trastuzumab. Drug Saf. 2008;31:459–67.
47. Smith I, Procter M, Gelber RD, Guillaume S, Feyereislova A, Dowsett M, Goldhirsch A, Untch M, Mariani G, Baselga J, Kaufmann M, Cameron D, Bell R, Bergh J, Coleman R, Wardley A, Harbeck N, Lopez RI, Mallmann P, Gelmon K, Wilcken N, Wist E, Sanchez Rovira P, Piccart-Gebhart MJ, team Hs. 2-year follow-up of trastuzumab after adjuvant chemotherapy in her2-positive breast cancer: a randomised controlled trial. Lancet. 2007;369:29–36.
48. Procter M, Suter TM, de Azambuja E, Dafni U, van Dooren V, Muehlbauer S, Climent MA, Rechberger E, Liu WT, Toi M, Coombes RC, Dodwell D, Pagani O, Madrid J, Hall M, Chen SC, Focan C, Muschol M, van Veldhuisen DJ, Piccart-Gebhart MJ. Longer-term assessment of

trastuzumab-related cardiac adverse events in the herceptin adjuvant (hera) trial. J Clin Oncol. 2010;28:3422–8.

49. Piccart-Gebhart MJ, Procter M, Leyland-Jones B, Goldhirsch A, Untch M, Smith I, Gianni L, Baselga J, Bell R, Jackisch C, Cameron D, Dowsett M, Barrios CH, Steger G, Huang CS, Andersson M, Inbar M, Lichinitser M, Lang I, Nitz U, Iwata H, Thomssen C, Lohrisch C, Suter TM, Ruschoff J, Suto T, Greatorex V, Ward C, Straehle C, McFadden E, Dolci MS, Gelber RD, Herceptin Adjuvant Trial Study T. Trastuzumab after adjuvant chemotherapy in her2-positive breast cancer. New Engl J Med. 2005;353:1659–72.

50. Romond EH, Jeong JH, Rastogi P, Swain SM, Geyer CE, Jr., Ewer MS, Rathi V, Fehrenbacher L, Brufsky A, Azar CA, Flynn PJ, Zapas JL, Polikoff J, Gross HM, Biggs DD, Atkins JN, Tan-Chiu E, Zheng P, Yothers G, Mamounas EP, Wolmark N. Seven-year follow-up assessment of cardiac function in nsabp b-31, a randomized trial comparing doxorubicin and cyclophosphamide followed by paclitaxel (acp) with acp plus trastuzumab as adjuvant therapy for patients with node-positive, human epidermal growth factor receptor 2-positive breast cancer. J Clin Oncol. 2012;30:3792–99.

51. Serrano C, Cortes J, De Mattos-Arruda L, Bellet M, Gomez P, Saura C, Perez J, Vidal M, Munoz-Couselo E, Carreras MJ, Sanchez-Olle G, Tabernero J, Baselga J, Di Cosimo S. - Trastuzumab-related cardiotoxicity in the elderly: a role for cardiovascular risk factors. Ann Oncol. 2012;23:897–902.

52. Fox KF. The evaluation of left ventricular function for patients being considered for, or receiving trastuzumab (herceptin) therapy. Br J Cancer. 2006;95:1454.

53. Romond EH, Perez EA, Bryant J, Suman VJ, Geyer Jr CE, Davidson NE, Tan-Chiu E, Martino S, Paik S, Kaufman PA, Swain SM, Pisansky TM, Fehrenbacher L, Kutteh LA, Vogel VG, Visscher DW, Yothers G, Jenkins RB, Brown AM, Dakhil SR, Mamounas EP, Lingle WL, Klein PM, Ingle JN, Wolmark N. Trastuzumab plus adjuvant chemotherapy for operable HER2-positive breast cancer. N Engl J Med. 2005;353:1673–84.

54. Cardinale D, Colombo A, Torrisi R, Sandri MT, Civelli M, Salvatici M, Lamantia G, Colombo N, Cortinovis S, Dessanai MA, Nole F, Veglia F, Cipolla CM. Trastuzumab-induced cardiotoxicity: clinical and prognostic implications of troponin i evaluation. J Clin Oncol. 2010;28:3910–6.

55. Seicean S, Seicean A, Alan N, Plana JC, Budd GT, Marwick TH. Cardioprotective effect of beta-adrenoceptor blockade in patients with breast cancer undergoing chemotherapy: follow-up study of heart failure. Circ Heart Fail. 2013;6:420–6.

56. Pituskin E, Mackey JR, Koshman S, et al. Prophylactic beta-blockade preserves left ventricular ejection fraction in HER2-overexpressing breast cancer patients receiving trastuzumab: Primary results of the manticore randomized controlled trial. 2015 San Antonio Breast Cancer Symposium. Abstract S1-05. Presented December 9, 2015.

57. Arnold JM, Liu P, Demers C, Dorian P, Giannetti N, Haddad H, Heckman GA, Howlett JG, Ignaszewski A, Johnstone DE, Jong P, McKelvie RS, Moe GW, Parker JD, Rao V, Ross HJ, Sequeira EJ, Svendsen AM, Teo K, Tsuyuki RT, White M, Canadian CS. Canadian Cardio-vascular Society consensus conference recommendations on heart failure 2006: diagnosis and management. Can J Cardiol. 2006;22:23–45.

58. Yancy CW, Jessup M, Bozkurt B, Butler J, Casey DE, Jr., Drazner MH, Fonarow GC, Geraci SA, Horwich T, Januzzi JL, Johnson MR, Kasper EK, Levy WC, Masoudi FA, McBride PE, McMurray JJ, Mitchell JE, Peterson PN, Riegel B, Sam F, Stevenson LW, Tang WH, Tsai EJ, Wilkoff BL, American College of Cardiology F, American Heart Association Task Force on Practice G. 2013 ACCF/AHA guideline for the management of heart failure: A report of the American College of Cardiology Foundation/American Heart Association Task Force on Practice Guidelines. J Am Coll Cardiol. 2013;62:e147–239.

59. McMurray JJ, Adamopoulos S, Anker SD, Auricchio A, Bohm M, Dickstein K, Falk V, Filippatos G, Fonseca C, Gomez-Sanchez MA, Jaarsma T, Kober L, Lip GY, Maggioni AP, Parkhomenko A, Pieske BM, Popescu BA, Ronnevik PK, Rutten FH, Schwitter J, Seferovic P, Stepinska J, Trindade PT, Voors AA, Zannad F, Zeiher A, Guidelines ESCCfP. ESC

guidelines for the diagnosis and treatment of acute and chronic heart failure 2012: The Task Force for the Diagnosis and Treatment of Acute and Chronic Heart Failure 2012 of the European Society of Cardiology. Developed in collaboration with the Heart Failure Association (HFA) of the ESC. Eur Heart J. 2012;33:1787–847.

60. Effect of enalapril on survival in patients with reduced left ventricular ejection fractions and congestive heart failure. The SOLVD investigators. New Engl J Med. 1991;325:293–302.

61. Effect of enalapril on mortality and the development of heart failure in asymptomatic patients with reduced left ventricular ejection fractions. The SOLVD investigators. New Engl J Med. 1992;327:685–91.

62. Effects of enalapril on mortality in severe congestive heart failure. Results of the COoperative North Scandinavian ENalapril SUrvival Study (CONSENSUS). The CONSENSUS trial study group. New Engl J Med. 1987;316:1429–35.

63. Al Khalaf MM, Thalib L, Doi SA. Cardiovascular outcomes in high-risk patients without heart failure treated with arbs: a systematic review and meta-analysis. Am J Cardiovasc Drugs. 2009;9:29–43.

64. Taylor AL, Sabolinski ML, Tam SW, Ziesche S, Ghali JK, Archambault WT, Worcel M, Cohn JN, Investigators AH. Effect of fixed-dose combined isosorbide dinitrate/hydralazine in elderly patients in the African-American heart failure trial. J Card Fail. 2012;18:600–6.

65. Kostis JB, Shelton BJ, Yusuf S, Weiss MB, Capone RJ, Pepine CJ, Gosselin G, Delahaye F, Probstfield JL, Cahill L, et al. Tolerability of enalapril initiation by patients with left ventricular dysfunction: results of the medication challenge phase of the studies of left ventricular dysfunction. Am Heart J. 1994;128:358–64.

66. Ahmed A. Use of angiotensin-converting enzyme inhibitors in patients with heart failure and renal insufficiency: how concerned should we be by the rise in serum creatinine? J Am Geriatr Soc. 2002;50:1297–300.

67. Packer M, Poole-Wilson PA, Armstrong PW, Cleland JG, Horowitz JD, Massie BM, Ryden L, Thygesen K, Uretsky BF. Comparative effects of low and high doses of the angiotensin-converting enzyme inhibitor, lisinopril, on morbidity and mortality in chronic heart failure. Atlas study group. Circulation. 1999;100:2312–8.

68. Brophy JM, Joseph L, Rouleau JL. Beta-blockers in congestive heart failure. A bayesian meta-analysis. Ann Intern Med. 2001;134:550–60.

69. Kukin ML, Mannino MM, Freudenberger RS, Kalman J, Buchholz-Varley C, Ocampo O. Hemodynamic comparison of twice daily metoprolol tartrate with once daily metoprolol succinate in congestive heart failure. J Am Coll Cardiol. 2000;35:45–50.

70. Wikstrand J, Hjalmarson A, Waagstein F, Fagerberg B, Goldstein S, Kjekshus J, Wedel H, Group M-HS. Dose of metoprolol cr/xl and clinical outcomes in patients with heart failure: analysis of the experience in MEtoprolol cr/xl Randomized Intervention Trial in chronic Heart Failure (MERIT-HF). J Am Coll Cardiol. 2002;40:491–8.

71. Zannad F, McMurray JJ, Krum H, van Veldhuisen DJ, Swedberg K, Shi H, Vincent J, Pocock SJ, Pitt B, Group E-HS. Eplerenone in patients with systolic heart failure and mild symptoms. N Engl J Med. 2011;364:11–21.

72. Pitt B, Zannad F, Remme WJ, Cody R, Castaigne A, Perez A, Palensky J, Wittes J. The effect of spironolactone on morbidity and mortality in patients with severe heart failure. Randomized aldactone evaluation study investigators. N Engl J Med. 1999;341:709–17.

73. Cohn JN, Archibald DG, Ziesche S, Franciosa JA, Harston WE, Tristani FE, Dunkman WB, Jacobs W, Francis GS, Flohr KH, et al. Effect of vasodilator therapy on mortality in chronic congestive heart failure. Results of a Veterans Administration cooperative study. N Engl J Med. 1986;314:1547–52.

74. Cohn JN, Johnson G, Ziesche S, Cobb F, Francis G, Tristani F, Smith R, Dunkman WB, Loeb H, Wong M, et al. A comparison of enalapril with hydralazine-isosorbide dinitrate in the treatment of chronic congestive heart failure. N Engl J Med. 1991;325:303–10.

75. Digitalis IG. The effect of digoxin on mortality and morbidity in patients with heart failure. N Engl J Med. 1997;336:525–33.

76. Rathore SS, Curtis JP, Wang Y, Bristow MR, Krumholz HM. Association of serum digoxin concentration and outcomes in patients with heart failure. JAMA. 2003;289:871–8.
77. Oliveira GH, Hardaway BW, Kucheryavaya AY, Stehlik J, Edwards LB, Taylor DO. Characteristics and survival of patients with chemotherapy-induced cardiomyopathy undergoing heart transplantation. J Heart Lung Transplant. 2012;31:805–10.
78. Oliveira GH, Dupont M, Naftel D, Myers SL, Yuan Y, Tang WH, Gonzalez-Stawinski G, Young JB, Taylor DO, Starling RC. Increased need for right ventricular support in patients with chemotherapy-induced cardiomyopathy undergoing mechanical circulatory support: outcomes from the INTERMACS registry (INTEragency Registry for Mechanically Assisted Circulatory Support). J Am Coll Cardiol. 2014;63:240–8.
79. DePasquale EC, Nasir K, Jacoby DL. Outcomes of adults with restrictive cardiomyopathy after heart transplantation. J Heart Lung Transplant. 2012;31:1269–75.
80. Chang AS, Smedira NG, Chang CL, Benavides MM, Myhre U, Feng J, Blackstone EH, Lytle BW. Cardiac surgery after mediastinal radiation: extent of exposure influences outcome. J Thorac Cardiovasc Surg. 2007;133:404–13.
81. Uriel N, Vainrib A, Jorde UP, Cotarlan V, Farr M, Cheema FH, Naka Y, Mancini D, Colombo PC. Mediastinal radiation and adverse outcomes after heart transplantation. J Heart Lung Transplant. 2010;29:378–81.

Chapter 5
Treatment of Hypertension in Patients Receiving Cancer Therapy

Aaron P. Kithcart, Giuseppe Curigliano, and Joshua A. Beckman

Introduction

Hypertension affects one in three adults in the United States. Epidemiological studies estimate that high blood pressure contributes to one out of every seven deaths and nearly half of all cardiovascular disease-related deaths in the United States [1]. Not surprisingly, hypertension is diagnosed commonly in the oncology population with important implications for both antineoplastic therapy and long-term prognosis. The presence of hypertension may be a negative predictor of morbidity and mortality [2].

High blood pressure is the most common comorbidity in patients with malignancy [3]. While the prevalence of hypertension in cancer patients is similar at the time of initial diagnosis, the prevalence increases to 37 % over the course of cancer therapy, especially those who have received chemotherapy [4, 5]. The increased prevalence stems from the effect of many antineoplastic agents on blood pressure, in part, due to their mechanisms of cancer treatment [6–8].

Electronic supplementary material: The online version of this chapter (doi:10.1007/978-3-319-43096-6_5) contains supplementary material, which is available to authorized users.

A.P. Kithcart (✉)
Cardiology, Brigham and Women's Hospital, Boston, MA, USA
e-mail: apkithcart@partners.org

G. Curigliano
Division of Early Drug Development for Innovative Therapies,
Istituto Europeo di Oncologia, Milano, Italy
e-mail: giuseppe.curigliano@ieo.it

J.A. Beckman
Vanderbilt Heart and Vascular Institute, Vanderbilt University Medical Center,
Nashville, TN, USA
e-mail: joshua.a.beckman@vanderbilt.edu

© Springer International Publishing Switzerland 2017
G.G. Kimmick et al. (eds.), *Cardio-Oncology*, DOI 10.1007/978-3-319-43096-6_5

The clinician caring for the oncologic patient has a constantly expanding requirement to be acquainted with the management of hypertension, the associated risks of antineoplastic therapy, and the impact of cancer therapy on cardiovascular disease to provide high-quality care. This chapter will define hypertension and describe a basic approach for management, provide an overview of the association between cancer and hypertension, review common chemotherapeutic agents that contribute to hypertension, and discuss the mechanisms by which these agents increase blood pressure thereby providing insight into the specific treatment of hypertension.

Hypertension

Hypertension is the most common cardiovascular comorbidity in the United States, found in nearly one third of all adults [1]. The prevalence among adults is 30.9 %, but among those greater than 65, the prevalence approaches 70 % [1]. Rates remain highest among African-Americans, with Mexican-Americans having the lowest rates of documented hypertension. Contemporary studies suggest there is no clear difference across socioeconomic status or education level, although it is worth noting that the highest rates of hypertension are found in those on Medicare compared to other forms of public or private insurance, confirming a clear age-associated risk for hypertension [1].

While the overall prevalence of hypertension has remained steady over the last 10 years, the proportion of those receiving antihypertensive treatment continues to rise [9]. Hypertension is the most common primary diagnosis, accounting for nearly 35 million office visits annually [10]. Many efforts, including those by the Joint National Committee, have contributed to the greater number of Americans receiving therapy. The widespread availability of generic medications has improved the accessibility and affordability of therapy. Yet, control to target still remains less than 50 % among patients with high blood pressure [1].

Definition

Hypertension has historically been defined as any sustained blood pressure greater than 140 mmHg of systolic blood pressure or 90 mmHg of diastolic blood pressure. Current guidelines recommend that the diagnosis be made when the mean of two or more properly measured seated blood pressure readings on each of two or more office visits are elevated. Practitioners are advised that patients should be in a quiet room for at least 5 min prior to taking any recordings. Notably, the US Preventive Services Task Force is currently reexamining recommendations for blood pressure screening, and their revised guidelines will likely include ambulatory blood pressure monitoring as a complement to office testing.

Publication of the Seventh Report of the Joint National Committee on Prevention, Evaluation, and Treatment of High Blood Pressure (JNC7) added an additional category, termed prehypertension, defined as 120–139 mmHg of systolic blood pressure or 80–89 mmHg of diastolic blood pressure (Table 5.1) [11]. The authors described two stages of hypertension: Stage 1, defined as a systolic blood pressure of 140–159 mmHg or a diastolic blood pressure of 90–99 mmHg, and Stage 2, defined as a systolic blood pressure greater than 160 mmHg or diastolic blood pressure greater than 100 mmHg. Recent studies, including the SPRINT trial published in late 2015, suggest that targeting an even lower blood pressure may lead to fewer events [12]. The method of achieving this level of blood pressure, the populations to whom to generalize the results, and the relevance to hypertension in malignancy are currently in development.

Within oncology, the Common Terminology Criteria for Adverse Events is a set of toxicity assessments during cancer research published by the National Cancer Institute that defines a number of complications of antineoplastic therapy, including hypertension. The most recent criteria published in 2009 define five grades of hypertension, ranging from 1 through 5 (Table 5.2) [13]. Grade 1 hypertension corresponds with prehypertension, as defined by JNC7 (SBP 120–139 mmHg and

Table 5.1 Classification of normal blood pressure and hypertension

Classification	Systolic BP (mmHg)	Diastolic BP (mmHg)
Normal	<120	<80
Prehypertension	120–139	80–89
Stage 1	140–159	90–99
Stage 2	>160	>100

Table 5.2 Common terminology criteria for adverse events for hypertension

Grade				
1	2	3	4	5
Prehypertension (systolic BP 120–139 mmHg or diastolic BP 80–89 mmHg)	Stage 1 hypertension (systolic BP 140–159 mmHg or diastolic BP 90–99 mmHg); medical intervention indicated; recurrent or persistent (>=24 h); symptomatic increase by >20 mmHg (diastolic) or to >140/90 mmHg if previously WNL; monotherapy indicated	Stage 2 hypertension (systolic BP >=160 mmHg or diastolic BP >=100 mmHg); medical intervention indicated; more than one drug or more intensive therapy than previously used indicated	Life-threatening consequences (e.g., malignant hypertension, transient or permanent neurologic deficit, hypertensive crisis); urgent intervention indicated	Death

DBP 80–89); Grade 2 and Grade 3 hypertension correspond with Stage 1 and Stage 2 hypertension, respectively. Grade 4 is defined as hypertension that results in a life-threatening condition, including malignant hypertension, transient or permanent neurologic deficit, and hypertensive crisis. Finally, Grade 5 hypertension includes blood pressure elevation leading to death. These standards are commonly used for reporting adverse events during clinical trials and thus will serve as a common reference point in this chapter.

Treatment

The benefits of treating hypertension are clear. Often described as the "silent killer," the immediate effects may not be apparent, but the long-term consequences are well known. The goal of hypertension therapy is to reduce end-organ damage associated with long-term high blood pressure. Clinical trials have shown that antihypertensive therapy is associated with marked reductions in stroke, myocardial infarction, heart failure, and renal failure [14]. Treating just 11 patients with Stage 1 hypertension over 10 years prevents one death [15].

The first line of therapy recommended for all levels of hypertension, whether prehypertension, Stage 1, or Stage 2, is lifestyle modification [11]. These modifications include weight reduction, adoption of the Dietary Approaches to Stop Hypertension (DASH) diet, dietary sodium reduction, physical activity, and moderate alcohol consumption [16–22]. Despite universal recommendation, these approaches commonly lead to a modest improvement, with the average reduction in systolic blood pressure between 2 and 20 mmHg [11].

For those who continue to have Stage 1 or Stage 2 high blood pressure despite lifestyle modification, the initiation of pharmacological therapy is indicated (Table 5.3). The most recent recommendations advise the use of either a thiazide-type diuretic, calcium channel blocker (CCB), angiotensin-converting enzyme inhibitor (ACEI), or angiotensin receptor blocker (ARB) [23]. Each of these medications has similar effects on mortality and cardiovascular outcomes, so none is preferred. However, there are certain populations in which specific therapy is recommended.

In the black population, thiazide-type diuretics and CCBs are preferred. These agents have been shown to have better outcomes than inhibition of the angiotensin-renin system in this population [23]. Furthermore, patients with chronic kidney disease, defined as a GFR of less than 30, should include an ACEI or ARB as part of their medication regimen. The combination of ACEI and ARB, however, should be avoided as this may lead to adverse effects on kidney function and a dangerous elevation in potassium.

When initiating pharmacological therapy, the clinician should begin with one of the classes of medications reviewed above. Blood pressure should continue to be assessed, and, if elevated after 1 month despite maximum therapy, a second agent should be added from a different class of medications. An additional agent should

Table 5.3 Oral antihypertension therapy

Drug class	Name	Dose range (mg/d)
Thiazide-type diuretics	Chlorothiazide	125–500
	Chlorthalidone	12.5–25
	Hydrochlorothiazide	12.5–50
	Metolazone	2.5–5
Calcium channel blockers	Amlodipine	2.5–10
Dihydropyridines	Nicardipine sustained release	60–120
	Nifedipine long-acting	30–60
Non-dihydropyridines	Diltiazem extended release	180–540
	Verapamil immediate release	80–320
	Verapamil long-acting	120–360
ACE inhibitors	Benazepril	10–40
	Captopril	25–100
	Enalapril	2.5–40
	Fosinopril	10–40
	Lisinopril	10–40
	Quinapril	10–40
	Ramipril	2.5–20
Aldosterone receptor blockers	Eplerenone	50–100
	Spironolactone	25–50

not be added, however, until the highest tolerated dose of the first agent is used. For instance, if an otherwise healthy patient is started on lisinopril and remains hypertensive even on 40 mg daily, then a thiazide-type diuretic or CCB may be considered. As with any new medication, drug-drug interactions should be evaluated, especially with concurrent chemotherapy.

If treatment remains insufficient with two medications at maximum tolerated doses, then a third agent should be added from the remaining classes of medications. Blood pressure that remains elevated despite three medications is defined as resistant and may require additional assessment by a specialist. Patients with cardiovascular comorbidities, including heart failure, coronary artery disease, chronic kidney disease, and diabetes, should be targeted to a lower systolic blood pressure.

Hypertension Associated with Antineoplastic Therapy

As discussed previously, hypertension is increasingly recognized as an important comorbidity in oncology. While some patients will have a history of hypertension at the time of their cancer diagnosis, others will develop hypertension over the course of antineoplastic therapy. An important subset of new cases of hypertension will be the direct result of the therapies they receive for cancer treatment.

Advances in cancer therapy have produced a number of new strategies for treating malignancy, some with serious cardiovascular side effects. One group of new chemotherapy agents in particular, agents that inhibit the vascular endothelial growth factor (VEGF) signaling pathway, is highly associated with hypertension. However other broad categories of chemotherapy may contribute to high blood pressure as well, including immunosuppressant agents used during the course of stem cell transplant. There are also several sporadic reports of other antineoplastic medications and alternative non-pharmacological therapies associated with hypertension that will be reviewed here.

Angiogenesis Inhibitors

The classic group of medications associated with hypertension is the angiogenesis (VEGF) inhibitors. This class of agents can include tyrosine kinase inhibitors (TKI) as well as monoclonal antibodies. Angiogenesis is a biological prerequisite for benign tumors to become malignant. Within the last two decades, highly specific agents, which encompass both small molecule TKIs and monoclonal antibodies, have proven to be important inhibitors of angiogenesis. These pharmacological agents function by inhibiting the steps of the signaling pathways necessary for vascular growth, which may include vascular endothelial growth factor and/or its receptor (VEGFR), epidermal growth factor receptor (EGFR), basic fibroblast growth factor (bFGF), and platelet-derived growth factor receptor (PDGFR) [24].

Bevacizumab is a monoclonal antibody that binds to and inhibits the activity of VEGF. It has approval for treatment of multiple solid tumors and is one of the more widely used antiangiogenic therapies [25]. Bevacizumab is prototypical in this class as a medication shown to cause hypertension. Several retrospective studies have estimated a prevalence of all-grade hypertension between 4 and 35 % with its use [26–33] and a rate of CTCAE Grade 3 hypertension in 11–18 % of patients [26–29, 34]. Rarely, hypertension associated with bevacizumab can be severe enough to require hospitalization or discontinuation of therapy. There may be a dose-dependent relationship with the degree of hypertension [29]

Tyrosine kinase inhibitors were first introduced as inhibitors of highly specific signal transduction in the 1980s and 1990s [35]. Imatinib, released in 2000, was the first TKI introduced to clinical practice. Antiangiogenic TKIs may target VEGFR, EGFR, and PDGFR and have been strongly associated with hypertension. Multiple TKIs targeting angiogenesis have been developed; examples of hypertensive effects are described below.

Sunitinib is a small molecule TKI used to treat renal cell carcinoma and imatinib-resistant gastrointestinal stromal tumor (GIST). It is a potent inhibitor of VEGFR-1, VEGFR-2, and PDGFR. In the initial Phase I and II clinical trials, it was associated with an overall rate of hypertension of 17 %, and at least one patient developed Grade 4 hypertension [36, 37]. Other rarely observed cardiovascular complications included myocardial infarction and impaired systolic function. In larger Phase III clinical trials of sunitinib, a lower risk of hypertension was observed, with Grade 3 hypertension in 2–8 % of patients [37–41]. Hypertension was typically diagnosed within the first 4 weeks of therapy in this group of patients [42].

Sorafenib is a small molecule TKI also used to treat advanced renal cell carcinoma [6]. Like sunitinib, it inhibits VEGFR-2 as well as PDGFR. Initial Phase I and II clinical trials showed comparable rates of hypertension as sunitinib. The overall rate of all-grade hypertension was 17 %, with a very low rate of Grade 4 hypertension, at 1 % [6]. Across all clinical trials, the rates of all-grade hypertension observed in patients receiving sorafenib were moderate, occurring in 17–43 % of patients [6, 43–46]. Rates of Grade 3/Grade 4 hypertension were variable, occurring in 1.4–38 % of patients. A meta-analysis showed the incidence of Stage 3 or higher hypertension with sorafenib to be 2.1–30.7 % [47].

Pazopanib, a recently approved oral TKI for advanced renal cell cancer, is also associated with hypertension. One meta-analysis showed an incidence of all-grade hypertension of 35.9 %, with a rate of severe hypertension of 6.5 % [48]. Like the other VEGFR inhibitors, close monitoring is recommended for any patients initiating pazopanib therapy.

Significant work has investigated the mechanisms for hypertension when the VEGF pathway is inhibited [49]. The most likely explanation for TKI-associated hypertension is the impact on nitric oxide bioavailability. VEGF stimulates endothelial nitric oxide synthase (eNOS), increasing NO production and arterial vasodilation. Inhibition of VEGF signaling reduces eNOS activity and decreases NO levels, leading to vasoconstriction and hypertension (Fig. 5.1) [49]. Nitric oxide is a potent vasodilator, so any inhibition of its production will lead to an increase in vascular tone [50]. Increases in blood pressure have been shown to correlate with VEGFR-2 inhibition [51].

Other downstream effects of VEGF inhibition include stimulation of plasminogen activator inhibitor-1 expression and increased vascular and renal endothelin production [50, 52]. Vascular rarefaction is an additional proposed mechanism by which these angiogenesis inhibitors can cause hypertension through the loss of peripheral microvessels [53].

Fig. 5.1 Vandetanib reduced plasma nitrite levels (Adapted from Mayer et al. 2011)

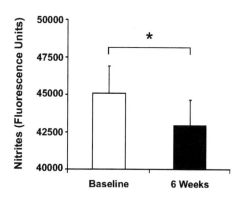

VEGF may also have a role within the renin-angiotensin system, which is a well-known regulator of blood pressure, although the evidence for this is conflicting [54, 55]. Finally, inhibition of VEGF may lead to damage of the glomerulus through cholesterol emboli syndrome or renal thrombotic microangiopathy [56, 57]. In reality, a combination of all of the above mechanisms likely contributes to hypertension in patients receiving this class of antineoplastic therapy.

Alkylating Agents

Alkylating agents were among the first antineoplastic medications associated with hypertension. One retrospective study studied the rates of cardiovascular disease in testicular cancer patients at least 10 years after receiving ifosfamide-containing chemotherapy. Their analysis showed a higher rate of hypertension (39 %) and hypercholesterolemia (79 %) compared with similar stage I controls [7]. These patients also had higher rates of coronary artery disease and diastolic dysfunction.

Another study looked at patients receiving multiple alkylating agents following bone marrow transplant and showed hypertension developing in 15 of 18 patients [58]. Busulfan, an alkylating agent used in chronic myelogenous leukemia (CML) prior to bone marrow transplant, has a reported frequency of hypertension of 36 % [3].

Taxanes

The taxane family of chemotherapy agents, including paclitaxel and docetaxel, derives from the *Taxus* genus of plants [59]. They are effective through inhibition of microtubule function and have been used since the 1990s to treat a number of solid tumors, including breast cancer, ovarian cancer, and non-small cell lung cancer [59].

When co-administered with doxorubicin, docetaxel has been shown to have a number of cardiovascular complications, including arrhythmias and hypertension, although the incidence of these findings is still rare [60]. Up to 3 % of patients receiving paclitaxel have been shown to have severe cardiovascular complications, including chest pain, cardiac arrest, supraventricular arrhythmias, and hypertension [2, 61]. The package insert for paclitaxel lists a frequency of hypertension of 1–10 % [3]. Notably, some patients have been shown to exhibit orthostatic hypotension, likely due to autonomic dysfunction [62]. These effects appear to be related to administration of the drug and typically resolve with cessation of therapy [59].

Neuroendocrine Agents

Certain types of cancers can be targeted through blockage of specific neuroendocrine pathways. Since many of these same hormones participate in blood pressure regulation, there is an association with hypertension with some of these agents.

Men receiving androgen deprivation therapy for prostate cancer are occasionally found to have worsening high blood pressure. For instance, nilutamide, an antiandrogen agent, has a reported frequency of hypertension of 1–10 % [3]. Another example is octreotide, a somatostatin inhibitor used in carcinoid disease, has a reported frequency of hypertension of 5–15 % [3]. Most of the hypertension associated with these agents is transitory and resolves with cessation of therapy.

Immunosuppression Agents

Hypertension is a well-known complication of bone marrow transplantation, especially with the introduction of cyclosporine for graft-versus-host prophylaxis [63–66].

Early clinical trials comparing cyclosporine versus methotrexate showed rates of high blood pressure of 57 % versus 4 %, respectively [63]. These rates were in stark contrast to the relatively normotensive state of most patients prior to transplant. The effect was compounded by the addition of glucocorticoids, which are commonly used during and posttransplant [63, 66].

Hypertension occurs in at least 20 % of patients receiving glucocorticoids, and the degree of high blood pressure is typically dose dependent. A dose of 80–200 mg of cortisol a day can increase systolic blood pressure by 15 mmHg [67]. The combination of steroids with natural licorice candy or even certain topical agents, include hemorrhoid creams, can potentiate this effect and lead to further hypertension [68].

Other Chemotherapy Agents

There are a number of additional chemotherapeutic agents that have been associated with observational reports of hypertension but do not fit into a single category. One review identified several drugs whose package inserts included hypertension as a known side effect [3]. These included alemtuzumab, arsenic, clofarabine, daunorubicin, gemtuzumab, goserelin, interferon, pentostatin, tretinoin, vinblastine, and vincristine [3]. The use of these agents should prompt close monitoring for rises in blood pressure.

Symptomatic Agents

While the adverse effects of antineoplastic agents are well known, one area in which toxicities may be underappreciated is those medications used to treat the complications of chemotherapy.

Several commonly used antiemetics, including metoclopramide, alizapride, and prochlorperazine, are all associated with a transient rise in blood pressure [67]. There may be a synergistic relationship between metoclopramide and cisplatin as the elevation in blood pressure was particularly profound in patients receiving both these medications [68].

Recombinant erythropoietin is an agent commonly used to treat profound anemia secondary to malignancy and antineoplastic therapy [69]. While effective at stimulating hematopoiesis, it has the side effect of hypertension. Up to 20–30 % of patients receiving erythropoietin will develop or have a worsening of high blood pressure [70]. This effect may be dose dependent and can be seen as early as 2 weeks or as late as 4 months following therapy [67]. Hypertension due to erythropoietin is not often serious, although hypertensive urgency has been reported [71].

Surgery and Irradiation

Although beyond the scope of this chapter, surgery and radiation therapy can also contribute to hypertension in the oncology patient who may receive a full range of treatment modalities in addition to pharmacotherapy.

Disruption of the patient's native baroreflex system can lead to refractory hypertension that is often difficult to manage. This can be due to direct tumor invasion of regions within the baroreflex arc, including the carotid sinus, glossopharyngeal nerve, and vagus nerve [72]. Also, surgical resection and radiation therapy to these regions can lead to refractory hypertension, especially in the setting of head and neck cancers [72, 73].

Patients with baroreflex failure often present dramatically, typically with profound hypertensive crisis with systolic blood pressures exceeding 250 mmHg or particularly volatile hypertension with wide variations in blood pressure [72]. Orthostatic tachycardia, while a common problem, is not typically due to baroreflex failure but rather neuropathic postural tachycardia syndrome [74]. Management of high blood pressure in patients with baroreflex dysfunction often requires multiple antihypertensive medications and consultation with a specialist.

A Focused Strategy for Treatment

Today's oncologist will increasingly encounter hypertension, regardless of his or her practice setting, whether ambulatory or inpatient. With the increasing ability of antineoplastic therapies to manage malignancy, the burden of cardiovascular disease, including hypertension, may continue to rise, both in patients undergoing active treatment and in cancer survivors. The mechanism by which blood pressure rises varies based on the type of antineoplastic therapy. Thus, a focused approach to the treatment of hypertension must be utilized. We will introduce a basic framework with which to approach newly diagnosed hypertension. In some cases, however, hypertension may be multifactorial, a result of prior risk factors, genetic predisposition, and the initiation of cancer therapy.

In 2010, the Cardiovascular Toxicities Panel, convened by the Angiogenesis Task Force of the National Cancer Institute Investigational Drug Steering Committee, issued a set of recommendations for the approach to patients with hypertension secondary to VEGF signaling pathway inhibitors [5]. They stopped short of making guidelines, as the quantity of evidence was limited; however, these recommendations are a useful start for the management of hypertension related to cancer therapy. While specifically written for VEGF inhibitors, these recommendations can be broadened to any oncology patient presenting with hypertension.

Before any antineoplastic therapy is initiated, a comprehensive risk assessment should be made which includes measurement of blood pressure, review of known cardiovascular risk factors, and targeted laboratory studies. While not every patient requires electrocardiographic or echocardiographic evaluation, when indicated, these studies should be performed prior to initiating therapy. Careful consideration should be made for the use of known cardiotoxic therapies in patients who already have cardiovascular disease.

Blood pressure should be actively monitored following the initiation of VEGF inhibitors, as well as other chemotherapy agents associated with hypertension. There are no established guidelines; however, biweekly blood pressure checks while receiving potentially toxic agents would be reasonable. A rise in blood pressure is typically seen within the first cycle of therapy, and the risk may be highest in those with preexisting hypertension or known risk factors. The presentation of high blood pressure can be delayed, however, so monitoring should be ongoing throughout therapy. Routine screening every 2 to 3 weeks is appropriate.

The goals for hypertension control are based on the most recent recommendations from JNC 7 [11]. Most adults should have a treatment goal of less than 140 mmHg of systolic blood pressure and 90 mmHg of diastolic blood pressure. Patients with coronary disease and/or heart failure should be targeted to a lower blood pressure and may require the assistance of a specialist [75].

When the decision to begin pharmacotherapy is made, careful consideration regarding drug choice should be made based on a number of factors. The mechanism by which chemotherapy increases blood pressure may be directly related to the mechanism of action against malignancy. Thus, when an oncologist is treating a patient with hypertension, it is important to first determine what agents may be contributing to the patient's high blood pressure.

Angiogenesis Inhibitors

As discussed above, treatment with angiogenesis inhibitors, including both bevacizumab and the VEGFR TKIs, can frequently lead to the development of hypertension. Patients receiving angiogenesis inhibitor therapy who develop hypertension may benefit from early initiation of pharmacotherapy. Clinicians should consider an ACEI or ARB as a first line of therapy, as there is some evidence that these classes of medications may be more effective than others [47, 50]. ACEI, specifically, are preferred as there are in vivo studies demonstrating a reduction in microcirculatory changes, decreased catabolism of bradykinin, and increased production of nitric oxide with ACEI exposure [30].

Selection of an antihypertensive medication also requires careful examination for drug-drug interactions. Sorafenib, for example, is metabolized by the cytochrome p450 system. Thus, non-dihydropyridine calcium channel blockers which also inhibit cytochrome p450, including diltiazem and verapamil, should not be used in combination with sorafenib [76]. It has been observed that development of hypertension with VEGF antagonist exposure may be associated with greater response from therapy; therefore, efforts should be made to continue therapy if hypertension can be controlled and an anticancer effect is observed [77]. Routine surveillance is recommended for any patient receiving anti-VEGF therapy, with blood pressure checks at least once every 2 to 3 weeks [67].

Taxanes

Both paclitaxel and docetaxel are generally well tolerated; however, toxicities can occur which include peripheral neuropathy, neutropenia, alopecia, and hypersensitivity reactions [78]. Hypertension is a rare complication, possibly related to endothelial damage during drug administration [79]. Thus, unlike other classes of chemotherapeutic agents, there is no targeted therapy for the management of blood pressure elevation. Hypertension will typically resolve with the cessation of drug; however, if symptoms persist, a general approach including CCBs, thiazide-type diuretics, ACEI, or ARB can be utilized [59].

Immunosuppression Agents

Of all the agents used in conjunction with bone marrow transplantation, perhaps the most studied and linked to high blood pressure is cyclosporine [80]. It also happens to be one of the widest studied agents for control of hypertension.

The mechanism by which cyclosporine causes hypertension is likely multifactorial and includes renal afferent vasoconstriction, stimulation of endothelin, and increase in intracellular calcium [80–82]. For these reasons, the majority of studies have examined what role calcium channel blockers may have in the amelioration of cyclosporine-induced hypertension. Some studies have suggested that the addition of verapamil improves the efficacy of immunosuppression with cyclosporine in transplant recipients [81, 82]. Thus, CCBs should be considered as a first line of therapy in patients receiving cyclosporine.

Notably, most patients with cyclosporine-induced hypertension have disturbed circadian rhythms in which the blood pressure does not exhibit typical diurnal variation with a decrease at night [83]. This is particularly problematic as the degree of end-organ damage is worsened with persistently high blood pressure.

Hypertension typically resolves after cessation of therapy, although this is not usually necessary with appropriate pharmacotherapy [84]. Other immunosuppressive agents, including tacrolimus, rapamycin, and mycophenolate mofetil, have a modest effect on blood pressure and, if appropriate, may be considered as a substitute for cyclosporine [85, 86]

Symptomatic Agents

With any of the symptomatic agents, cessation of the offending medication is typically sufficient to improve blood pressure.

In cases where therapy is indicated, such as recombinant erythropoietin, conventional antihypertensive therapy is usually effective. Risk factors associated with worsening hypertension in conjunction with erythropoietin include the presence of preexisting hypertension, a rapid increase in hematocrit, low baseline hematocrit, high doses of erythropoietin, genetic predisposition to hypertension, and younger age [87]. Phlebotomy of 500 mL of blood may be considered for those with refractory hypertension despite medical therapy [68].

A final note should be made regarding the choice of antihypertension therapy in those patients with serious comorbidities, including cardiovascular disease. For instance, although beta-blockers are not a first-line therapy in the most recent guidelines, they should be considered in patients with a history of coronary artery disease, heart failure, and myocardial infarction. Furthermore, contraindications should also be considered, including drug-drug interactions or combination ACEI/ARB therapy.

Certain populations also require particularly close attention. Patients with diabetes and chronic kidney disease should have aggressive blood pressure management, and, if refractory, selection of a chemotherapeutic agent that does not increase blood pressure should be considered. Many practitioners will target a lower blood pressure in these populations, and combination therapy is often required. Referral to a specialist may be necessary.

Conclusion

While the prevalence of hypertension has remained constant over the last 10 years, the rate of treatment continues to rise [1]. As discussed above, management of hypertension is a critical component of a comprehensive approach to the oncology patient. As cancer therapies improve, the number of long-term survivors is increasing, creating a large population at risk for cardiovascular disease [88]. The overarching goal of hypertension therapy is to reduce end-organ damage, including kidney disease, heart disease, and stroke. Thus, a proactive approach in the oncology patient must be taken, which includes careful monitoring for rises in blood pressure and focused treatment when necessary.

Contemporary cardio-oncologists must consider the patient's entire health, and not just their oncologic diagnosis, when making management decisions. This necessitates early identification and treatment of known cardiovascular risk factors, including hypertension. In those patients at the highest risk for developing hypertension, or those who already have hypertension, careful consideration should be made before starting agents that are associated with high blood pressure.

Once hypertension has been diagnosed, a rational approach should be made to guide therapy, keeping in mind the underlying mechanism of the disease and contribution from concomitant anticancer therapy. Careful consideration includes not only the choice of initial therapy but also comorbidities such as coronary artery disease, chronic kidney disease, diabetes, or heart failure. The management of patients with hypertension may follow several paths: upon recognition by an oncologist, the patient can be treated by the oncologist, may be referred to the patient's primary care physician, or may be referred to an expert in hypertension. The last option may be particularly relevant for patients who require more than monotherapy for blood pressure control.

References

1. Centers for Disease C, Prevention. Vital signs: prevalence, treatment, and control of hypertension–United States, 1999–2002 and 2005–2008. MMWR Morb Mortal Wkly Rep. 2011;60(4):103–8.
2. Solimando DA. Paclitaxel package insert. Cancer Invest. 1997;15(5):503.
3. Jain M, Townsend RR. Chemotherapy agents and hypertension: a focus on angiogenesis blockade. Curr Hypertens Rep. 2007;9(4):320–8.
4. Piccirillo JF, Tierney RM, Costas I, Grove L, Spitznagel Jr EL. Prognostic importance of comorbidity in a hospital-based cancer registry. JAMA. 2004;291(20):2441–7.
5. Maitland ML, Bakris GL, Black HR, Chen HX, Durand JB, Elliott WJ, et al. Initial assessment, surveillance, and management of blood pressure in patients receiving vascular endothelial growth factor signaling pathway inhibitors. J Natl Cancer Inst. 2010;102(9):596–604.
6. Escudier B, Eisen T, Stadler WM, Szczylik C, Oudard S, Siebels M, et al. Sorafenib in advanced clear-cell renal-cell carcinoma. N Engl J Med. 2007;356(2):125–34.

7. Meinardi MT, Gietema JA, van der Graaf WT, van Veldhuisen DJ, Runne MA, Sluiter WJ, et al. Cardiovascular morbidity in long-term survivors of metastatic testicular cancer. J Clin Oncol. 2000;18(8):1725–32.

8. Bursztyn M, Zelig O, Or R, Nagler A. Isradipine for the prevention of cyclosporine-induced hypertension in allogeneic bone marrow transplant recipients: a randomized, double-blind study. Transplantation. 1997;63(7):1034–6.

9. Yoon SS, Ostchega Y, Louis T. Recent trends in the prevalence of high blood pressure and its treatment and control, 1999–2008. NCHS Data Brief. 2010;48:1–8.

10. Cherry DK, Woodwell DA. National ambulatory medical care survey: 2000 summary. Adv Data. 2002;(328):1–32.

11. Chobanian AV, Bakris GL, Black HR, Cushman WC, Green LA, Izzo Jr JL, et al. The seventh report of the joint national committee on prevention, detection, evaluation, and treatment of high blood pressure: the JNC 7 report. JAMA. 2003;289(19):2560–72.

12. SPRINT Research Group, Wright Jr JT, Williamson JD, Whelton PK, Snyder JK, Sink KM, Rocco MV, Reboussin DM, Rahman M, Oparil S, Lewis CE, Kimmel PL, Johnson KC, Goff Jr DC, Fine LJ, Cutler JA, Cushman WC, Cheung AK, Ambrosius WT. A randomized trial of intensive versus standard blood-pressure control. N Engl J Med. 2015;373(22):2103–16.

13. National Cancer Institute (U.S.). Common terminology criteria for adverse events (CTCAE), Rev ed. Bethesda, MD: U.S. Dept. of Health and Human Services, National Institutes of Health, National Cancer Institute; 2009. 194p.

14. Neal B, MacMahon S, Chapman N, Blood Pressure Lowering Treatment Trialists C. Effects of ACE inhibitors, calcium antagonists, and other blood-pressure-lowering drugs: results of prospectively designed overviews of randomised trials. Blood Pressure Lowering Treatment Trialists' Collaboration. Lancet. 2000;356(9246):1955–64.

15. Ogden LG, He J, Lydick E, Whelton PK. Long-term absolute benefit of lowering blood pressure in hypertensive patients according to the JNC VI risk stratification. Hypertension. 2000;35(2):539–43.

16. Effects of weight loss and sodium reduction intervention on blood pressure and hypertension incidence in overweight people with high-normal blood pressure. The Trials of Hypertension Prevention, phase II. The Trials of Hypertension Prevention Collaborative Research Group. Archiv Intern Med. 1997;157(6):657–67.

17. He J, Whelton PK, Appel LJ, Charleston J, Klag MJ. Long-term effects of weight loss and dietary sodium reduction on incidence of hypertension. Hypertension. 2000;35(2):544–9.

18. Vollmer WM, Sacks FM, Ard J, Appel LJ, Bray GA, Simons-Morton DG, et al. Effects of diet and sodium intake on blood pressure: subgroup analysis of the DASH-sodium trial. Ann Intern Med. 2001;135(12):1019–28.

19. Chobanian AV, Hill M. National Heart, Lung, and Blood Institute Workshop on sodium and blood pressure : a critical review of current scientific evidence. Hypertension. 2000;35 (4):858–63.

20. Kelley GA, Kelley KS. Progressive resistance exercise and resting blood pressure: a meta-analysis of randomized controlled trials. Hypertension. 2000;35(3):838–43.

21. Whelton SP, Chin A, Xin X, He J. Effect of aerobic exercise on blood pressure: a meta-analysis of randomized, controlled trials. Ann Intern Med. 2002;136(7):493–503.

22. Xin X, He J, Frontini MG, Ogden LG, Motsamai OI, Whelton PK. Effects of alcohol reduction on blood pressure: a meta-analysis of randomized controlled trials. Hypertension. 2001;38 (5):1112–7.

23. James PA, Oparil S, Carter BL, Cushman WC, Dennison-Himmelfarb C, Handler J, et al. 2014 evidence-based guideline for the management of high blood pressure in adults: report from the panel members appointed to the Eighth Joint National Committee (JNC 8). JAMA. 2014;311 (5):507–20.

24. Folkman J. Angiogenesis: an organizing principle for drug discovery? Nat Rev Drug Discov. 2007;6(4):273–86.

25. Ferrara N, Hillan KJ, Novotny W. Bevacizumab (Avastin), a humanized anti-VEGF mono-clonal antibody for cancer therapy. Biochem Biophys Res Commun. 2005;333(2):328–35.
26. Miller K, Wang M, Gralow J, Dickler M, Cobleigh M, Perez EA, et al. Paclitaxel plus bevacizumab versus paclitaxel alone for metastatic breast cancer. N Engl J Med. 2007;357 (26):2666–76.
27. Miller KD, Chap LI, Holmes FA, Cobleigh MA, Marcom PK, Fehrenbacher L, et al. Ran-domized phase III trial of capecitabine compared with bevacizumab plus capecitabine in patients with previously treated metastatic breast cancer. J Clin Oncol. 2005;23(4):792–9.
28. Hurwitz H, Fehrenbacher L, Novotny W, Cartwright T, Hainsworth J, Heim W, et al. Bevacizumab plus irinotecan, fluorouracil, and leucovorin for metastatic colorectal cancer. N Engl J Med. 2004;350(23):2335–42.
29. Kabbinavar FF, Schulz J, McCleod M, Patel T, Hamm JT, Hecht JR, et al. Addition of bevacizumab to bolus fluorouracil and leucovorin in first-line metastatic colorectal cancer: results of a randomized phase II trial. J Clin Oncol. 2005;23(16):3697–705.
30. Pande A, Lombardo J, Spangenthal E, Javle M. Hypertension secondary to anti-angiogenic therapy: experience with bevacizumab. Anticancer Res. 2007;27(5B):3465–70.
31. Cobleigh MA, Langmuir VK, Sledge GW, Miller KD, Haney L, Novotny WF, et al. A phase I/II dose-escalation trial of bevacizumab in previously treated metastatic breast cancer. Semin Oncol. 2003;30(5 Suppl 16):117–24.
32. Johnson DH, Fehrenbacher L, Novotny WF, Herbst RS, Nemunaitis JJ, Jablons DM, et al. Randomized phase II trial comparing bevacizumab plus carboplatin and paclitaxel with carboplatin and paclitaxel alone in previously untreated locally advanced or metastatic non-small-cell lung cancer. J Clin Oncol. 2004;22(11):2184–91.
33. Yang JC, Haworth L, Sherry RM, Hwu P, Schwartzentruber DJ, Topalian SL, et al. A randomized trial of bevacizumab, an anti-vascular endothelial growth factor antibody, for metastatic renal cancer. N Engl J Med. 2003;349(5):427–34.
34. Shih T, Lindley C. Bevacizumab: an angiogenesis inhibitor for the treatment of solid malig-nancies. Clin Ther. 2006;28(11):1779–802.
35. Levitzki A. Tyrosine kinase inhibitors: views of selectivity, sensitivity, and clinical perfor-mance. Annu Rev Pharmacol Toxicol. 2013;53:161–85.
36. Fiedler W, Serve H, Dohner H, Schwittay M, Ottmann OG, O'Farrell AM, et al. A phase 1 study of SU11248 in the treatment of patients with refractory or resistant acute myeloid leukemia (AML) or not amenable to conventional therapy for the disease. Blood. 2005;105 (3):986–93.
37. Motzer RJ, Hutson TE, Tomczak P, Michaelson MD, Bukowski RM, Rixe O, et al. Sunitinib versus interferon alfa in metastatic renal-cell carcinoma. N Engl J Med. 2007;356(2):115–24.
38. Burstein HJ, Elias AD, Rugo HS, Cobleigh MA, Wolff AC, Eisenberg PD, et al. Phase II study of sunitinib malate, an oral multitargeted tyrosine kinase inhibitor, in patients with metastatic breast cancer previously treated with an anthracycline and a taxane. J Clin Oncol. 2008;26 (11):1810–6.
39. Motzer RJ, Michaelson MD, Redman BG, Hudes GR, Wilding G, Figlin RA, et al. Activity of SU11248, a multitargeted inhibitor of vascular endothelial growth factor receptor and platelet-derived growth factor receptor, in patients with metastatic renal cell carcinoma. J Clin Oncol. 2006;24(1):16–24.
40. Demetri GD, van Oosterom AT, Garrett CR, Blackstein ME, Shah MH, Verweij J, et al. Efficacy and safety of sunitinib in patients with advanced gastrointestinal stromal tumour after failure of imatinib: a randomised controlled trial. Lancet. 2006;368(9544):1329–38.
41. Motzer RJ, Rini BI, Bukowski RM, Curti BD, George DJ, Hudes GR, et al. Sunitinib in patients with metastatic renal cell carcinoma. JAMA. 2006;295(21):2516–24.
42. Chu TF, Rupnick MA, Kerkela R, Dallabrida SM, Zurakowski D, Nguyen L, et al. Cardiotoxicity associated with tyrosine kinase inhibitor sunitinib. Lancet. 2007;370 (9604):2011–9.

43. Procopio G, Verzoni E, Gevorgyan A, Mancin M, Pusceddu S, Catena L, et al. Safety and activity of sorafenib in different histotypes of advanced renal cell carcinoma. Oncology. 2007;73(3–4):204–9.

44. Furuse J, Ishii H, Nakachi K, Suzuki E, Shimizu S, Nakajima K. Phase I study of sorafenib in Japanese patients with hepatocellular carcinoma. Cancer Sci. 2008;99(1):159–65.

45. Ratain MJ, Eisen T, Stadler WM, Flaherty KT, Kaye SB, Rosner GL, et al. Phase II placebo-controlled randomized discontinuation trial of sorafenib in patients with metastatic renal cell carcinoma. J Clin Oncol. 2006;24(16):2505–12.

46. Riechelmann RP, Chin S, Wang L, Tannock IF, Berthold DR, Moore MJ, et al. Sorafenib for metastatic renal cancer: the Princess Margaret experience. Am J Clin Oncol. 2008;31 (2):182–7.

47. Wu S, Chen JJ, Kudelka A, Lu J, Zhu X. Incidence and risk of hypertension with sorafenib in patients with cancer: a systematic review and meta-analysis. Lancet Oncol. 2008;9(2):117–23.

48. Qi WX, Lin F, Sun YJ, Tang LN, He AN, Yao Y, et al. Incidence and risk of hypertension with pazopanib in patients with cancer: a meta-analysis. Cancer Chemother Pharmacol. 2013;71 (2):431–9.

49. Mayer EL, Dallabrida SM, Rupnick MA, Redline WM, Hannagan K, Ismail NS, et al. Contrary effects of the receptor tyrosine kinase inhibitor vandetanib on constitutive and flow-stimulated nitric oxide elaboration in humans. Hypertension. 2011;58(1):85–92.

50. Dincer M, Altundag K. Angiotensin-converting enzyme inhibitors for bevacizumab-induced hypertension. Ann Pharmacother. 2006;40(12):2278–9.

51. Kamba T, McDonald DM. Mechanisms of adverse effects of anti-VEGF therapy for cancer. Br J Cancer. 2007;96(12):1788–95.

52. Dhaun N, Webb DJ. Receptor tyrosine kinase inhibition, hypertension, and proteinuria: is endothelin the smoking gun? Hypertension. 2010;56(4):575–7.

53. Aparicio-Gallego G, Afonso-Afonso FJ, Leon-Mateos L, Firvida-Perez JL, Vazquez-Estevez-S, Lazaro-Quintela M, et al. Molecular basis of hypertension side effects induced by sunitinib. Anticancer Drugs. 2011;22(1):1–8.

54. Sane DC, Anton L, Brosnihan KB. Angiogenic growth factors and hypertension. Angiogenesis. 2004;7(3):193–201.

55. Veronese ML, Mosenkis A, Flaherty KT, Gallagher M, Stevenson JP, Townsend RR, et al. Mechanisms of hypertension associated with BAY 43-9006. J Clin Oncol. 2006;24(9):1363–9.

56. Mir O, Mouthon L, Alexandre J, Mallion JM, Deray G, Guillevin L, et al. Bevacizumab-induced cardiovascular events: a consequence of cholesterol emboli syndrome? J Natl Cancer Inst. 2007;99(1):85–6.

57. Eremina V, Jefferson JA, Kowalewska J, Hochster H, Haas M, Weisstuch J, et al. VEGF inhibition and renal thrombotic microangiopathy. N Engl J Med. 2008;358(11):1129–36.

58. Graves SW, Eder JP, Schryber SM, Sharma K, Brena A, Antman KH, et al. Endogenous digoxin-like immunoreactive factor and digitalis-like factor associated with the hypertension of patients receiving multiple alkylating agents as part of autologous bone marrow transplantation. Clin Sci. 1989;77(5):501–7.

59. Sereno M, Brunello A, Chiappori A, Barriuso J, Casado E, Belda C, et al. Cardiac toxicity: old and new issues in anti-cancer drugs. Clin Transl Oncol. 2008;10(1):35–46.

60. Salvatorelli E, Menna P, Cascegna S, Liberi G, Calafiore AM, Gianni L, et al. Paclitaxel and docetaxel stimulation of doxorubicinol formation in the human heart: implications for cardiotoxicity of doxorubicin-taxane chemotherapies. J Pharmacol Exp Ther. 2006;318 (1):424–33.

61. Gradishar WJ, Tjulandin S, Davidson N, Shaw H, Desai N, Bhar P, et al. Phase III trial of nanoparticle albumin-bound paclitaxel compared with polyethylated castor oil-based paclitaxel in women with breast cancer. J Clin Oncol. 2005;23(31):7794–803.

62. Jerian SM, Sarosy GA, Link Jr CJ, Fingert HJ, Reed E, Kohn EC. Incapacitating autonomic neuropathy precipitated by taxol. Gynecol Oncol. 1993;51(2):277–80.

63. Loughran Jr TP, Deeg HJ, Dahlberg S, Kennedy MS, Storb R, Thomas ED. Incidence of hypertension after marrow transplantation among 112 patients randomized to either cyclosporine or methotrexate as graft-versus-host disease prophylaxis. Br J Haematol. 1985;59 (3):547–53.
64. June CH, Thompson CB, Kennedy MS, Loughran Jr TP, Deeg HJ. Correlation of hypomagnesemia with the onset of cyclosporine-associated hypertension in marrow transplant patients. Transplantation. 1986;41(1):47–51.
65. Kone BC, Whelton A, Santos G, Saral R, Watson AJ. Hypertension and renal dysfunction in bone marrow transplant recipients. Q J Med. 1988;69(260):985–95.
66. Textor SC, Forman SJ, Bravo EL, Carlson J. De novo accelerated hypertension during sequential cyclosporine and prednisone therapy in normotensive bone marrow transplant recipients. Transplant Proc. 1988;20(3 Suppl 3):480–6.
67. Grossman E, Messerli FH. Secondary hypertension: interfering substances. J Clin Hypertens. 2008;10(7):556–66.
68. Grossman E, Messerli FH. High blood pressure. A side effect of drugs, poisons, and food. Arch Intern Med. 1995;155(5):450–60.
69. Bokemeyer C, Aapro MS, Courdi A, Foubert J, Link H, Osterborg A, et al. EORTC guidelines for the use of erythropoietic proteins in anaemic patients with cancer. Eur J Cancer. 2004;40 (15):2201–16.
70. Smith KJ, Bleyer AJ, Little WC, Sane DC. The cardiovascular effects of erythropoietin. Cardiovasc Res. 2003;59(3):538–48.
71. Novak BL, Force RW, Mumford BT, Solbrig RM. Erythropoietin-induced hypertensive urgency in a patient with chronic renal insufficiency: case report and review of the literature. Pharmacotherapy. 2003;23(2):265–9.
72. Ketch T. Four faces of baroreflex failure: hypertensive crisis, volatile hypertension, orthostatic tachycardia, and malignant vagotonia. Circulation. 2002;105(21):2518–23.
73. Shapiro MH, Ruiz-Ramon P, Fainman C, Ziegler MG. Light-headedness and defective cardiovascular reflexes after neck radiotherapy. Blood Press Monit. 1996;1(1):81–5.
74. Jacob G, Costa F, Shannon JR, Robertson RM, Wathen M, Stein M, et al. The neuropathic postural tachycardia syndrome. N Engl J Med. 2000;343(14):1008–14.
75. Rosendorff C, Lackland DT, Allison M, Aronow WS, Black HR, Blumenthal RS, et al. Treatment of hypertension in patients with coronary artery disease: a scientific statement from the American Heart Association, American College of Cardiology, and American Society of Hypertension. J Am Coll Cardiol. 2015;9(6):453–98.
76. Yeh ET, Bickford CL. Cardiovascular complications of cancer therapy: incidence, pathogenesis, diagnosis, and management. J Am Coll Cardiol. 2009;53(24):2231–47.
77. Rixe O, Billemont B, Izzedine H. Hypertension as a predictive factor of Sunitinib activity. Ann Oncol. 2007;18(6):1117.
78. Markman M. Management of toxicities associated with the administration of taxanes. Expert Opin Drug Saf. 2003;2(2):141–6.
79. Hung CH, Chan SH, Chu PM, Tsai KL. Docetaxel facilitates endothelial dysfunction through oxidative stress via modulation of protein kinase C beta: the protective effects of sotrastaurin. Toxicol Sci. 2015;145(1):59–67.
80. Porter GA, Bennett WM, Sheps SG. Cyclosporine-associated hypertension. National High Blood Pressure Education Program. Arch Intern Med. 1990;150(2):280–3.
81. Dawidson I, Rooth P, Fisher D, Fry WR, Alway C, Coorpender L, et al. Verapamil ameliorates acute cyclosporine A (CsA) nephrotoxicity and improves immunosuppression after cadaver renal transplantation. Transplant Proc. 1989;21(1 Pt 2):1511–3.
82. Textor SC, Canzanello VJ, Taler SJ, Wilson DJ, Schwartz LL, Augustine JE, et al. Cyclosporine-induced hypertension after transplantation. Mayo Clin Proc. 1994;69 (12):1182–93.
83. Cifkova R, Hallen H. Cyclosporin-induced hypertension. J Hypertens. 2001;19(12):2283–5.

84. Rodicio JL. Calcium antagonists and renal protection from cyclosporine nephrotoxicity: long-term trial in renal transplantation patients. J Cardiovasc Pharmacol. 2000;35(3 Suppl 1):S7–11.

85. Manzia TM, De Liguori CN, Orlando G, Toti L, De Luca L, D'Andria D, et al. Use of mycophenolate mofetil in liver transplantation: a literature review. Transplant Proc. 2005;37 (6):2616–7.

86. Morales JM, Andres A, Rengel M, Rodicio JL. Influence of cyclosporin, tacrolimus and rapamycin on renal function and arterial hypertension after renal transplantation. Nephrol Dial Transplant. 2001;16 Suppl 1:121–4.

87. Luft FC. Erythropoietin and arterial hypertension. Clin Nephrol. 2000;53(1 Suppl):S61–4.

88. Schultz PN, Beck ML, Stava C, Vassilopoulou-Sellin R. Health profiles in 5836 long-term cancer survivors. Int J Cancer. 2003;104(4):488–95.

Chapter 6
Preoperative and Pre-transplant Cardiac Evaluation in the Cancer Patient

Stacey Goodman, Robert Frank Cornell, Gregg F. Rosner, and Daniel S. O'Connor

Part I: Preoperative Cardiac Evaluation in the Cancer Patient

Introduction

Background

Perioperative assessment and management of cancer patients is an integral part of successful patient outcomes. There are many unique issues that arise prior to surgery in cancer patients, making clinical management complex. Cancer-related

_____

Electronic supplementary material: The online version of this chapter (doi:10.1007/978-3-319-43096-6_6) contains supplementary material, which is available to authorized users.

S. Goodman
Vanderbilt Blood Disorders, Vanderbilt University Medical Center, Nashville, TN, USA
e-mail: stacey.goodman@Vanderbilt.Edu

R.F. Cornell
Division of Hematology and Oncology, Vanderbilt University Medical Center, 777 Preston Research Building, Nashville, TN 37232, USA
e-mail: robert.f.cornell@Vanderbilt.Edu

G.F. Rosner
Cardiology & Cardiac Intensive Care, Columbia University Medical Center, Herbert Irving Pavilion - Suite 6-636, 161 Fort Washington Avenue, New York, NY 10032, USA
e-mail: gfr2107@cumc.columbia.edu

D.S. O'Connor (✉)
Division of Cardiology, Columbia College of Physicians and Surgeons, New York Presbyterian Hospital, New York, NY, USA
e-mail: dso2112@cumc.columbia.edu

processes can affect blood counts and the immune system and involve multiple organs which can impact a patient's functional status and therefore impact surgical risk and perioperative management. A timely evaluation and management strategy is also imperative as delaying surgeries or procedures can adversely affect patient prognosis.

Clinical Assessment

History

Highest yield information obtained from patient history centers around questions pertaining to active or unstable cardiac syndromes. Most important are those that include unstable angina, decompensated heart failure and critical valve disease. Functional capacity is a proven component of surgical risk assessment; however for cancer patients, functional capacity can be limited secondary to concomitant treatment (i.e., chemotherapy) or cancer burden. Therefore in this patient population, functional capacity provides only a small portion of overall surgical risk assessment.

Physical

Key components of the physical exam in the preoperative period are hemodynamic assessments (blood pressure, heart rate, and heart rhythm), volume status, and the evaluation for heart valve disease. Blood pressures should be checked in both arms from the sitting and standing positions. Peripheral pulses are manually palpated and rhythm checked by electrocardiogram. Determinants of clinical decompensated heart failure are investigated by jugular venous pressure assessment, pulmonary auscultation, liver palpation, lower extremity palpation, and cardiac auscultation for S3 gallop. Aortic valve stenosis represents the most crucial valve disease to evaluate. Cues to severity of aortic stenosis arise from quality and timing of the systolic ejection murmur, the intensity and timing of A2 component of S2.

Cardiology Consultation

Patient history and physical exam findings that are concerning for angina, clinical heart failure, or severe aortic or mitral valve stenosis indicate that the patient should be referred to a cardiologist for further evaluation. Any prior history of ventricular arrhythmias, new-onset atrial arrhythmias, or conduction defects should also prompt referral. A thorough consultative report should include an assessment of perioperative risk, a management plan to evaluate and stabilize any active cardiac conditions, and postoperative recommendations.

Cardiac Risk Indexes

The Goldman Cardiac Risk Index

The Goldman Cardiac Risk Index is an established model to determine cardiac risk in noncardiac surgery with a point-based system of nine independent variables obtained from patient cardiac history, physical exam findings, laboratory results, and type of planned surgery [1].

Revised Goldman Cardiac Risk Index

This is a simplified version of the original Goldman Cardiac Risk Index and uses six risk factors. Currently, it is the most widely used index and is incorporated in the ACC/AHA guidelines for perioperative cardiac evaluation (Table 6.1) [2].

Clinical Assessment of Risk

Active cardiac conditions that include unstable coronary syndromes, decompensated heart failure, cardiac arrhythmias, and severe valve disease should be further evaluated and managed preoperatively with treatment plans in place for the postoperative period. The ACC/AHA Task Force has developed a stepwise algorithm to frame clinical decision making in the preoperative period (Table 6.2) [3].

Cardiac Risk with Type and Timing of Surgery

The type of planned surgery is an important determinant of cardiac risk (Table 6.3). *Low-risk* procedures are those that are defined by combined surgical and patient

Table 6.1 Goldman revised cardiac risk index

Risk factor	
High risk surgery[a]	
History of heart failure	
History of cerebrovascular disease	
History of ischemic heart disease	
Preoperative creatinine >2 mg/dL	
Preoperative treatment with insulin	
# of risk factors	Event rate %
0	0.4
1	1
2	2.4
3 or more	5.4

[a]Intrathoracic, intraperitoneal, or suprainguinal vascular procedures
Event = perioperative cardiac death, nonfatal MI, or nonfatal cardiac arrest

Table 6.2 Stepwise approach to perioperative cardiac assessment for coronary artery diseases (CAD)

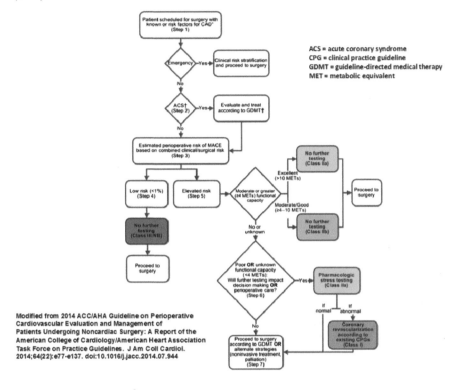

ACS = acute coronary syndrome
CPG = clinical practice guideline
GDMT = guideline-directed medical therapy
MET = metabolic equivalent

Modified from 2014 ACC/AHA Guideline on Perioperative Cardiovascular Evaluation and Management of Patients Undergoing Noncardiac Surgery: A Report of the American College of Cardiology/American Heart Association Task Force on Practice Guidelines. J Am Coll Cardiol. 2014;64(22):e77-e137. doi:10.1016/j.jacc.2014.07.944

Table 6.3 Risk estimation by procedure

A *low-risk* procedure is one in which the combined patient and surgical characteristics predict a risk of a major adverse cardiac event (MACE = death or myocardial infarction) of <1 %. Examples include: endoscopy, cataract surgery, plastic surgery, superficial skin and oral mucosa procedures, breast surgery

Procedures with a risk of MACE of ≥1 % are considered *elevated risk*

characteristics which predict the risk for a major adverse cardiac event (MACE) of death or myocardial infarction <1 %. *Elevated-risk* procedures are those whose risk for MACE is >1 %. Elevated-risk procedures can be further divided into *intermediate* and *high risk* and are usually managed similarly.

High-risk surgery includes aortic and major vascular surgery including peripheral vascular surgery and prolonged surgical procedures with large fluid shifts, blood loss, or both. Endovascular abdominal aortic aneurysm repair and carotid endarterectomy are excluded from the high-risk category and are both considered intermediate risk. Intermediate-risk and low-risk surgeries are the more common surgical occurrences when caring for cancer patients. Preoperative cardiac testing should be limited to those that affect management and reduce perioperative risk for cardiac events. An example is a preoperative echocardiogram in a patient with preoperative exam findings concerning for volume overload in order to assist perioperative fluid management and reduced risk for postoperative acute clinical heart failure.

Emergent surgery is usually defined as a treatment of a life-threatening illness and should proceed to the operating room within 6 h without delay of preoperative testing. *Urgent* surgeries typically proceed within 6–24 h and therefore allow limited time for clinical evaluation. A *time-sensitive* surgery is surgery that if delayed greater than >1–6 weeks would negatively affect patient outcomes. Most oncological procedures fall into this category. An *elective* surgery is one that can be delayed by up to a year.

Approach to Preoperative Cardiac Testing

Functional Capacity Assessment

Functional capacity is an established predictor of perioperative cardiac events, with poor functional capacity correlating to increased adverse events. Functional capacity is often defined in terms of metabolic equivalents (METS) and ranges from 1, which is defined as a resting state, to >10. Perioperative risk for cardiac events increases if an individual cannot achieve 4 METS which is defined as climbing a flight of stairs, walking up a hill, walking on level ground at >4 mph, or heavy house or yard work [4].

Preoperative Electrocardiogram

The prognostic significance of a preoperative electrocardiogram is unclear; however, it provides a baseline standard that can be compared to in the postoperative period. Timing should be approximately one to three months prior to the planned procedure. A 12-lead electrocardiogram is reasonable in patients undergoing *elevated-risk* procedures with history of coronary artery disease, arrhythmias, structural heart disease, or peripheral/neurovascular disease. There is no benefit of routine preoperative electrocardiograms in asymptomatic patients undergoing *low-risk* procedures.

Left Ventricular Function Evaluation

Reduced left ventricular function with ejection fraction <35 % correlates with a significant increase in perioperative events, particularly with risk for postoperative acute decompensated heart failure [5]. It is reasonable to evaluate left ventricular function preoperatively in patients who report dyspnea of unclear etiology or if there is evidence of clinical heart failure on preoperative examination. For patients with known left ventricular dysfunction and no assessment within the past 1 year, an echocardiogram is also reasonable prior to surgery. There is no evidence that routine echocardiogram is useful prior to surgery in other patient groups and is not recommended.

Pharmacological Stress Testing

Pharmacological stress testing may be useful in patients with poor functional capacity (<4 METS) in which clinical history and physical findings are concerning for an active or unstable coronary syndrome prior to surgery. Both dobutamine stress echocardiogram testing and pharmacological stress nuclear perfusion imaging have been studied in numerous studies prior to elevated-risk surgery; however, no randomized controlled trials exist. Regardless of the modality chosen, the presence of a moderate to large area of ischemia is associated with increased risk of perioperative myocardial infarction and/or death [6]. Evidence of prior myocardial infarct on rest imaging, however, is of little predictive value for perioperative cardiac events. A normal pharmacologic stress test has a high negative predictive value for myocardial infarction or cardiac death during the perioperative period.

Coronary Angiogram

Routine coronary angiogram is not recommended for patients undergoing elevated-risk noncardiac surgery. The indication for coronary angiogram in the preoperative period is the same as the indication in the nonoperative period, i.e., unstable and active coronary syndromes.

Coronary Revascularization

Preoperative risk stratification may lead the identification of obstructive coronary artery disease. Many factors play a role in deciding whether preoperative coronary revascularization should be performed and via which approach, i.e., surgical versus percutaneous coronary intervention (PCI). PCI should be performed in patients with high-risk coronary artery anatomy (left main disease) and prohibitive risk for surgical revascularization and those patients that have active unstable coronary syndromes and are candidates for revascularization. For patients with planned time-sensitive surgery, bare-metal stents (BMS) or balloon angioplasty is favorable. In these circumstances, preferably 4–6 weeks of aspirin and P2Y-12 platelet receptor blockers are given followed by aspirin perioperatively. If noncardiac surgery can be delayed >12 months, then drug-eluting stents (DESs) are a therapeutic option and allow 1 year of aspirin and P2Y-12 receptor blocker therapy. Some data demonstrate safety in termination of dual antiplatelet therapy with the use of newer-generation DESs at 6 months. Average recovery times for surgical revascularization need to be considered when considering preoperative surgical revascularization strategy. Currently, there are no randomized controlled trials demonstrating that coronary revascularization (either surgical or PCI) reduces hard end points of postoperative mortality or cardiac events. The Coronary Artery Revascularization Prophylaxis (CARP) trial is the largest available trial of 510 patients that were

randomized to either surgical/percutaneous revascularization or medical management with the exclusion of urgent/emergent surgery, unstable angina, left main
disease, severe left ventricular function (EF <20%), or aortic stenosis prior to
elevated high-risk vascular surgery [7]. The CARP trial demonstrated no difference
in postoperative death or myocardial infarctions at 30 days but did show that
coronary revascularization led to longer delays in patients getting their planned
surgical procedure.

Perioperative Beta-Blocker Therapy

Patients already receiving long-term beta-blocker treatment should continue in the
perioperative period; this is supported by multiple retrospective and observational
studies [8–10]. If beta-blockers are to be initiated prior to surgery, it is important to
allow sufficient time to assess patient tolerability and safety. It is our practice to
start patients on beta blockade 1 week prior to their surgery. For patients with
moderate- to high-risk myocardial ischemia on preoperative testing, it is reasonable
to start beta-blockers regardless of whether or not a coronary revascularization
approach is decided. In addition, for a patient with greater than three cardiac risk
factors of either coronary artery disease, heart failure, diabetes, chronic renal
disease, or history of cerebrovascular accident, it is reasonable to start a beta-
blocker if not previously prescribed.

Specific Disease States

Several specific disease states warrant detailed review in terms of cardiovascular
preoperative assessment.

Heart Failure

Heart failure is a very common disease which is more prevalent in the elderly.
Estimates are that >10% of patients older than 65 years of age suffer from the
condition [11]. Congestive heart failure is a clinical syndrome characterized by the
heart's inability to meet the metabolic demands of the body at normal ventricular
filling pressures. Heart failure can be classified according to the predominant
ventricle involved: left ventricular (LV), right ventricular (RV), or mixed LV/RV
failure. In LV heart failure, patients present with shortness of breath, fatigue,
exercise intolerance, and/or signs of RV failure. In RV heart failure, patients
present with lower extremity edema, early satiety, abdominal distension, fatigue,
and exercise intolerance. Heart failure can also be categorized into systolic, diastolic, or mixed systolic/diastolic. In systolic heart failure, there is evidence of
reduced LV function manifest by a reduced EF. In diastolic heart failure, the LV is
non-dilated with normal or near-normal systolic function but may shows signs of
structural changes (i.e., hypertrophy) and/or diastolic dysfunction.

Heart failure is a well-recognized risk factor for perioperative morbidity and
mortality [1, 12]. The single most important piece of information to be obtained

Table 6.4 New York Heart Association (NYHA) functional classification

Class	Symptoms
I (Minimal)	No symptoms and no limitation in ordinary physical activity
II (Mild)	No symptoms at rest. Mild symptoms and slight limitation during ordinary activity
III (Marked)	Marked limitation in activity due to symptoms, even during less than ordinary activity. Comfortable only at rest
IV (Severe)	Severe limitations. Experiences symptoms even while at rest

Symptoms include: fatigue, shortness of breath, angina, palpitations

from a patient with a history of heart failure is their preoperative symptom complex. Using the standard New York Heart Association scale (Table 6.4) for symptoms, patient's status and risk can be determined. The higher the NYHA class, the higher the risk for perioperative complications.

Transthoracic echocardiography (TTE) is the single most important diagnostic tool used preoperatively to assess patients with known or suspected heart failure. Parameters which can be determined on TTE include LV size, wall thickness, LVEF, right and left atrial size, and RV size and function, as well as assessment for any significant valvular lesions. Additional information which can be obtained on a standard 2D TTE include diastolic function, estimated central venous pressure, and estimated pulmonary artery systolic pressures (PASP). It is our practice to obtain a preoperative TTE in all patients with a history of HF undergoing elevated-risk noncardiac surgery.

In addition to TTE, there is significant literature to support the use of perioperative levels of natriuretic peptides (BNP or NTproBNP) in the risk stratification of heart failure patients undergoing noncardiac surgery [13]. Elevated natriuretic peptide levels are strongly correlated to perioperative morbidity and mortality.

All patients with HF who are scheduled to undergo elective noncardiac surgery should be "optimized" from a medical standpoint. This includes diuresis to achieve a euvolemic volume status, stable heart rates, and adequate blood pressures with optimal end-organ perfusion. Patients should be instructed to continue their HF medications (beta-blockers, ACE inhibitors/angiotensin receptor blockers, aldosterone antagonists, diuretics) until the day of surgery. In patients with heart failure, judicious use of fluids in the perioperative period is required to avoid issues of volume overload and pulmonary edema. In patients with advanced heart failure, it is reasonable to have a cardiac anesthesiologist (if available) to perform anesthesia for the case using invasive monitoring with pulmonary artery catheter and/or transesophageal echocardiogram as needed. In all patients, HF medications should be reinstituted postoperatively as soon as clinically indicated.

Valvular Heart Disease

Patients with significant valvular heart disease (VHD) are at increased risk of perioperative morbidity and mortality [1, 12]. The risk is dependent upon the type and severity of VHD and the nature of the procedure being performed.

As with HF, a comprehensive history and physical exam (looking for overt signs/symptoms of HF or angina) is the first step in assessing a patient with VHD. The NYHA HF scale is a useful tool to determine a patient's functional status. TTE should be performed in any patient with known or suspected VHD. A high index of suspicion for VHD should be present in any patient with a history of cardiac murmur.

Aortic stenosis (AS) is the most common VHD particularly among the elderly [14]. AS causes a fixed obstruction at the aortic valve level resulting in pressure overload of the left ventricle resulting in concentric hypertrophy of the LV. Valvular AS has several causes including congenital, rheumatic, bicuspid, and calcific (senile). In the USA, severe AS in the elderly (>70 years of age) is most commonly related to calcific degeneration, while severe AS in younger patients (50–70) is typically related to the bicuspid aortic valve (1–2 % of the general population). Severe aortic stenosis is defined as an aortic valve area (AVA) <1 cm^2, Vmax >4 m/s, and/or a mean aortic valve gradient >40 mmHg [15].

In patients with severe AS, determination of symptoms directly attributable to the valve is critical. Cardinal symptoms of AS include angina, HF, and syncope. In patients with severe symptomatic AS who are scheduled for elective surgery, serious consideration must be made to intervening upon the AV prior to noncardiac surgery to lower the risk of perioperative complications. There are essentially three different interventions that can be performed in a patient with severe symptomatic AS: balloon valvuloplasty (BAV), percutaneous valve replacement (TAVR), or surgical valve replacement (SAVR). Balloon valvuloplasty is used as a bridging strategy aimed at temporarily improving hemodynamics by reducing the severity of AS. A successful BAV results in a 50 % improvement in AVA and a 50 % reduction in pressure gradients [16]. Risks of BAV include stroke (up to 10 % of patients), acute aortic regurgitation, and vascular access site complications [17]. BAV is not an effective long-term therapy for severe AS, as 50% of patients will have restenosis of the AV within 6 months [18]. TAVR is a newer procedure that has a proven mortality benefit in inoperable patients with severe AS and is an attractive alternative for high-risk patients with severe AS [19]. The recovery from TAVR is significantly shorter than with SAVR, which can require 2–3 months for an elderly patient to return to their baseline. Uncomplicated TAVR patients are typically discharged from the hospital within 2–3 days and are back to their baseline with 2–3 weeks post-procedure.

In patients with severe asymptomatic AS, the decision to intervene upon the AV prior to elective surgery is more difficult and requires a case-by-case analysis. The absence of symptoms should be confirmed with exercise stress testing. In those patients with severe symptomatic AS who must undergo an urgent or emergent noncardiac surgery, if BAV is not available, invasive hemodynamic monitoring, avoidance of rapid volume shifts/loads, careful administration of vasodilators, and maintenance of normal sinus rhythm are all essential.

Mitral stenosis (MS) secondary to rheumatic heart disease was once the most common form of VHD worldwide and is still the leading cause of VHD in developing nations [20]. With the introduction of rapid screening for strep infections and prompt antibiotic treatment, the incidence of rheumatic fever and its sequelae is now exceedingly rare in the USA except for in patients who have emigrated from endemic areas [21]. MS can also occur secondary to congenital malformation, prior mitral valve surgery (including repaired and replaced valves), and from systemic diseases which can cause valvular fibrosis (e.g., carcinoid, lupus, rheumatoid arthritis). The normal mitral valve has an orifice which is 4–5 cm^2. As the mitral orifice narrows, a pressure gradient between the left atrium (LA) and LV develops. This pressure gradient is added to the LV diastolic pressure causing an increase in the LA pressure which leads to LA dilatation, elevated pulmonary arterial pressures, and pulmonary congestion. As the severity of MS progresses, LV diastolic filling is impaired, ultimately resulting in reduced cardiac output. Symptoms of severe MS mimic symptoms of combined LV systolic/diastolic HF. Severe MS is defined as an MV area (MVA) <1.5 cm^2 which corresponds to a transmitral gradient of >5–10 mmHg at a normal heart rate [15]. In general, noncardiac surgery can be performed safely in patients with MS with an MVA >1.5 cm^2 and in asymptomatic patients with severe MS and estimated PASP <50 mmHg. As with asymptomatic AS, if feasible, the absence of symptoms should be confirmed with exercise stress testing. In asymptomatic patients with severe MS and estimated PASP >50 mmHg and in symptomatic patients with severe MS, the risk of perioperative morbidity and/or mortality is significantly increased, and consideration for mitral valve intervention (either percutaneous BAV or open surgical repair) must be entertained. Medical management of all patients with significant MS includes optimization of volume status, avoidance of volume shifts/loads, and maintenance of normal sinus rhythm with a slow heart rate to allow for diastolic filling.

In general, nonsignificant regurgitant valvular disease (aortic insufficiency or mitral regurgitation) is well tolerated and does not increase the risk of perioperative complications as the LV is conditioned to tolerate typical volume shifts associated with perioperative care. Patients with severe asymptomatic regurgitant valvular disease (aortic insufficiency or mitral regurgitation) and preserved LVEF can safely be sent to the operating room for noncardiac surgery. For patients with severe asymptomatic regurgitant valvular disease and reduced LVEF ($<30\%$) or for those patients with severe symptomatic regurgitant valvular disease, there is an increased risk of cardiac complications, and management must be tailored based upon a risk-benefit analysis for the proposed noncardiac procedure [22]. If a patient requires noncardiac surgery, pharmacologic optimization (with the use of diuretics and afterload-reducing agents) prior to the OR can lower the cardiac risk.

In patients with a history of prosthetic valve replacement or repair, there is no additional risk for noncardiac surgery provided there is no evidence of valvular and/or ventricular dysfunction. The major risk associated with a history of valve replacement comes from the perioperative management of anticoagulation (discussed separately below) in patients who are chronically anticoagulated.

Antithrombotic Therapy

Management of antithrombotic (antiplatelet ± anticoagulation) therapy in patients undergoing noncardiac surgery is a common situation facing clinicians. Physicians must decide upon the safety of interruption of antithrombotic therapy, optimal timing of preoperative cessation and postoperative resumption of these medications, as well as bridging strategy (if any). Safety of interruption of antiplatelet therapy hinges upon the indication for antiplatelet therapy (recent coronary stenting vs. primary risk reduction in an asymptomatic patient with coronary artery disease) and the type of procedure being planned. Procedural risk is determined by the anatomic site and propensity for bleeding (Table 6.5). Similarly, the approach to anticoagulation is determined by both the indication for anticoagulation (low-risk atrial fibrillation vs. mechanical heart valves/rheumatic heart disease/recent venous thromboembolism) and type of procedure being planned.

Antiplatelet agents include aspirin, nonsteroidal anti-inflammatory drugs, platelet P2Y12 receptor inhibitors including thienopyridines (clopidogrel, prasugrel) and the cyclopentyltriazolopyrimidine (ticagrelor), phosphodiesterase inhibitors (dipyridamole, cilostazol), and glycoprotein IIb/IIIa receptor inhibitors (abciximab,

Table 6.5 Procedural risk according to anatomic site, severity of tissue trauma and the risk of peri-procedural bleeding

Minimal procedures (little tissue trauma)
Superficial skin and oral mucosal surgery, including skin biopsies
Wound revisions
Non-extraction dental treatment
Minor procedures (little tissue trauma, but relevant bleeding risk)
Transluminal cardiac, arterial, and venous interventions
Pacemaker-related surgery
Pleura and ascites puncture
Cataract surgery
Arthoscopy, endoscopy, laparoscopy
Organ biopsies
Dental extraction
Hernia repair
Intramuscular and paravertebral injections
Major procedures (relevant tissue trauma and high bleeding risk)
Open pelvic, abdominal and thoracic surgery
Brain surgery
Major orthopaedic and trauma surgery
Vascular surgery

Adapted from: J. Beyer-Westendorf, V. Gelbricht, K. Forster, et al., "Peri-interventional management of novel oral anticoagulants in daily care: results from the prospective Dresden NOAC registry," *European Heart Journal*, 2014

eptifibatide, tirofiban). Platelets have a 10-day life span in the blood. As such the entire platelet pool can be regenerated after 10 days. Aspirin, prasugrel, and ticagrelor are all inhibitors of platelets. Aspirin and prasugrel are both irreversible inhibitors of platelet function, while ticagrelor is a potent reversible inhibitor of platelet function.

In patients (excluding those with a history of coronary stents or recent acute coronary syndrome) who are taking aspirin monotherapy for cardiovascular risk reduction, we recommend that aspirin be held for 5–7 days prior to noncardiac/ vascular surgery. Aspirin should be resumed postoperatively once the patient is tolerating oral intake and the risk of major surgical bleeding has passed. This recommendation is based largely upon the results of the POISE 2 trial [23]. Briefly, in POISE 2, investigators used a 2×2 factorial design that compared clonidine to placebo and aspirin to placebo in 10,010 patients who were undergoing noncardiac surgery (excluding carotid endarterectomy, retinal surgery, or intracranial surgery) and were at risk for vascular complications. Patients were stratified according to whether they had been taking aspirin (continuation stratum; $n = 4382$) or not (starting stratum; $n = 5628$) prior to the study. Patients in the initiation stratum started taking aspirin (at a dose of 200 mg) or placebo just before surgery and continued it daily (at a dose of 100 mg) for 30 days in the initiation stratum and for 7 days in the continuation stratum; after which, patients resumed their regular aspirin dosing. The primary outcome of death or nonfatal myocardial infarction (MI) at 30 days was similar in both the aspirin and placebo group (7.0 vs. 7.1%, respectively; hazard ratio [HR] 0.99, 95% CI, 0.86–1.15). As expected, major bleeding was more common in the aspirin group (4.6 vs. 3.8%; HR 1.23, 95% CI, 1.01–1.49).

The approach to perioperative management of antiplatelet therapy in patients with prior percutaneous coronary intervention (PCI) with stenting warrants specific discussion (Table 6.6). Each year, approximately 500,000 patients in the USA undergo cardiac stent implantation [24]. It has been estimated that up to 10% of patients with coronary stents undergo noncardiac surgery within a year of stent implantation [25]. Following coronary stent implantation, patients are given aspirin and a second antiplatelet agent (clopidogrel, prasugrel, or ticagrelor). This is termed dual antiplatelet therapy (DAPT). The concern over premature cessation of DAPT following coronary stenting is in-stent thrombosis (acute occlusion of the stent). In-stent thrombosis is a condition that carries a high degree of morbidity and mortality. The highest risk for stent thrombosis following either bare-metal stent (BMS) or drug-eluting stent (DES) is in the first 4–6 weeks after stent implantation [26]. Discontinuation of DAPT during this high-risk period is a strong risk factor for in-stent thrombosis. The "recommended" waiting time prior to proceeding with noncardiac surgery is typically 2–4 weeks following balloon angioplasty (PCI without stent implantation), 4–6 weeks following BMS, and 12 months following DES. In those patients who require noncardiac surgery within the recommended waiting time, strong consideration should be given for continuation of DAPT whenever feasible. If the risk of bleeding with DAPT is considered prohibitive, every attempt possible should be made to continue aspirin throughout the operative

Table 6.6 Perioperative management of antiplatelet therapy in patients post percutaneous coronary intervention

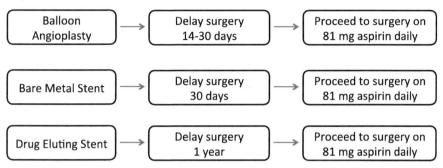

For patients who require non-cardiac surgery within the "optimal" time frame that requires dual antiplatelet therapy (DAPT) and cannot be delayed, strong consideration should be given to continuation of DAPT. If the risk of bleeding on DAPT outweighs the benefit, aspirin monotherapy should be continued unless there is a compelling contraindication (ie. neurosurgery). DAPT should be resumed as soon as surgically safe – typically within 24 hours of the procedure.

period. Once the surgical risk of bleeding has stabilized, the second antiplatelet agent should be resumed. It is critical to note that the recommended time frames for DAPT following coronary stenting are somewhat arbitrary (e.g., in Europe, there are certain DESs which have a recommended DAPT time frame of only 3 months compared to 12 months recommended by the FDA for the same stent) and are based on expert opinions, and thus decisions regarding perioperative management of DAPT must be individualized on a case-by-case basis. With current third-generation DES, our practice is to avoid discontinuing DAPT prior to 6 months post-implantation whenever feasible. To date, there is a lack of evidence to support "bridging" a patient with anticoagulation or IV glycoprotein IIb/IIIa inhibitor following discontinuation of DAPT prior to surgery. The specific antiplatelet management strategy should be communicated and discussed among the cardiologist, surgeon, anesthesiologist, and patient.

Anticoagulants include warfarin, heparin (unfractionated or low-molecular-weight), fondaparinux, direct thrombin inhibitors (recombinant hirudins, bivalirudin, argatroban, dabigatran), and direct Xa inhibitors (rivaroxaban, apixaban, edoxaban). It has been estimated that over 6 million Americans are on chronic anticoagulation for prevention of thromboembolism for atrial fibrillation (AF), mechanical heart valve, or treatment of a thromboembolic disorder. The risks of bleeding for any procedure must be weighed against the benefit of remaining on anticoagulation on a case-by-case basis.

The first step is to determine the risk of thromboembolic event during the period when anticoagulation is to be held. For patients with atrial fibrillation, the daily risk associated with cessation of anticoagulation is extrapolated from yearly risks outside of the surgical period. Two commonly used risk prediction calculators are the CHADS2 and CHA2DS2-VASc score, which can be used to estimate the yearly

Table 6.7 CHADS2 and CHA2DS2-VASc

Risk factor	CHADS2	CHA2DS2-VASc
Congestive heart failure/LV dysfunction	1	1
Hypertension	1	1
Age > 75	1	2
Diabetes	1	1
Stroke/TIA/thromboembolism	2	2
Vascular disease	–	1
Age 65–74	–	1
Sex category (female)	–	1
Maximum Score	6	9

Table 6.8 Estimated yearly risk of stroke

	Patients ($n = 1733$)	Stroke rate (%)/year
CHADS2 score		
0	120	1.9
1	463	2.8
2	523	4
3	337	5.9
4	220	8.5
5	65	12.5
6	5	18.2
CHA2DS2-VASc score		
0	1	0
1	422	1.3
2	1230	2.2
3	1730	3.2
4	1718	4
5	1159	6.7
6	679	9.8
7	294	9.6
8	82	6.7
9	14	15.2

risk of stroke in patients with non-valvular AF (AF in the absence of rheumatic mitral stenosis, a mechanical or bioprosthetic heart valve, or mitral valve repair) [27, 28] (Table 6.7). In both of these scoring systems, the higher the total score, the greater the yearly risk of stroke (Table 6.8).

In patients with mechanical heart valves, the risk of thromboembolism is determined by the type, number, and location of mechanical valves as well as the presence or absence of any additional risk factors (i.e., heart failure, prior stroke, AF) [29] (Table 6.9). In general, mechanical valves in the mitral position portend a higher risk of embolism compared to the aortic position.

Table 6.9 Risk estimation for thromboembolic event in patients with a mechanical heart value

Low Risk
Bileaflet aortic-valve prosthesis without any concomitant risk factors[a]
High Risk
Any prosthesis in the mitral position
Prosthetic valve in the presence of 1 or more risk factors[a]
Caged-ball or tilting-disk aortic valve prosthesis
Double mechanical valve

[a]Risk factors: atrial fibrillation, LV ejection fraction ≤35%, left atrial dilation (diameter ≥50 mm), previous thromboembolism, spontaneous echocardiographic contrast, or hypercoagulable condition

Table 6.10 Risk Estimation for Thromboembolic Event in Patients with a History of Venous Thromboembolism (VTE)

Low annual risk (<5%)
Provoked VTE >12 months prior
Moderate annual risk (5–10%)
Provoked VTE within 3–12 months
Heterozygote for factor V Leiden or prothrombin mutation
Recurrent VTE
High annual risk (>10%)
VTE within the prior 3 months
Unprovoked VTE
Active cancer
Protein C, Protein S or anti-thrombin deficiency
Homozygote for factor V Leiden or prothrombin mutation
Anti-phospholipid antibody

Adapted from: T. Baron, P. Kamath, and R. McBane. "Management of Antithrombotic Therapy in Patients Undergoing Invasive Procedures," *N Engl J Med* 2013;368:2113–24

In patients with a history of thromboembolic disease, the risk of recurrent thromboembolism is determined by how recently a clinical event occurred and whether or not the thromboembolism was "provoked" [30] (Table 6.10). The risk of recurrent thromboembolism is greatest within 3 months of a blood clot, and the risk rises in cases of idiopathic thromboembolism. In patients with a history of provoked thromboembolism, risk of recurrence diminishes greatly once the underlying risk factor is corrected.

Cancer patients represent a group with elevated risk for thromboembolism during the perioperative period. Several factors are thought to elevate the risk of clot including prothrombotic activity, cancer therapies (hormonal, radiation, angiogenesis inhibitors), and decreased mobility, as well as the presence of an indwelling central venous catheter (i.e., Mediport) which is common in cancer patients. Many cancer patients are also at increased risk of bleeding due to cancer or treatment-related thrombocytopenia, chemo-related hepatic and renal dysfunction, and tumor friability.

After the risk of thromboembolic event during the period when anticoagulation is to be held is determined, the second step for peri-procedural management of anticoagulation is to determine the risk of bleeding due to the planned procedure. As stated previously, procedural risk is determined by the anatomic site and propensity for bleeding (Table 6.5).

In patients at low risk for thromboembolism undergoing high-risk surgery or patients at high risk for thromboembolism undergoing low-risk procedures, the management is relatively straightforward. The number of days prior to surgery that anticoagulation must be held is determined principally by two factors: the pharmacokinetics of the specific anticoagulant and the patient's renal function (Table 6.11).

Patients at highest risk for a thromboembolic complication due to cessation of anticoagulation can be "bridged" with an alternative anticoagulant with rapid onset

Table 6.11 Overview of anticoagulants

Agent	Administration	Dosing	Mechanism of action	When to discontinue preoperatively
Heparin	IV or Subcutaneous	PTT-based or fixed dose	Antithrombin activation	IV—2–6 h SC—12–24 h
Warfarin	Oral	Per INR	Inhibition of vitamin K-dependent factors	1–5 days (typically 3 days)
Enoxaparin	Subcutaneous	Weight-based	Antithrombin activation	1 day (CrCl 30–90) 2 days (CrCl < 30)
Dalteparin	Subcutaneous	Weight-based	Antithrombin activation	1 day (CrCl 30–90) 2 days (CrCl < 30)
Fondaparinux	Subcutaneous	Fixed dose	Factor Xa inhibitor	1 day (CrCl > 90) 2 days (CrCl 50–90) 3 days (CrCl < 50)
Dabigatran	Oral	Fixed dose	Direct thrombin inhibitor	1–2 days (CrCl > 50) 3–5 days (CrCl < 50)
Rivaroxaban	Oral	Fixed dose	Direct factor Xa inhibitor	1 day (CrCl > 90) 3 days (CrCl 30–90) 5 days (CrCl < 30)
Apixiban	Oral	Fixed dose	Direct factor Xa inhibitor	1–2 days (CrCl > 60) 3 days (Cr Cl 50–59) 5 days (Cr Cl < 50)
Edoxaban	Oral	Fixed dose	Direct factor Xa inhibitor	1 day

Table 6.12 General approach to bridging therapy

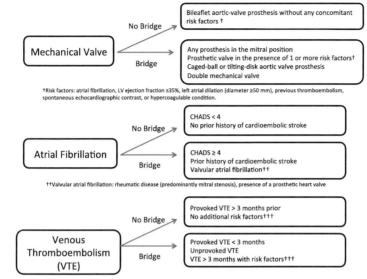

†Risk factors: atrial fibrillation, LV ejection fraction ≤35%, left atrial dilation (diameter ≥50 mm), previous thromboembolism, spontaneous echocardiographic contrast, or hypercoagulable condition.

††Valvular atrial fibrillation: rheumatic disease (predominantly mitral stenosis), presence of a prosthetic heart valve

†††Risk factors: Protein C, Protein S or anti-thrombin deficiency, factor V Leiden or prothrombin mutation, Anti-phospholipid antibody, Active Cancer

and shorter duration of action to minimize time without anticoagulation (Table 6.12). It is important to note that despite this common practice, there is a lack of clear data showing a reduction in adverse events associated with a bridging strategy. Common approaches for bridging include stopping Coumadin 5 days prior to a planned procedure and bringing the patient into the hospital (when the INR is <2) to initiate an unfractionated heparin drip until the time of surgery. Alternatively, for those patients able to inject themselves (or have somebody else inject them), LMWH can be used allowing the patient to be bridged in the outpatient setting. The bridging agent is stopped prior to the procedure, with the timing based on whether unfractionated heparin or LMWH is used, and is usually resumed within 48 h after the procedure, once hemostasis is secured.

An additional consideration is duration of action and reversibility of the anticoagulant. In cases where urgent or emergent surgery is a distinct possibility, Coumadin or LMWH may be preferred over the longer-acting novel oral anticoagulants (NOACs).

Cardiovascular Implantable Electronic Device

The number of patients with a cardiovascular implantable electronic device (CIED) continues to rise. Perioperative management requires a rudimentary understanding of these devices and forethought for their management. There are two categories of CIED: (1) implantable cardioverter-defibrillator (ICD) and (2) pacemaker (PM).

All ICDs can also function as a PM; however, isolated PMs do not have ICD capabilities. The main concern in the perioperative management of CIEDs is the potential for "cross-talk" or interference between the CIED and electromagnetic interference (EMI), typically from electrocautery (monopolar >>> bipolar) [31].

In patients who are PM dependent, EMI can result in temporary inhibition of PM function leaving a patient vulnerable for asystole. In patients who have an ICD, EMI can lead to inappropriate shocks. Prior to elective surgery, reprogramming of the CIED should be performed to render a PM or ICD "OR ready." In patients who are PM dependent, this involves reprogramming the PM into an asynchronous mode (VOO or DOO). A PM in an asynchronous mode paces at a set rate which limits the ability of the PM to misinterpret EMI. Reprogramming of ICDs involves temporarily inhibiting all tachyarrhythmia therapy. This will prevent any ICD shock from occurring in the OR.

All patients with CIEDs should have continuous monitoring of the heart rhythm throughout the perioperative period. In those cases where ICD function has been inhibited, an external defibrillator should be readily available should a life-threatening arrhythmias arise. The CIED setting should be returned to its preoperative state as soon as possible to prevent accidentally discharging a patient with an inappropriate CIED setting. In emergency cases where the CIED cannot be reprogrammed, placement of a magnet over the CIED generator will cause a PM to switch to an asynchronous mode and will inhibit ICD shocks.

Congenital Heart Disease

Congenital heart disease (CHD) covers a wide spectrum of heart defects ranging from small defects which are inconsequential and cause no hemodynamic effect to more severe forms which are incompatible with life if not for various interventions. As our ability to treat these more serious forms of CHD continues to progress, the number of adult survivors of complex CHD rises. The risk that CHD imposes upon an individual undergoing noncardiac surgery is dependent entirely upon the nature of the CHD lesion and its resultant morbidities. Severe CHD is manifest by HF, arrhythmia, pulmonary hypertension, and/or systemic deoxygenation. For all but the most basic CHD lesions, we recommend patients undergoing elective noncardiac surgery be evaluated in a center with expertise in the care of the CHD patient.

Part II: Cardiac Evaluation in Stem Cell Transplantation

Introduction

Cardiovascular complications pose a significant challenge in patients that undergo hematopoietic stem cell transplantation (HSCT). In a retrospective single institution analysis of 2821 patients, Murdych et al. reported that 26 patients (0.9%) developed early cardiotoxicity in the first 100 days following HSCT [32]. Analysis of long-term (2 or more years post-transplant) survivors revealed that 5.6–13.1% of patient deaths were attributed to cardiotoxicity following autologous or allogeneic HSCT [33, 34]. Furthermore, arterial vascular events (i.e., cerebrovascular, coronary artery, and/or peripheral artery) were found to affect as many as 22% of long-term survivors that had undergone HSCT [35].

Over the past decade, the chemotherapy and/or radiation regimens given to patients pre-HSCT have become less myelosuppressive (i.e., reduced intensity or non-ablative) and more immunosuppressive. Reduced-intensity chemotherapy regimens decrease the risk of organ toxicity. Consequently, organ function eligibility criteria for HSCT have become less stringent. Enhanced immunosuppressive therapies have allowed for use of partial HLA-matched stem cell donors. Partial HLA-matched donors and alternative stem cell sources, such as umbilical cord blood and haploidentical donors, have greatly expanded the potential of HSCT. The use of post-HSCT cyclophosphamide for haploidentical HSCT has resulted in low rates of transplant-related mortality and reduced incidence of acute and chronic GVHD [36]. These changes have led to a broader use of HSCT in patients of advanced age and those with advanced disease that have undergone multiple lines of standard-dose chemotherapy. In addition, patients with nonmalignant diseases such as sickle cell and autoimmune disease are now candidates for HSCT. As the eligible patient population becomes more diverse and as HSCT technology advances, new guidelines are necessary to identify patients that exhibit high risk for cardiac and cardiovascular complications. Careful pre-HSCT screening and post-HSCT monitoring may reduce the incidence of cardiovascular events and improve outcomes.

Cardiovascular Stress Associated with HSCT

The cardiovascular system may be exposed to a number of stressors during HSCT, requiring enhanced function, or cardiac reserve. Changes in volume status, with shifts both up and down, may occur as a result of chemotherapy infusion, stem cell mobilization and isolation, stem cell infusion, hematopoietic cell reconstitution, gastrointestinal loss, or insensible loss due to fever. Prior to red blood cell reconstitution, patients are anemic and require increased cardiac output. During periods of pancytopenia and neutropenia, patients are susceptible to infections and life-threatening sepsis, which may lead to severe vasodilation and left ventricular dysfunction [37, 38]. Furthermore, pre-HSCT therapies (i.e., anthracyclines and radiation therapy) can be directly cytotoxic to the heart, affecting organ function [39–41].

Risk Factors for Early Cardiovascular Complications Following HSCT

Cardiovascular complications that occur early, within 100 days, after transplant are usually attributed to the condition of the patient prior to transplant and cardiac comorbidity, the patient's primary diagnosis and history of disease (Table 6.13), and transplant-related factors including mobilization, conditioning, and transplant complications [42].

Pre-transplant Cardiovascular Comorbidities

Pre-existing cardiovascular comorbidities should be considered in determining HSCT eligibility. An HSCT-specific comorbidity index (Table 6.14), developed by Sorror et al. in 2005, was shown to be useful in predicting non-relapse mortality and overall survival following allogeneic transplant [43]. This index includes arrhythmia, coronary artery disease, congestive heart failure, myocardial infarction, decreased ejection fraction, heart valve disease, and cerebrovascular disease as significant risk factors for non-relapse mortality in HSCT.

Risk Factors Related to the Primary Disease

Several autoimmune conditions may predispose HSCT patients to cardiac risk. In patients with *systemic sclerosis*, pulmonary hypertension is evident in 7–12% of patients, and 10% display diastolic dysfunction [44–46]. In early HSCT studies in

Table 6.13 Cardiovascular risk factors in patients undergoing HSCT

Clinical indication for HSCT	Cardiovascular concern

Autoimmune conditions:
    Systemic lupus erythematosus
    Dermatomyositis
    Polymyositis
    Systemic sclerosis
	PHT, PC, VD, CAD, CD, AR
	PHT, MCD
	PHT, MCD
	PCT, DD

Sickle cell disease	PHT, LD, RF
Thalassemia	MCD, AR, PHT, SCT
Amyloidosis	MCD, CHF, CAD, VD, AR

Cancer patients:
    Anthracycline therapy
    Mediastinal or chest radiation
	DSLV, CHF
	PC, MF, CAD, VD, CD

PHT pulmonary hypertension, *PC* pericarditis, *MCD* myocardial disease, *PC* pericarditis, *VD* valvular disease, *CAD* coronary artery disease, *CD* conduction disturbance, *AR* arrhythmia, *DD* diastolic dysfunction, *LD* lung disease, *RF* respiratory failure, *SCT* sudden cardiac tamponade, *CHF* congestive heart failure, *DSLV* decreased systolic left ventricular function, *MF* myocardial fibrosis

Table 6.14 Hematopoietic cell transplant comorbidity index

Comorbidity	Score	Comorbidity	Score

Arrhythmia
  Atrial fibrillation
  Atrial flutter
  Supraventricular tachycardia
  Sick sinus syndrome
  Heart block
  Ventricular arrhythmia
	1	Rheumatologic
		  Systemic lupus erythematosus
		  Rheumatoid arthritis
		  Polymyositis
		  Mixed connective tissue disease
		  Polymyalgia rheumatica
			2

Cardiovascular
  Coronary artery disease
  Congestive heart failure
  Ejection fraction ($\leq$50)
  Shortening fraction ($\leq$26)
	1	Infection
		  Documented infection
		  Fever of unknown origin
		  Pulmonary nodules (pneumonia)
		  PPD positive (tuberculosis)
			1

Inflammatory bowel disease
  Crohn's disease
  Ulcerative colitis
	1	Peptic ulcer
		  Gastric
		  Duodenal
			2

Diabetes
  Diabetes
  Steroid-induced
hyperglycemia
	1	Renal
		  Serum creatinine
		  Current dialysis
		  Prior renal transplantation
			2

Cerebrovascular disease
  Transient ischemic attack
  Subarachnoid hemorrhage
  Cerebral thrombosis
  Cerebral embolism
  Cerebral hemorrhage
	1	Pulmonary
		  Diffusion capacity of carbon mon-
		oxide
		  Forced expiratory volume
		  Shortness of breath (active)
		  Shortness of breath (resting)
		  Oxygen supplementation
			2–3

Hepatic Comorbidity
  Bilirubin
  Aspartate transaminase
  Alanine transaminase
  Hepatitis B
  Hepatitis C
  Liver cirrhosis
	1–3	Heart valve disease
		  Valve stenosis
		  Valve insufficiency
		  Prosthetic valve
		  Symptomatic mitral valve prolapse
			3

Psychiatric disturbance
  Depression
  Anxiety
	1	Prior solid tumor	3

		Age 40 or older	1
		Obesity (BMI)	1

This summary was generated from the HCT Comorbidity Index Calculator (http://www.hctci.org/)

patients with sclerosis, a 17% mortality rate was reported, and death was attributed, in subset of cases, to advanced pulmonary and cardiac fibrosis [45, 47]. Pulmonary hypertension and myocardial disease have been reported in patients with *dermatomyositis* and *polymyositis*, and these conditions have been associated with cardiac mortality in HSCT [48, 49]. Pericarditis, valvular disease, conduction disease and arrhythmias, coronary artery disease, pulmonary arterial hypertension, and myocarditis have been reported in patients with *systemic lupus erythematosus* (SLE) [49–52]. Of note, cardiac symptoms have been shown to stabilize or improve following successful HSCT in association with SLE remission, suggesting that the benefits of transplant outweigh the risks [53].

Sickle cell disease, especially in cases with recurrent vaso-occlusive crises in the lungs, can result in restrictive and obstructive lung disease and respiratory failure [54]. Hypertension also occurs in 30% of these patients [55, 56]. Such patients require a thorough evaluation before HSCT.

Thalassemia patients may be at higher risk for cardiac complications in HSCT. Chronic intravascular hemolysis and regular red blood cell transfusions can lead to iron deposition within the myocardium, particularly in patients who are poorly compliant with chelation treatment. This can lead to restrictive or dilated cardiomyopathy and cardiac arrhythmias. Chronic hemolysis, a high-output state, tissue hypoxia, and the procoagulant effects of splenectomy may also lead to pulmonary hypertension in these patients [57]. Patients that present with extensive damage to the liver due to high levels of iron fare poorly after allogeneic HSCT [32, 58]. Sudden cardiac tamponade occurred in 8 of 400 patients with thalassemia either during pre-transplant conditioning or within 1 month following the transplant, leading to death in 6 patients [59].

Amyloidosis commonly involves protein deposition and accumulation in the heart, leading to cardiomyopathy, congestive heart failure, coronary heart disease, valvular heart disease, or arrhythmia [60]. Historically, transplant-related mortality (TRM) rates of 15–43% have been reported in patients with amyloid light chain (AL) amyloidosis [61, 62]. Patients with amyloidosis represent a high-risk population for cardiac complications following HSCT. More recent data incorporating better selection criteria and more modern transplant practices have resulted in a reduction in TRM. D'Souza et al. compared mortality rates in patients that underwent autotransplant in 1995–2000, 2001–2006, or 2007–2012 and found that rates fell from 11–20% to 5–11% and 2–5%, while 5-year survival rates increased from 55 to 61% and 77%, respectively [63]. Two additional studies revealed 3-year survival rates as high as 83 and 88% [64, 65]. To aid in determining patients at high risk for cardiac complications, the Mayo cardiac staging system is used, which classifies patients into stages I–IV based on elevations in the cardiac biomarkers troponin T (cTnT) and N-terminal pro-B-type brain natriuretic peptide (NTproBNP) and the difference between serum levels of involved and uninvolved light chain (FLC-diff) [66]. In patients with advanced amyloid-associated cardiomyopathy for which HSCT is not feasible, orthotopic heart transplantation may be used prior to HSCT with success [67].

Transplant-Related Risk Factors

Peri-transplant Cardiovascular Risks

Cardiovascular-related deaths in a subset of high-risk sclerosis and amyloidosis patients occurred during stem cell mobilization or infusion [59, 68]. High-dose cyclophosphamide, which is commonly used as a mobilizing agent in autologous

HSCT, can be cardiotoxic. Acute toxicity, ranging from electrocardiographic changes to severe pericarditis and myocarditis, was reported in 17–28% of patients following cyclophosphamide conditioning for HSCT [69, 70]. Early post-transplant infections are common in HSCT prior to neutrophil recovery. Endocarditis, involving valves in the left side of the heart, occurs rarely after HSCT but has been associated with high mortality [71]. In severe cases of infection, sepsis may lead to organ failure syndrome with cardiopulmonary decompensation [42].

Cardiac Graft-Versus-Host Disease (GVHD)

Although rare, the heart may be a target of GVHD following allogeneic HSCT [72–79]. Cardiac GVHD is diagnosed by histological evidence of lymphocytic infiltration, when a biopsy is feasible, or responsiveness to immunosuppressive treatments. Coronary artery vessel involvement and myocardial infarction, bradycardia, cardiomyolysis, third-degree atrioventricular block, pericardial effusion, and acute heart failure have been associated with cardiac GVHD. While the cardiac GVHD is most common within 100 days after HCT, cardiac effects can manifest later (e.g., 20 months post-transplant) in cases of chronic GVHD [78]. In two case reports, cardiac GVHD was fatal [73, 74]. A more recent retrospective analysis of 205 HSCT patients found that nine patients (4.4 %) developed pericardial effusions between 18 and 210 days post-transplant [76]. Seven of the nine patients received an allogeneic transplant and developed acute or advanced GVHD. Although cardiac GVHD was not confirmed in these patients, this study suggests that GVHD is associated with cardiac complications.

Risk Factors for Late Cardiovascular Complications Following HSCT

Cardiovascular complications that are delayed (i.e., 3 months to 2 years) or occur late (i.e., 2 years to decades) after transplant have been associated with the conditioning regimen, previous cardiotoxic chemotherapy or mediastinal radiation therapy, chronic GVHD and its treatment, and pre-transplant comorbidities [42, 80].

Cardiotoxic Therapies Prior to HSCT

Anthracyclines, a class of cell cycle-nonspecific drugs commonly used in cancer chemotherapy (e.g., doxorubicin, daunorubicin, and mitoxantrone), are known to cause cardiotoxicity [40, 41]. Increasing doses of anthracycline have been associated with a decrease in systolic left ventricular function and an increased incidence of congestive heart failure (Table 6.13) [41, 81]. Of note, cardiac function may be compromised immediately, within the first year or as late as 10–20 years after anthracycline treatment [82, 83].

Previous mediastinal or chest radiation in young patients with Hodgkin's lymphoma and early-stage breast cancer can lead to pericarditis, myocardial fibrosis, coronary artery disease, valvular abnormalities, and conduction disturbances (Table 6.13) [40]. Cardiovascular disease is the leading cause of non-relapse morbidity and mortality in long-term survivors of Hodgkin's lymphoma. The incidence of congestive heart failure in survivors of Hodgkin's lymphoma after mediastinal radiotherapy and anthracyclines was 7.9 %, and the risk of cardiovascular disease was increased threefold to fivefold over that of the general population [84].

Hydroxychloroquine, which is commonly used in the long-term treatment of malaria, SLE, and rheumatoid arthritis, has been associated with cardiac toxicities, including conduction disorders, restrictive cardiomyopathy, and arterial ventricular block [85]. There are no studies to date that have investigated the contribution of hydroxychloroquine in HSCT-associated cardiac risk. We suggest that a history of prolonged hydroxychloroquine therapy may increase the risk of cardiac complications, especially in patients with SLE where underlying cardiac dysfunction may be exacerbated, and should be considered when determining HSCT eligibility and monitoring strategy.

Allogeneic HSCT and Chronic GVHD

In a retrospective analysis of 265 long-term survivors that had undergone HSCT, 22 % of patients had experienced a cardiovascular event (e.g., cerebrovascular disease, coronary artery disease, or peripheral artery disease) [35]. Cardiovascular risk was higher in patients that underwent an allogeneic HSCT (6.8 %) compared to those that received an autologous HSCT (2.1 %). It has been proposed that persistent vascular inflammation and endothelial cell death in the context of GVHD may elicit atherosclerosis, putting long-term survivors of HSCT with GVHD at a higher risk for cardiovascular events [42]. Although acute and/or chronic GVHD was evident in 14 of the 18 allogeneic HSCT recipients that developed a cardiovascular event, no statistically significant correlation was found between GVHD and cardiovascular disease.[11] Of note, endothelial cell damage is known to occur during the first 21 days after both autologous and allogeneic HSCT and, in combination with other cardiovascular risk factors, could contribute to the development of late cardiovascular complications [86–88].

Metabolic Syndrome and Cardiovascular Risk

Metabolic syndrome, the development of obesity, insulin resistance, glucose intolerance, dyslipidemia, and hypertension, is growing in both the general population and in HSCT survivors and is associated with a higher risk for type 2 diabetes and cardiovascular disease [89, 90]. HSCT patients were shown to have a higher incidence of hyperinsulinemia, impaired glucose tolerance, hypertriglyceridemia, low HDL cholesterol, and abdominal obesity compared to non-HSCT patients or healthy controls [91]. More recently, HSCT survivors were found to have a higher risk for diabetes and hypertension compared to sibling controls [92]. Another large study surveyed HSCT survivors compared to normal controls, using the National Health and Nutrition Examination Survey, and found higher rates of cardiomyopathy (4.0 % vs. 2.6 %), stroke (4.8 % vs. 3.3 %), dyslipidemia (33.9 % vs. 22.3 %), and diabetes (14.3 vs. 11.7), but not hypertension, in HSCT survivors [93]. Obesity and poor diet were associated with a higher risk of dyslipidemia and diabetes, suggesting that lifestyle is an important factor in cardiovascular risk after HSCT. Patients that adhered to the recommended lifestyle choices had a reduced risk for cardiovascular events after HSCT [93]. Of note, the presence of at least two cardiovascular risk factors (i.e., hypertension, diabetes, dyslipidemia, obesity) has been associated with an increased risk of cardiovascular events following HSCT [35].

Advanced Age

The age of a patient at the time of HSCT has been associated with morbidity and mortality. Specifically, in patients receiving allogeneic HSCT for chronic myeloid leukemia between 1989 and 1997, patients 40 years of age or older had a higher risk of transplant-related death compared to patients 20–40 or less than 20 years of age [94]. A more recent study of patients that underwent allogeneic HSCT for acute myeloid leukemia, acute lymphocytic leukemia, or myelodysplastic syndromes between 1997 and 2005 found that patients 40 years of age or older had a significantly higher risk of mortality (hazard ratio = 1.8; $p = 0.001$) [95]. Tichelli et al. specifically investigated the role of age in cardiovascular complications (i.e., cerebrovascular disease, coronary heart disease, and peripheral arterial disease) following HSCT and found that the cumulative incidences after 20 years of follow-up were 8.7%, 20.2%, and 50.1% in patients 20, 20–40, and 40–60 years of age at the time of transplant, respectively [35].

Prevention, Monitoring, and Treatment of Cardiovascular Complications with HSCT

Pre-transplant Evaluation

Judicious patient selection is crucial in prevention of cardiovascular events following HSCT. Prior to HSCT, all patients should undergo a full clinical examination, including evaluation of recent chest pain, dyspnea, heart palpitations, and syncope. A history of cardiovascular disease, cardiovascular events and risk factors (i.e., familial risk, hypertension, diabetes, lifestyle), and exposure to cardiotoxic therapies (e.g., cyclophosphamide, anthracyclines, radiation) should be obtained. Cardiac function should be assessed by chest X-ray, electrocardiogram (ECG), and echocardiogram (ECHO). Cardiac risk can be determined by the presence of cardiomyopathy, heart failure, coronary artery disease, hypertension, arrhythmia/syncope, and QTc prolongation (>500 ms) [96].

Evaluation of High-Risk Patients

High-risk patients with evident cardiac abnormalities or a history of cardiovascular events require consultation with a cardiology or cardio-oncology specialist and further testing (i.e., NTproBNP, ECHO, 24-h Holter monitoring, and/or exercise stress test) before proceeding with HSCT (Fig. 6.1). In addition to direct cardiovascular screening, patients with an underlying disease that poses enhanced cardiovascular risk should undergo testing to determine the severity of their disease. Renal function should be assessed, including glomerular filtration rate, in patients with systemic sclerosis, lupus, or amyloidosis [48]. International guidelines advise exclusion of high-risk patients with systemic sclerosis that display elevated pulmonary artery pressure (>50 mmHg), exhibit advanced myocardial disease (>50% reduction in ventricular ejection fraction and/or uncontrolled dysrhythmias), or suffer from lung disease or gastrointestinal involvement [47]. Patients with amyloidosis are eligible if they maintain a cardiac ejection fraction of 40% or higher and show no symptoms of pleural effusion, heart failure, treatment-resistant dysrhythmias, or elevated blood pressure (≥90 mmHg diastolic) [97]. Iron overload should be evaluated in patients with thalassemia and sickle cell anemia. These patients can develop hemochromatosis from their underlying condition or from a multitude of red cell transfusions over many years. The initial evaluations for iron overload include serum or plasma ferritin and transferrin saturation. A noninvasive T2* liver MRI may confirm the initial findings [98, 99]. A cardiac T2* by MRI <20 ms is consistent with cardiac iron overload. If further confirmation is necessary, a liver biopsy should be performed. Hepatic iron levels >2 mg/g are consistent with iron overload [100].

Pre-transplant Cardiac Intervention

In patients for whom HSCT is essential for a chance of survival, the benefits of transplant may outweigh the cardiac risk. For example, for a patient with high-risk acute myeloid leukemia that has achieved remission, the only hope for cure is an allogeneic HSCT. If the cardiac risk was considered manageable, the patient would proceed with the transplant. In contrast, other patients may be advised to postpone HSCT and placed on a regimen to reduce existing cardiovascular risk factors. For example, a patient with multiple myeloma that is undergoing autologous HSCT as part of a salvage therapy could be medically managed to optimize cardiac function

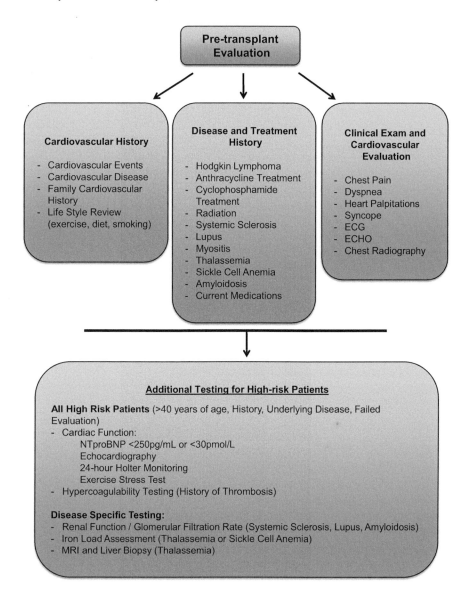

Fig. 6.1 Proposed algorithm for pre-HSCT cardiac assessment

prior to transplant. Medical modification of cardiovascular risks (i.e., diabetes mellitus, hypertension, hyperlipidemia, smoking), reduced EF, or arrhythmias should be carried out under the direction of a cardiologist or cardio-oncologist using standard practices. Patients requiring coronary angioplasty prior to transplant should be given a bare-metal stent and dual antiplatelet therapy for 30 days prior to transplant [101].

Preventative Measures

A number of guidelines have been proposed to prevent cardiovascular events in high-risk patients that are deemed eligible for HSCT. During stem cell mobilization for autologous HSCT in patients with amyloidosis, granulocyte colony-stimulating factor (G-CSF) should be used alone if possible, to avoid the cytotoxic effect of cyclophosphamide. Similarly, reduced-intensity conditioning (e.g., melphalan only) is preferred in these high-risk patients [62]. Patients that have thalassemia or have undergone multiple transfusions should be monitored and treated for iron overload (i.e., >7 mg/g dry weight in the liver or >1000–2000 ug/L serum ferritin) by regular phlebotomy or chelation therapy to reduce iron deposition in the myocardium [102]. Long-term cancer survivors (i.e., Hodgkin's lymphoma and breast cancer) that develop valvular disease following radiation should be treated prophylactically to prevent endocarditis [103].

Monitoring of Pre-transplant and Peri-transplant Complications

All patients should be monitored carefully with particular attention paid to fluid balance during mobilization, conditioning, and stem cell infusion processed. Many commonly used drugs, including *antiemetics* and *antimicrobials,* can prolong the QT interval, increasing the risk of tachyarrhythmias and sudden death [104]. A careful review of the patient's medications and potential drug interactions is critical throughout the HSCT process. Alternative agents with less effect on QT should be considered in patients with borderline or prolonged QT. However if this is not possible, an ECG should be repeated within 1 week. In some cases, patients require a high-dose cyclophosphamide-containing regimen for conditioning and closer monitoring of ECG and brain natriuretic peptide (BNP) should be considered [80]. BNP is released from the ventricles in response to cardiac stress, and levels of BNP in the plasma are inversely related to cardiac function. Increased plasma BNP levels were found to correlate with impaired left ventricular function in patients that underwent HSCT [105]. Peripheral increases were evident days to weeks prior to clinical manifestation, suggesting that BNP levels may have prognostic value for cardiac events in patients undergoing HSCT. In support of this hypothesis, BNP levels were an indicator of myocardial dysfunction in patients with amyloidosis [106]. Patients that develop GVHD following HSCT should be monitored for the development of dysrhythmia and pericardial effusion [42].

Monitoring and Detection of Late Complications

Guidelines have been proposed for screening and prevention in long-term survivors after HSCT [42, 80, 107]. All patients undergoing HSCT should be monitored annually to assess their history of cardiovascular disease and to discuss any lifestyle changes since their last visit. A full clinical evaluation should be performed to address their compliance with any ongoing cardiovascular therapy and to uncover any new cardiovascular risk factors (e.g., dyslipidemia). Patients in the high-risk category may require exercise tolerance testing, echocardiography, 24-h electro-cardiogram, and radiological and echocardiographic assessment of vascular disease. Ten years of annual follow-up is recommended for autologous HSCT, but assessment may continue in patients that warrant longer follow-up based on age, clinical complaints, and history. Allogeneic HSCT patients should continue life-long annual screening, including clinical assessment and screening for preexisting cardiovascular risk factors. Patients with thalassemia should be assessed for iron overload at least one year after HSCT, until transfusions are no longer necessary.

Therapeutic Intervention Following HSCT

The incidence of congestive heart failure associated with anthracycline toxicity may be reduced following HSCT with angiotensin-converting enzyme (ACE) inhibitors, which reduce left ventricular end-systolic wall stress [108]. While the long-term efficacy of ACE inhibitors is controversial, these initial findings warrant further investigation [109, 110]. In patients with unexplained dysrhythmias, coronary heart disease, or polyserositis following HSCT, GVHD should be considered as a possible cause. These patients should undergo a GVHD evaluation in a subspecialty clinic, preferably a long-term follow-up HSCT clinic. If GVHD is confirmed, standard treatment for GVHD should be initiated with careful monitoring by the treating physician and cardiologist or cardio-oncologist. Finally, effective management of existing cardiovascular conditions, such as arterial hypertension, diabetes, and dyslipidemia, is essential in reducing the comorbidity-associated risk of cardiovascular complications after HSCT. Lifestyle risk factors (i.e., diet, sedentary lifestyle, and smoking) should be discussed, and healthy choices should be encouraged to reduce cardiovascular risk in long-term survivors [42, 107].

References

1. Goldman L, Caldera DL, Nussbaum SR, et al. Multifactorial index of cardiac risk in noncardiac surgical procedures. N Engl J Med. 1977;297:845–50.
2. Lee TH, Marcantonio ER, Mangione CM, et al. Derivation and prospective validation of a simple index for prediction of cardiac risk of major noncardiac surgery. Circulation. 1999;100(10):1043–9.
3. Fleisher LA, Fleischman KE, Auerbach AD, et al. 2014 ACC/AHA guideline on preoperative cardiac evaluation and management of patients undergoing noncardiac surgery. J Am Coll Cardiol. 2014;64(22):e77–137.
4. Girish M, Trayner Jr E, Dammann O, et al. Symptom-limited stair climbing as a predictor of postoperative cardiopulmonary complications after high-risk surgery. Chest. 2001;120 (4):1147.

5. Xu-Cai YO, Brotman DJ, Philips CO, et al. Outcomes of patients with stable heart failure undergoing elective noncardiac surgery. Mayo Clin Proc. 2008;83:280–8.
6. Brown KA, Rowen M. Extent of jeopardized myocardium determined by myocardial perfusion imaging best predicts perioperative cardiac events in patients undergoing noncardiac surgery. J Am Coll Cardiol. 1993;21:325–30.
7. McFalls MO, et al. Coronary-artery revascularization before elective major vascular surgery. N Engl J Med. 2004;351:2795–804.
8. Devereaux PJ, Yang H, Guyatt GH, et al. Rationale, design, and organization of the PeriOperative Ischemic Evaluation (POISE) trial: a randomized controlled trial of metoprolol versus placebo in patients undergoing noncardiac surgery. Am Heart J. 2006;152:223–30.
9. Lindenauer PK, Pekow P, Wang K, et al. Perioperative beta-blocker therapy and mortality after major noncardiac surgery. N Engl J Med. 2005;353:349–61.
10. Shammash JB, Trost JC, Gold JM, et al. Perioperative beta-blocker withdrawal and mortality in vascular surgical patients. Am Heart J. 2001;141:148–53.
11. Viana de Freitas E, Batlouni M, Gamarsky R. Heart failure in the elderly. J Geriatr Cardiol. 2012;9:101–7.
12. Detsky AS, Abrams HB, McLaughlin JR, et al. Predicting cardiac complications in patients undergoing non-cardiac surgery. J Gen Intern Med. 1986;1:211–9.
13. Karthikeyan G, Moncur RA, Levine O, et al. Is a pre-operative brain natriuretic peptide or N-terminal pro–B-type natriuretic peptide measurement an independent predictor of adverse cardiovascular outcomes within 30 days of noncardiac surgery? A systematic review and meta-analysis of observational studies. J Am Coll Cardiol. 2009;54:1599–606.
14. Eveborn GW, Schirmer H, Heggelund G, et al. The evolving epidemiology of valvular aortic stenosis. the Tromsøstudy. Heart. 2013;99:396–400.
15. Nishimura RA, Otto CM, Bonow RO, et al. 2014 ACC/AHA guideline for the management of patients with valvular heart disease. Circulation. 2014;129:2440–92.
16. Desnoyers MR, Isner JM, Pandian NG, et al. Clinical and noninvasive hemodynamic results after aortic balloon valvuloplasty for aortic stenosis. Am J Cardiol. 1988;62:1078–84.
17. Badheka AO, Patel NJ, Singh V, et al. Percutaneous aortic balloon valvotomy in the United States: a 13-year perspective. Am J Med. 2014;127:744–53.
18. Lieberman EB, Bashore TM, Hermiller JB, et al. Balloon aortic valvuloplasty in adults: failure of procedure to improve long-term survival. J Am Coll Cardiol. 1995;26:1522–8.
19. Leon MB, Smith CR, Mack M, et al. Transcatheter aortic-valve implantation for aortic stenosis in patients who cannot undergo surgery. N Engl J Med. 2010;363:1597–607.
20. Seckeler MD, Hoke TR. The worldwide epidemiology of acute rheumatic fever and rheumatic heart disease. Clin Epidemiol. 2011;3:67–84.
21. Shulman ST, Stollerman G, Beall B, et al. Temporal changes in streptococcal m protein types and the near-disappearance of acute rheumatic fever in the United States. Clin Infect Dis. 2006;42:441–7.
22. Lai HC, Lai HC, Lee WL, Wang KY, et al. Mitral regurgitation complicates postoperative outcome of noncardiac surgery. Am Heart J. 2007;153:712–7.
23. Devereaux PJ, Mrkobrada M, Sessler DI, et al. Aspirin in patients undergoing noncardiac surgery. N Engl J Med. 2014;370:1494–503.
24. National Hospital Discharge Survey: 2010 table, Procedures by selected patient characteristics—number by procedure category and age. 30 June 2015. Available from: http://www.cdc.gov/nchs/fastats/inpatient-surgery.htm.
25. Hawn MT, Graham L, Richman J, et al. The incidence and timing of noncardiac surgery after cardiac stent implantation. J Am Coll Cardiol. 2012;214:658–66.
26. Kałuza GL, Joseph J, Lee JR, Raizner ME, et al. Catastrophic outcomes of noncardiac surgery soon after coronary stenting. J Am Coll Cardiol. 2000;35:1288–94.
27. Gage BF, Waterman AD, Shannon W, et al. Validation of clinical classification schemes for predicting stroke: results from the National Registry of Atrial Fibrillation. JAMA. 2001;285:2864–70.

28. Lip GY, Nieuwlaat R, Pisters R, et al. Refining clinical risk stratification for predicting stroke and thromboembolism in atrial fibrillation using a novel risk factor-based approach: the Euro Heart Survey on atrial fibrillation. Chest. 2010;137:263–72.
29. Ruel M, Masters RG, Rubens FD, et al. Late incidence and determinants of stroke after aortic and mitral valve replacement. Ann Thorac Surg. 2004;78:77–83.
30. Kearon C, Akl EA, Comerota AJ, et al. Antithrombotic therapy for VTE disease: Antithrombotic Therapy and Prevention of Thrombosis, 9th ed: American College of Chest Physicians Evidence-Based Clinical Practice Guidelines. Chest. 2012;141:e419S–94.
31. Crossley GH, Poole JE, Rozner MA, et al. The Heart Rhythm Society (HRS)/American Society of Anesthesiologists (ASA) Expert Consensus Statement on the perioperative management of patients with implantable defibrillators, pacemakers and arrhythmia monitors: facilities and patient management this document was developed as a joint project with the American Society of Anesthesiologists (ASA), and in collaboration with the American Heart Association (AHA), and the Society of Thoracic Surgeons (STS). Heart Rhythm. 2011;8:1114–54.
32. Murdych T, Weisdorf DJ. Serious cardiac complications during bone marrow transplantation at the University of Minnesota, 1977–1997. Bone Marrow Transplant. 2001;28:283–7.
33. Bhatia S, Robison LL, Francisco L, Carter A, Liu Y, Grant M, et al. Late mortality in survivors of autologous hematopoietic-cell transplantation: report from the Bone Marrow Transplant Survivor Study. Blood. 2005;105:4215–22.
34. Bhatia S, Francisco L, Carter A, Sun CL, Baker KS, Gurney JG, et al. Late mortality after allogeneic hematopoietic cell transplantation and functional status of long-term survivors: report from the Bone Marrow Transplant Survivor Study. Blood. 2007;110:3784–92.
35. Tichelli A, Bucher C, Rovo A, Stussi G, Stern M, Paulussen M, et al. Premature cardiovascular disease after allogeneic hematopoietic stem-cell transplantation. Blood. 2007;110:3463–71.
36. Brunstein CG, Fuchs EJ, Carter SL, Karanes C, Costa LJ, Wu J, et al. Alternative donor transplantation after reduced intensity conditioning: results of parallel phase 2 trials using partially HLA-mismatched related bone marrow or unrelated double umbilical cord blood grafts. Blood. 2011;118:282–8.
37. Artucio H, Digenio A, Pereyra M. Left ventricular function during sepsis. Crit Care Med. 1989;17:323–7.
38. Glauser MP, Zanetti G, Baumgartner JD, Cohen J. Septic shock: pathogenesis. Lancet. 1991;338:732–6.
39. Carver JR, Shapiro CL, Ng A, Jacobs L, Schwartz C, Virgo KS, et al. American Society of Clinical Oncology clinical evidence review on the ongoing care of adult cancer survivors: cardiac and pulmonary late effects. J Clin Oncol. 2007;25:3991–4008.
40. Curigliano G, Cardinale D, Suter T, Plataniotis G, de Azambuja E, Sandri MT, et al. Cardiovascular toxicity induced by chemotherapy, targeted agents and radiotherapy: ESMO Clinical Practice Guidelines. Ann Oncol. 2012;23 Suppl 7:vii155–66.
41. Lefrak EA, Pitha J, Rosenheim S, Gottlieb JA. A clinicopathologic analysis of adriamycin cardiotoxicity. Cancer. 1973;32:302–14.
42. Tichelli A, Bhatia S, Socie G. Cardiac and cardiovascular consequences after haematopoietic stem cell transplantation. Br J Haematol. 2008;142:11–26.
43. Sorror ML, Maris MB, Storb R, Baron F, Sandmaier BM, Maloney DG, et al. Hematopoietic cell transplantation (HCT)-specific comorbidity index: a new tool for risk assessment before allogeneic HCT. Blood. 2005;106:2912–9.
44. Mukerjee D, St George D, Coleiro B, Knight C, Denton CP, Davar J, et al. Prevalence and outcome in systemic sclerosis associated pulmonary arterial hypertension: application of a registry approach. Ann Rheum Dis. 2003;62:1088–93.
45. Rosen O, Massenkeil G, Hiepe F, Pest S, Hauptmann S, Radtke H, et al. Cardiac death after autologous stem cell transplantation (ASCT) for treatment of systemic sclerosis (SSc): no

evidence for cyclophosphamide-induced cardiomyopathy. Bone Marrow Transplant. 2001;27:657–8.

46. Tyndall A, Passweg J, Gratwohl A. Haemopoietic stem cell transplantation in the treatment of severe autoimmune diseases 2000. Ann Rheum Dis. 2001;60:702–7.

47. Binks M, Passweg JR, Furst D, McSweeney P, Sullivan K, Besenthal C, et al. Phase I/II trial of autologous stem cell transplantation in systemic sclerosis: procedure related mortality and impact on skin disease. Ann Rheum Dis. 2001;60:577–84.

48. Saccardi R, Tyndall A, Coghlan G, Denton C, Edan G, Emdin M, et al. Consensus statement concerning cardiotoxicity occurring during haematopoietic stem cell transplantation in the treatment of autoimmune diseases, with special reference to systemic sclerosis and multiple sclerosis. Bone Marrow Transplant. 2004;34:877–81.

49. Yoshida S, Katayama M. Pulmonary hypertension in patients with connective tissue diseases. Nihon Rinsho. 2001;59:1164–7.

50. Law WG, Thong BY, Lian TY, Kong KO, Chng HH. Acute lupus myocarditis: clinical features and outcome of an oriental case series. Lupus. 2005;14:827–31.

51. Mandell BF. Cardiovascular involvement in systemic lupus erythematosus. Semin Arthritis Rheum. 1987;17:126–41.

52. Winslow TM, Ossipov MA, Fazio GP, Simonson JS, Redberg RF, Schiller NB. Five-year follow-up study of the prevalence and progression of pulmonary hypertension in systemic lupus erythematosus. Am Heart J. 1995;129:510–5.

53. Loh Y, Oyama Y, Statkute L, Traynor A, Satkus J, Quigley K, et al. Autologous hematopoietic stem cell transplantation in systemic lupus erythematosus patients with cardiac dysfunction: feasibility and reversibility of ventricular and valvular dysfunction with transplant-induced remission. Bone Marrow Transplant. 2007;40:47–53.

54. Santoli F, Zerah F, Vasile N, Bachir D, Galacteros F, Atlan G. Pulmonary function in sickle cell disease with or without acute chest syndrome. Eur Respir J. 1998;12:1124–9.

55. Ataga KI, Sood N, De Gent G, Kelly E, Henderson AG, Jones S, et al. Pulmonary hypertension in sickle cell disease. Am J Med. 2004;117:665–9.

56. Gladwin MT, Sachdev V, Jison ML, Shizukuda Y, Plehn JF, Minter K, et al. Pulmonary hypertension as a risk factor for death in patients with sickle cell disease. N Engl J Med. 2004;350:886–95.

57. Coghlan JG, Handler CE, Kottaridis PD. Cardiac assessment of patients for haematopoietic stem cell transplantation. Best Pract Res Clin Haematol. 2007;20:247–63.

58. Lucarelli G, Galimberti M, Polchi P, Angelucci E, Baronciani D, Giardini C, et al. Bone marrow transplantation in patients with thalassemia. N Engl J Med. 1990;322:417–21.

59. Angelucci E, Mariotti E, Lucarelli G, Baronciani D, Cesaroni P, Durazzi SM, et al. Sudden cardiac tamponade after chemotherapy for marrow transplantation in thalassaemia. Lancet. 1992;339:287–9.

60. Kholova I, Niessen HW. Amyloid in the cardiovascular system: a review. J Clin Pathol. 2005;58:125–33.

61. Moreau P, Leblond V, Bourquelot P, Facon T, Huynh A, Caillot D, et al. Prognostic factors for survival and response after high-dose therapy and autologous stem cell transplantation in systemic AL amyloidosis: a report on 21 patients. Br J Haematol. 1998;101:766–9.

62. Sanchorawala V, Wright DG, Seldin DC, Dember LM, Finn K, Falk RH, et al. An overview of the use of high-dose melphalan with autologous stem cell transplantation for the treatment of AL amyloidosis. Bone Marrow Transplant. 2001;28:637–42.

63. D'Souza A, Dispenzieri A, Wirk B, Zhang MJ, Huang J, Gertz MA, et al. Improved outcomes after autologous hematopoietic cell transplantation for light chain amyloidosis: a center for international blood and marrow transplant research study. J Clin Oncol. 2015.

64. Girnius S, Seldin DC, Meier-Ewert HK, Sloan JM, Quillen K, Ruberg FL, et al. Safety and efficacy of high-dose melphalan and auto-SCT in patients with AL amyloidosis and cardiac involvement. Bone Marrow Transplant. 2014;49:434–9.

65. Kongtim P, Qazilbash MH, Shah JJ, Hamdi A, Shah N, Bashir Q, et al. High-dose therapy with auto-SCT is feasible in high-risk cardiac amyloidosis. Bone Marrow Transplant. 2015;50:668–72.
66. Kumar S, Dispenzieri A, Lacy MQ, Hayman SR, Buadi FK, Colby C, et al. Revised prognostic staging system for light chain amyloidosis incorporating cardiac biomarkers and serum free light chain measurements. J Clin Oncol. 2012;30:989–95.
67. Davis MK, Kale P, Liedtke M, Schrier S, Arai S, Wheeler M, et al. Outcomes after heart transplantation for amyloid cardiomyopathy in the modern era. Am J Transplant. 2015;15:650–8.
68. Saba N, Sutton D, Ross H, Siu S, Crump R, Keating A, et al. High treatment-related mortality in cardiac amyloid patients undergoing autologous stem cell transplant. Bone Marrow Transplant. 1999;24:853–5.
69. Goldberg MA, Antin JH, Guinan EC, Rappeport JM. Cyclophosphamide cardiotoxicity: an analysis of dosing as a risk factor. Blood. 1986;68:1114–8.
70. Gottdiener JS, Appelbaum FR, Ferrans VJ, Deisseroth A, Ziegler J. Cardiotoxicity associated with high-dose cyclophosphamide therapy. Arch Intern Med. 1981;141:758–63.
71. Kuruvilla J, Forrest DL, Lavoie JC, Nantel SH, Shepherd JD, Song KW, et al. Characteristics and outcome of patients developing endocarditis following hematopoietic stem cell transplantation. Bone Marrow Transplant. 2004;34:969–73.
72. Gilman AL, Kooy NW, Atkins DL, Ballas Z, Rumelhart S, Holida M, et al. Complete heart block in association with graft-versus-host disease. Bone Marrow Transplant. 1998;21:85–8.
73. Platzbecker U, Klingel K, Thiede C, Freiberg-Richter J, Schuh D, Ehninger G, et al. Acute heart failure after allogeneic blood stem cell transplantation due to massive myocardial infiltration by cytotoxic T cells of donor origin. Bone Marrow Transplant. 2001;27:107–9.
74. Prevost D, Taylor G, Sanatani S, Schultz KR. Coronary vessel involvement by chronic graft-versus-host disease presenting as sudden cardiac death. Bone Marrow Transplant. 2004;34:655–6.
75. Rackley C, Schultz KR, Goldman FD, Chan KW, Serrano A, Hulse JE, et al. Cardiac manifestations of graft-versus-host disease. Biol Blood Marrow Transplant. 2005;11:773–80.
76. Rhodes M, Lautz T, Kavanaugh-Mchugh A, Manes B, Calder C, Koyama T, et al. Pericardial effusion and cardiac tamponade in pediatric stem cell transplant recipients. Bone Marrow Transplant. 2005;36:139–44.
77. Seber A, Khan SP, Kersey JH. Unexplained effusions: association with allogeneic bone marrow transplantation and acute or chronic graft-versus-host disease. Bone Marrow Transplant. 1996;17:207–11.
78. Toren A, Nagler A. Massive pericardial effusion complicating the course of chronic graft-versus-host disease (cGVHD) in a child with acute lymphoblastic leukemia following allogeneic bone marrow transplantation. Bone Marrow Transplant. 1997;20:805–7.
79. Ueda T, Manabe A, Kikuchi A, Yoshino H, Ebihara Y, Ishii T, et al. Massive pericardial and pleural effusion with anasarca following allogeneic bone marrow transplantation. Int J Hematol. 2000;71:394–7.
80. Tichelli A, Passweg J, Wojcik D, Rovo A, Harousseau JL, Masszi T, et al. Late cardiovascular events after allogeneic hematopoietic stem cell transplantation: a retrospective multicenter study of the Late Effects Working Party of the European Group for Blood and Marrow Transplantation. Haematologica. 2008;93:1203–10.
81. Jensen BV, Skovsgaard T, Nielsen SL. Functional monitoring of anthracycline cardiotoxicity: a prospective, blinded, long-term observational study of outcome in 120 patients. Ann Oncol. 2002;13:699–709.
82. Grenier MA, Lipshultz SE. Epidemiology of anthracycline cardiotoxicity in children and adults. Semin Oncol. 1998;25:72–85.
83. Lipshultz SE, Lipsitz SR, Sallan SE, Dalton VM, Mone SM, Gelber RD, et al. Chronic progressive cardiac dysfunction years after doxorubicin therapy for childhood acute lymphoblastic leukemia. J Clin Oncol. 2005;23:2629–36.

84. Aleman BM, van den Belt-Dusebout AW, De Bruin ML, van't Veer MB, Baaijens MH, de Boer JP, et al. Late cardiotoxicity after treatment for Hodgkin lymphoma. Blood. 2007;109:1878–86.

85. Tonnesmann E, Kandolf R, Lewalter T. Chloroquine cardiomyopathy—a review of the literature. Immunopharmacol Immunotoxicol. 2013;35:434–42.

86. Palomo M, Diaz-Ricart M, Carbo C, Rovira M, Fernandez-Aviles F, Escolar G, et al. The release of soluble factors contributing to endothelial activation and damage after hematopoietic stem cell transplantation is not limited to the allogeneic setting and involves several pathogenic mechanisms. Biol Blood Marrow Transplant. 2009;15:537–46.

87. Palomo M, Diaz-Ricart M, Carbo C, Rovira M, Fernandez-Aviles F, Martine C, et al. Endothelial dysfunction after hematopoietic stem cell transplantation: role of the conditioning regimen and the type of transplantation. Biol Blood Marrow Transplant. 2010;16:985–93.

88. Woywodt A, Scheer J, Hambach L, Buchholz S, Ganser A, Haller H, et al. Circulating endothelial cells as a marker of endothelial damage in allogeneic hematopoietic stem cell transplantation. Blood. 2004;103:3603–5.

89. Ford ES, Giles WH, Dietz WH. Prevalence of the metabolic syndrome among US adults: findings from the third National Health and Nutrition Examination Survey. JAMA. 2002;287:356–9.

90. Talvensaari KK, Lanning M, Tapanainen P, Knip M. Long-term survivors of childhood cancer have an increased risk of manifesting the metabolic syndrome. J Clin Endocrinol Metab. 1996;81:3051–5.

91. Taskinen M, Saarinen-Pihkala UM, Hovi L, Lipsanen-Nyman M. Impaired glucose tolerance and dyslipidaemia as late effects after bone-marrow transplantation in childhood. Lancet. 2000;356:993–7.

92. Baker KS, Ness KK, Steinberger J, Carter A, Francisco L, Burns LJ, et al. Diabetes, hypertension, and cardiovascular events in survivors of hematopoietic cell transplantation: a report from the bone marrow transplantation survivor study. Blood. 2007;109:1765–72.

93. Chow EJ, Baker KS, Lee SJ, Flowers ME, Cushing-Haugen KL, Inamoto Y, et al. Influence of conventional cardiovascular risk factors and lifestyle characteristics on cardiovascular disease after hematopoietic cell transplantation. J Clin Oncol. 2014;32:191–8.

94. Gratwohl A, Hermans J, Goldman JM, Arcese W, Carreras E, Devergie A, et al. Risk assessment for patients with chronic myeloid leukaemia before allogeneic blood or marrow transplantation. Chronic Leukemia Working Party of the European Group for Blood and Marrow Transplantation. Lancet. 1998;352:1087–92.

95. Armand P, Kim HT, Cutler CS, Ho VT, Koreth J, Ritz J, et al. A prognostic score for patients with acute leukemia or myelodysplastic syndromes undergoing allogeneic stem cell transplantation. Biol Blood Marrow Transplant. 2008;14:28–35.

96. Herrmann J, Lerman A, Sandhu NP, Villarraga HR, Mulvagh SL, Kohli M. Evaluation and management of patients with heart disease and cancer: cardio-oncology. Mayo Clin Proc. 2014;89:1287–306.

97. Skinner M, Sanchorawala V, Seldin DC, Dember LM, Falk RH, Berk JL, et al. High-dose melphalan and autologous stem-cell transplantation in patients with AL amyloidosis: an 8-year study. Ann Intern Med. 2004;140:85–93.

98. Ooi GC, Khong PL, Chan GC, Chan KN, Chan KL, Lam W, et al. Magnetic resonance screening of iron status in transfusion-dependent beta-thalassaemia patients. Br J Haematol. 2004;124:385–90.

99. Wood JC, Otto-Duessel M, Aguilar M, Nick H, Nelson MD, Coates TD, et al. Cardiac iron determines cardiac T2*, T2, and T1 in the gerbil model of iron cardiomyopathy. Circulation. 2005;112:535–43.

100. Jensen PD. Evaluation of iron overload. Br J Haematol. 2004;124:697–711.

101. Levine GN, Bates ER, Blankenship JC, Bailey SR, Bittl JA, Cercek B, et al. 2011 ACCF/ AHA/SCAI Guideline for Percutaneous Coronary Intervention: a report of the American College of Cardiology Foundation/American Heart Association Task Force on Practice

Guidelines and the Society for Cardiovascular Angiography and Interventions. Circulation. 2011;124:e574–651.
102. Rizzo JD, Wingard JR, Tichelli A, Lee SJ, Van Lint MT, Burns LJ, et al. Recommended screening and preventive practices for long-term survivors after hematopoietic cell transplantation: joint recommendations of the European Group for Blood and Marrow Transplantation, Center for International Blood and Marrow Transplant Research, and the American Society for Blood and Marrow Transplantation (EBMT/CIBMTR/ASBMT). Bone Marrow Transplant. 2006;37:249–61.
103. Friedlander AH, Sung EC, Child JS. Radiation-induced heart disease after Hodgkin's disease and breast cancer treatment: dental implications. J Am Dent Assoc. 2003;134:1615–20.
104. Yap YG, Camm AJ. Drug induced QT prolongation and torsades de pointes. Heart. 2003;89:1363–72.
105. Snowden JA, Hill GR, Hunt P, Carnoutsos S, Spearing RL, Espiner E, et al. Assessment of cardiotoxicity during haemopoietic stem cell transplantation with plasma brain natriuretic peptide. Bone Marrow Transplant. 2000;26:309–13.
106. Palladini G, Campana C, Klersy C, Balduini A, Vadacca G, Perfetti V, et al. Serum N-terminal pro-brain natriuretic peptide is a sensitive marker of myocardial dysfunction in AL amyloidosis. Circulation. 2003;107:2440–5.
107. Majhail NS, Rizzo JD, Lee SJ, Aljurf M, Atsuta Y, Bonfim C, et al. Recommended screening and preventive practices for long-term survivors after hematopoietic cell transplantation. Biol Blood Marrow Transplant. 2012;18:348–71.
108. Silber JH, Cnaan A, Clark BJ, Paridon SM, Chin AJ, Rychik J, et al. Enalapril to prevent cardiac function decline in long-term survivors of pediatric cancer exposed to anthracyclines. J Clin Oncol. 2004;22:820–8.
109. Jong P, Yusuf S, Rousseau MF, Ahn SA, Bangdiwala SI. Effect of enalapril on 12-year survival and life expectancy in patients with left ventricular systolic dysfunction: a follow-up study. Lancet. 2003;361:1843–8.
110. Lipshultz SE, Lipsitz SR, Sallan SE, Simbre 2nd VC, Shaikh SL, Mone SM, et al. Long-term enalapril therapy for left ventricular dysfunction in doxorubicin-treated survivors of childhood cancer. J Clin Oncol. 2002;20:4517–22.

Chapter 7
Radiation Therapy and Cardiotoxicity

Manisha Palta, Chang-Lung Lee, Syed Wamique Yusuf, and David G. Kirsch

Introduction

Radiotherapy is an integral part of achieving long-term cure in a number of intrathoracic malignancies. In this chapter the authors provide an overview of the epidemiology of heart disease after radiotherapy, with specific focus on data from Hodgkin lymphoma and breast cancer survivors. As clinical manifestation of heart disease can take years, if not decades, to manifest, animal models can assist in our understanding of the pathogenesis as well as the cellular and molecular mechanisms of radiation-induced heart disease, elucidating opportunities for intervention and prevention. Finally, recommendations for monitoring patients after radiotherapy and management of cardiac disease in patients with prior thoracic/breast neoplasms will be discussed.

Electronic supplementary material: The online version of this chapter (doi:10.1007/978-3-319-43096-6_7) contains supplementary material, which is available to authorized users.

M. Palta (✉)
Department of Radiation Oncology, Duke University Medical Center, Morris Clinic Building, DUMC 3085, Research Drive, Durham, NC 27710, USA
e-mail: manisha.palta@duke.edu

C.-L. Lee • D.G. Kirsch
Department of Radiation Oncology, Duke University Medical Center, 450 Research Drive, LSRC Building, Rm. B324, Durham, NC 27708, USA
e-mail: chang-lung.lee@duke.edu; david.kirsch@dm.duke.edu

S.W. Yusuf
Department of Cardiology, University of Texas MD Anderson Cancer Center, Houston, TX 77030, USA
e-mail: syusuf@mdanderson.org

© Springer International Publishing Switzerland 2017
G.G. Kimmick et al. (eds.), *Cardio-Oncology*, DOI 10.1007/978-3-319-43096-6_7

Pathogenesis of Radiation-Induced Heart Disease in Experimental Animals

The pathological effects of ionizing radiation on the heart have been studied in different species of laboratory animals including mice, rats, rabbits, and dogs [1–8]. Sequential necropsies to evaluate histological changes to the heart were performed after either a single fraction (single dose of ≥ 15 Gy) or multiple fractions (cumulative dose of ≥ 36 Gy) of radiation to the thorax. Results from these animal studies demonstrate that focal irradiation results in time-dependent structural damage in various anatomical areas of the heart. Here, we will focus on animal studies that examine pathogenesis of radiation-associated cardiovascular problems commonly observed in the clinic, including pericarditis, cardiomyopathy, and coronary artery disease [9, 10].

Pericarditis

Acute pericarditis can develop in experimental animals within days to weeks after irradiation with 20–40 Gy due to inflammation [2, 3, 8]. Although acute inflammation may resolve with time, chronic changes have been observed over 20 months, which include a thickened pericardium with edema, inflammatory cells, fibroblast proliferation, and collagen deposition [5, 6]. The underlying mechanism of chronic pericarditis is not well understood, but it may be associated with increased inflammation secondary to microvascular injury [11].

Cardiomyopathy

Radiation-induced cardiomyopathy results from severe injury to the myocardium that subsequently impairs global function of the heart [9]. Animal studies reveal that radiation causes long-term tissue remodeling of the myocardium [1–3, 6]. For example, a large cohort study of radiation-induced heart disease (RIHD) using New Zealand white rabbits exposed to a single dose of 20 Gy showed progressive pericardial fibrosis, pericardial effusion, myocardial degeneration, and diffuse myocardial fibrosis 70 days after irradiation [1, 2]. Myocardial injury after irradiation is known to be associated with damage to the microvasculature, which is demonstrated by decreased microvessel density, focal loss of endothelial alkaline phosphatase, and increased expression of von Willebrand factor [1, 5]. In addition, infiltration of certain immune cells, such as mast cells, may also modulate the formation of myocardial degeneration and fibrosis [12]. The contribution of microvascular injury and mast cells to RIHD will be discussed in more detail later in this chapter.

Coronary Artery Disease

Epidemiological studies show that patients who received a mean radiation dose of 2 Gy to the heart have a significantly increased risk of developing ischemic heart disease more than 10 years after irradiation [10]. However, coronary artery disease associated with radiation exposure has not often been reported in animal studies of RIHD. This is likely because normal rodents are known to be relatively resistant to atherosclerosis as they have very low levels of low-density lipoprotein (LDL) in the plasma [10].

Several studies have used atherosclerosis-prone animal models to define the interaction of radiation with additional risk factors for cardiovascular disease, such as hypertension and hypercholesterolemia [13–16]. For example, Gabriels and colleagues studied RIHD in hypercholesterolemic and atherosclerosis-prone ApoE$^{-/-}$ mice, which received a single dose of focal heart irradiation up to 16 Gy. They found that radiation significantly increased the number of inflammatory cells, decreased microvascular density, and increased von Willebrand factor expression in the myocardium of the left ventricle. Most importantly, they found accelerated coronary atherosclerotic lesions that developed at 20 weeks after 16 Gy. Interestingly, despite these pronounced effects, cardiac gated SPECT and ultrasound measurements showed only minor changes in functional cardiac parameters at 20 weeks [15]. It is possible that surviving cardiomyocytes compensated for the radiation damage to the myocardium, and therefore these mice may slowly progress to develop cardiac dysfunction and heart failure with further follow-up.

Cellular and Molecular Mechanisms of Radiation-Induced Heart Disease

Endothelial Cells

Damage to vascular endothelial cells has generally been considered an underlying mechanism of RIHD [10, 17–19]. Radiation doses ≥ 2 Gy can substantially alter endothelial cell functions [10, 19]. After irradiation, endothelial cells significantly upregulate the expression of several cell adhesion molecules, including E-selectin, P-selectin, intercellular adhesion molecule-1 (ICAM-1), PECAM-1 (CD31), and CD44 [10, 20]. Increased expression of these adhesion molecules promotes leukocyte adhesion and transmigration, which subsequently elicits a pro-inflammatory response [10].

In addition to causing functional alterations to endothelial cells, radiation also leads to cell death of endothelial cells in vivo as radiation decreases microvessel density and increases permeability of microvessels in the heart. Several studies have used primary endothelial cells isolated from different types of blood vessels to study endothelial cell death after irradiation in vitro. Results from these studies indicate that radiation can trigger various forms of endothelial cell death in vitro including apoptosis [21], mitotic catastrophe [22], and senescence [20, 22–24]. It is possible that the spectrum of endothelial cell death observed in vitro might be influenced by the origin of the endothelial cells (species, anatomic location, etc) and the dose of radiation. Given the diversity of gene expression profiles in human endothelial cells isolated from different tissues [25], how endothelial cells in the heart die from radiation in vivo remains to be fully understood.

An important question in the field is whether endothelial cell damage following radiation triggers cardiomyocyte injury or whether cardiomyocyte injury occurs independently of endothelial cell death. To dissect the role of endothelial cells in mediating radiation-induced injury to the heart in vivo, investigators can use genetically engineered mice [26]. For example, Lee and colleagues have used the site-specific recombinase system, Cre-loxP, to study the role of the tumor suppressor p53 specifically in endothelial cells in a mouse model of RIHD [11]. The tumor suppressor p53 is a transcription factor that serves as a master regulator of cellular response to radiation [27–29]. Upon radiation exposure, activation of the DNA damage response increases the level of p53 protein to induce a variety of downstream signaling pathways that mediate cellular response to stress [30, 31]. After whole-heart irradiation, mice in which both alleles of p53 were deleted specifically in endothelial cells were sensitized to radiation-induced myocardial injury and compared to mice that retained one allele of p53 in endothelial cells [11]. After whole-heart irradiation, mice with endothelial cells lacking p53 showed a focal decrease in microvessel density in the myocardium, which led to cardiac ischemia and myocardial necrosis [11]. The progression of myocardial necrosis resulted in systolic dysfunction and heart failure. Together, these results not only demonstrate a critical role for p53 in protecting cardiac endothelial cells from radiation in vivo but also provide compelling genetic evidence to show that damage to the myocardial vasculature leads to cardiac ischemia and myocardial necrosis, which can cause systolic dysfunction and heart failure [11].

Mast Cells

In rat models of RIHD, focal irradiation to the heart induces infiltration of mast cells [32, 33], which are tissue-resident sentinel cells that can both positively and negatively regulate immune responses [34]. It has been shown that infiltration of mast cells is associated with coronary atherosclerosis and myocardial fibrosis in animal models [35, 36]. Interestingly, experiments using mast cell-deficient rats reveal that mast cells play a protective role in RIHD in rats [12, 37]. After focal heart irradiation, mast cell-deficient rats showed more severe changes in cardiac function with increased deposition of collagen type III compared to their mast cell-competent littermates. These results suggest that mast cells may regulate cardiac dysfunction after irradiation by modulating collagen type III deposition.

It has been hypothesized that mast cells may protect rats against RIHD by activating the kallikrein-kinin pathway [37], as mast cell-derived proteases have been shown to elicit the release of kinins from their precursors, kininogens. To test this hypothesis, kininogen-deficient rats have been used to investigate the role of the kallikrein-kinin pathway in RIHD [38]. In contrast to results from studies using mast cell-deficient mice, changes in cardiac function were less severe in kininogen-deficient rats after local heart irradiation compared to their kininogen-intact litter-mates. Irradiated kininogen-deficient rats also showed a significant decrease in the number of CD68-positive macrophages but showed no difference in the number of mast cells in the heart compared to their kininogen-intact littermates. These results suggest that the cardioprotective effect of mast cells is not mediated by the kallikrein-kinin pathway. Mechanisms by which mast cells protect rats from RIHD remain to be better defined.

Future Directions in Preclinical Study

Accumulating data from animal models of radiation-induced heart disease have significantly advanced our knowledge of the pathogenesis of cardiac complications associated with focal radiation to the thorax or to the whole heart. However, the etiology of radiation-induced heart disease after partial heart irradiation, which is more clinically relevant to patients treated for breast cancer and lung cancer, remains largely unexplored. With the development of image-guided irradiators for small laboratory animals, it is now possible to more precisely deliver radiation to part of the heart. For example, in a proof-of-concept study, Lee and colleagues have developed a mouse model of radiation-induced myocardial injury after partial heart irradiation [39]. They utilized novel dual-energy microCT and 4D microCT with nanoparticle-based contrast agents to noninvasively assess the change in myocardial vascular permeability and cardiac function of mice after irradiation. This study revealed that animal models of RIHD after partial heart irradiation can serve as a platform for the development of biomarkers for noninvasive imaging, such as echocardiography and CT scans, to identify surrogates of cardiac injury that can be measured in cancer survivors before severe heart disease occurs. Such studies may shed light on the critical clinical question of the relative importance of mean radiation dose to the entire heart versus a high radiation dose to part of the heart in mediating RIHD. Ultimately, findings from animal models of RIHD have the potential to define new approaches for assessing and treating heart disease from radiation therapy and to increase the quality and quantity of life for cancer survivors.

Epidemiology of Heart Disease After Radiotherapy

Radiotherapy can affect all cardiac structures, resulting in myocardial infarction (MI), valvular disease, pericardial disease, conduction abnormalities, and cardiomyopathy. While radiotherapy is associated with cardiac toxicity, various chemotherapeutic agents typically delivered sequentially may compound these effects on the heart. In addition patients with known cardiac comorbidities, such as hypertension, diabetes, smoking, and hyperlipidemia, are at higher risk of developing cardiac complications compared to patients with no known risk factors. The incidence of radiation-induced heart disease (RIHD) is best described from long-term clinical data in Hodgkin lymphoma and breast cancer survivors. Data suggest that CD and associated cardiac-related mortality does not manifest until nearly a decade posttreatment [40–42].

RIHD in Hodgkin Lymphoma Survivors

In Hodgkin lymphoma (HL), cardiac complications appear to be associated with radiotherapy (RT) dose and radiation field. Historically radiotherapy has been widely used in the treatment of lymphoma since the 1960s after promising data from Stanford University. Total nodal field radiotherapy included a classic mantle (treatment of the supradiaphragmatic nodes including cervical, supraclavicular, and mediastinal/hilar regions) and inverted Y field (encompassing para-aortic, pelvic, and inguinofemoral lymph nodes) was the definitive curative approach prior to utilization of systemic therapy [43]. Over time, systemic therapy has become more effective, and as a result the radiotherapy dose has reduced. In addition, the size of radiotherapy volumes have decreased over time from extended field to involved field (radiation to involved anatomic nodal region) and more recently involved site radiotherapy [44–47].

Five-year survivors of HL treated prior to age 40 were found to have a higher relative risk (RR) of 3–5 for cardiac disease (CD) compared with the general population [48]. A report from the US Childhood Cancer Survivor Study included 2717 5-year HL survivors, and the RR of death from all cardiac causes compared with the general population was 11.9. The RR of death from MI secondary to mediastinal RT was estimated to be as high as 41.5 with historically higher radiation doses [49]. More recent studies of low-dose thoracic RT are associated with a lower incidence of CD [50–52]. A study of 1132 HL survivors who received treatment before age 18 between the years 1978–1995 evaluated CD incidence. Although the dose of doxorubicin 160 mg/m^2 remained uniform during this time period, the mediastinal RT dose was 0, 20, 25, 30, or 36 Gray (Gy). A central, expert panel reviewed all reported cardiac abnormalities. CD was diagnosed in 50 patients, and valvular defects were reported most frequently, followed by CAD, cardiomyopathies, conduction disorders, and pericardial abnormalities. The 25-year cumulative incidence of CD was 21 % in the 36 Gy RT dose, decreasing to 10 %, 6 %, 5 %, and 3 % in the respective lower mediastinal RT dose cohorts ($p < 0.001$) [53].

Coinciding with decreasing RT dose, radiation fields have evolved from total nodal radiotherapy. With the use of combined modality therapy (chemotherapy and radiation), chemotherapy is paramount in eradicating subclinical disease. As such, there is now a shift toward involved field RT (IFRT) with randomized data demonstrating similar control rates with smaller treatment fields [46, 54, 55]. Ongoing studies are evaluating yet smaller treatment fields including involved site RT and involved nodal RT based on retrospective data suggesting equivalent outcomes compared to IFRT [56, 57]. As data emerge suggesting disease control with smaller RT fields, less heart in RT fields should result in a reduction of RIHD. This assertion has been corroborated by a series from Stanford in which 2232 HL patients from 1960 to 1991 were treated, and the associated RR for non-MI cardiac death fell from 5.3 to 1.4 once subcarinal blocking was introduced which decreased cardiac dose [50].

RIHD in Breast Cancer Survivors

Breast radiotherapy has evolved over time. Use of lower energy radiation, larger dose per fraction, and routine treatment of the internal mammary nodes were common practice in the 1970s and associated with increased risk of CD, but are no longer standard practice [40, 58]. In current treatment of breast cancer, the use of higher energy photons, CT-based planning to assess cardiac position, and techniques, such as prone positioning and breathing control (in breath hold the lungs insufflate and the heart is displaced away from the chest wall and inferiorly), help to minimize cardiac dose and thus decrease treatment-related toxicity. The long-term impact of these modifications on mitigating risk of CD is unknown as the associated cardiac-related mortality does not manifest until nearly a decade post-treatment. One key limitation of the data evaluating cardiovascular toxicity is that patients evaluated on these studies were typically treated decades ago with now antiquated techniques.

Long-term follow-up data from breast cancer randomized studies and large population databases demonstrate that RT can increase the risk of CD, specifically the risk of ischemic heart disease. A sample of over 4000 10-year breast cancer survivors treated in randomized studies prior to 1975 demonstrated no increased all-cause mortality rate; however, an increase in cardiac-related deaths was seen [58]. A large population-based case-control study of breast cancer patients in Denmark and Sweden assessed incidence of major coronary events in patients treated with radiotherapy between 1958 and 2001. Individual patient data were obtained from hospital records including the mean RT dose to the whole heart and left anterior descending (LAD) coronary artery. Major coronary events increased linearly with mean heart dose by 7.4 % per Gy [59].

Imaging tests have been utilized to objectively quantify RT effects on the heart. Single-photon emission computed tomography (SPECT) scans have been used to assess subclinical cardiac injury. A prospective study from Duke University assessed SPECT changes post-RT in women with left-sided breast cancer. SPECT abnormalities post-RT were visualized in 50 % of patients and were consistent with decreased perfusion in the volume of the irradiated left ventricle [60]. The clinical significance of these imaging findings, however, has not been fully elucidated. An analysis of a Swedish breast cancer cohort sought to determine the distribution of coronary artery stenosis and RT. Patients with a diagnosis of breast cancer were linked to registers of coronary angiography. The odds ratio of grade 3–5 stenosis (5 = complete occlusion) in the mid and distal LAD and distal diagonal for patients receiving left-sided radiotherapy was 4.38 compared to right-sided breast cancer treatment [61].

Although the aforementioned studies clearly suggest higher rates of cardiac disease associated with RT, additional data suggest that the incidence of RIHD has decreased over time with advances in RT planning and delivery. An analysis of patients treated at New York University calculated the excess absolute risk of radiation-induced coronary events as defined by Darby et al. with the use of more modern radiation techniques. For supine-positioned left breast RT, the cardiac dose was 2.17 Gray (Gy) and 1.03 Gy for prone positioning. Based on more modern data, the estimated lifetime risk of coronary events for patients receiving radiotherapy for breast cancer ranges from 0.05 to 3.5 % based on baseline risk (determined by total cholesterol, high-density lipoprotein, systolic blood pressure, and serum C-reactive protein) [62]. A Surveillance, Epidemiology, and End Results (SEER) analysis of patients treated between 1973 and 1989 estimated the risk of death from ischemic heart disease comparing women receiving left- to right-sided breast radiation. For women diagnosed between 1973 and 1979, there was a statistically significant 15-year mortality from ischemic heart disease of 13.1 % in left-sided patients compared to 10.2 % in right-sided. No differences between left- and right-sided cancers were seen in the cohorts of patients treated between 1980 and 1984 or 1985 and 1989 [40]. These data suggest that advances in radiation technique and delivery over time are responsible for the decline in late cardiac toxicities.

Advances in radiotherapy simulation and treatment planning have reduced the dose of radiation to the heart. In addition, radiation-associated CD is likely to be reduced by addressing concurrent cardiac risk factors through lifestyle modification and medication [62]. Understanding the pathophysiology of RIHD, particularly with the use of animal models may help clarify our understanding of this toxicity and create the opportunity for intervention and prevention.

Management of Cardiac Disease in Patients with Prior Radiotherapy

Pericarditis

In humans, acute pericarditis usually presents with chest pain and nonspecific ECG changes or classic ST elevation, while the patient is undergoing radiation therapy. Chronic pericardial disease may present with enlarging chronic pericardial effusion or constrictive pericarditis. Acute pericarditis is treated with conventional medical management including NSAIDs, colchicine, and steroids. For chronic pericardial effusion, pericardiocentesis may be needed. For symptomatic pericardial constriction, pericardial stripping may be indicated. However, among patients undergoing surgical pericardiectomy, previous radiotherapy is associated with a poorer outcome [63].

Cardiomyopathy

Cardiomyopathy and heart failure are treated with usual heart failure medical therapy, which includes beta-blockers, angiotensin-converting-enzyme inhibitors (ACE-I), angiotensin receptor blockers (ARB), and aldosterone antagonists, although mortality data on a large patient population with radiation-related cardiomyopathy is lacking. Individual cases may be offered pericardial stripping (in cases of constrictive pericarditis) and mechanical circulatory support. There are limited data with cardiac transplantation. In a small series of 12 patients undergoing cardiac transplantation, survival at 1, 5, and 10 years was 91.7 %, 75 %, and 46.7 %, respectively [64].

Coronary Artery Disease

The clinical presentation, diagnosis, and treatment of radiation-related CAD are similar to the general population. Patients commonly present with angina, myocardial infarction or sudden death [65]. There are no specific guidelines for the acute initial stabilization and subsequent management of these patients. Risk factors, e.g., hypertension and hyperlipidemia, should be treated as per American College of Cardiology/American Heart Association (ACC/AHA) guidelines.

For both acute and chronic radiation-induced CAD, treatment is similar to the atherosclerotic CAD in the general population, either with medical therapy or revascularization, considering the patient's symptoms, cancer stage, expected survival, and comorbidities. For patients with radiation-induced CAD, both percutaneous intervention and coronary artery bypass graft (CABG) have been used

[65]. Because of mediastinal fibrosis, surgical intervention and CABG may be associated with a higher incidence of complications [65]. In addition, the use of internal mammary artery as a graft may not always be possible due to radiation damage within this vessel itself [66]. A more recent study of 12 patients previously treated for Hodgkin lymphoma with mediastinal radiation therapy who underwent cardiac surgery, including two patients with coronary artery bypass grafting, showed that the early postoperative outcome in this population is reasonable [67].

Recommendations for Patient Monitoring After Radiotherapy

At baseline, in addition to obtaining a 12-lead ECG and an echocardiogram, risk factors like hyperlipidemia and diabetes mellitus should be identified and treated according to existing guidelines. At subsequent follow-up, chest x-ray and CT scan, if obtained, should be reviewed as chronic pericardial effusion (which can develop months to years after completion of radiation therapy) is usually picked up by findings of enlarging cardiac silhouette on chest x-ray or pericardial effusion on routine follow-up CT scan. Any finding of even minimal or small pericardial effusion should be followed at periodic intervals.

A follow-up echocardiogram should be done for any cardiac symptoms or signs that merit an echocardiogram. For high-risk asymptomatic patients (patients who have undergone anterior or left-sided chest radiation with >1 risk factors for radiation-induced heart disease), a screening echocardiogram should be done at 5 years after completion of radiation therapy, and in others a screening echocardiogram should be considered at 10 years after completion of radiation therapy [68]. A functional noninvasive stress test is recommended 5–10 years after completion of radiation in high-risk patients [68]. Recent data suggests that coronary CT scan is also a useful modality for identifying asymptomatic patients with radiation-induced CAD [69].

Conclusions

Epidemiologic data suggest an increasing risk of CD is patients treated with intrathoracic or breast radiotherapy. Newer radiation techniques may, in part, mitigate some of the potential late cardiac toxicities. Animal models can assist in our understanding of the pathogenesis as well as the cellular and molecular mechanisms of radiation-induced heart disease leading to opportunities for intervention and prevention. Management of pericarditis, cardiomyopathy, and coronary artery disease in patients with prior radiotherapy mirrors treatment in patients with no prior radiation therapy.

References

1. Fajardo LF, Stewart JR. Pathogenesis of radiation-induced myocardial fibrosis. Lab Invest. 1973;29(2):244–57.
2. Fajardo LF, Stewart JR. Experimental radiation-induced heart disease. I. Light microscopic studies. Am J Pathol. 1970;59(2):299–316.
3. Lauk S, Kiszel Z, Buschmann J, Trott KR. Radiation-induced heart disease in rats. Int J Radiat Oncol Biol Phys. 1985;11(4):801–8.
4. Yeung TK, Lauk S, Simmonds RH, Hopewell JW, Trott KR. Morphological and functional changes in the rat heart after X irradiation: strain differences. Radiat Res. 1989;119(3):489–99.
5. Seemann I, Gabriels K, Visser NL, Hoving S, Te Poele JA, Pol JF, et al. Irradiation induced modest changes in murine cardiac function despite progressive structural damage to the myocardium and microvasculature. Radiother Oncol. 2012;103(2):143–50. doi:10.1016/j.radonc.2011.10.011.
6. McChesney SL, Gillette EL, Powers BE. Radiation-induced cardiomyopathy in the dog. Radiat Res. 1988;113(1):120–32.
7. Gillette EL, McChesney SL, Hoopes PJ. Isoeffect curves for radiation-induced cardiomyopathy in the dog. Int J Radiat Oncol Biol Phys. 1985;11(12):2091–7.
8. McChesney SL, Gillette EL, Orton EC. Canine cardiomyopathy after whole heart and partial lung irradiation. Int J Radiat Oncol Biol Phys. 1988;14(6):1169–74.
9. Adams MJ, Lipshultz SE. Pathophysiology of anthracycline- and radiation-associated cardiomyopathies: implications for screening and prevention. Pediatr Blood Cancer. 2005;44 (7):600–6. doi:10.1002/pbc.20352.
10. Schultz-Hector S, Trott KR. Radiation-induced cardiovascular diseases: is the epidemiologic evidence compatible with the radiobiologic data? Int J Radiat Oncol Biol Phys. 2007;67 (1):10–8. doi:10.1016/j.ijrobp.2006.08.071.
11. Lee CL, Moding EJ, Cuneo KC, Li Y, Sullivan JM, Mao L, et al. p53 functions in endothelial cells to prevent radiation-induced myocardial injury in mice. Sci Signal. 2012;5(234):ra52. doi:10.1126/scisignal.2002918.
12. Boerma M, Wang J, Wondergem J, Joseph J, Qiu X, Kennedy RH, et al. Influence of mast cells on structural and functional manifestations of radiation-induced heart disease. Cancer Res. 2005;65(8):3100–7. doi:10.1158/0008-5472.CAN-04-4333.
13. Lauk S, Trott KR. Radiation induced heart disease in hypertensive rats. Int J Radiat Oncol Biol Phys. 1988;14(1):109–14.
14. Stewart FA, Heeneman S, Te Poele J, Kruse J, Russell NS, Gijbels M, et al. Ionizing radiation accelerates the development of atherosclerotic lesions in ApoE−/− mice and predisposes to an inflammatory plaque phenotype prone to hemorrhage. Am J Pathol. 2006;168(2):649–58. doi:10.2353/ajpath.2006.050409.
15. Gabriels K, Hoving S, Seemann I, Visser NL, Gijbels MJ, Pol JF, et al. Local heart irradiation of ApoE−/− mice induces microvascular and endocardial damage and accelerates coronary atherosclerosis. Radiother Oncol. 2012;105(3):358–64. doi:10.1016/j.radonc.2012.08.002.
16. Hoving S, Heeneman S, Gijbels MJ, Te Poele JA, Visser N, Cleutjens J, et al. Irradiation induces different inflammatory and thrombotic responses in carotid arteries of wildtype C57BL/6J and atherosclerosis-prone ApoE−/− mice. Radiother Oncol. 2012;105(3):365–70. doi:10.1016/j.radonc.2012.11.001.
17. Stewart FA, Hoving S, Russell NS. Vascular damage as an underlying mechanism of cardiac and cerebral toxicity in irradiated cancer patients. Radiat Res. 2010;174(6):865–9. doi:10.1667/RR1862.1.
18. Boerma M, Hauer-Jensen M. Preclinical research into basic mechanisms of radiation-induced heart disease. Cardiol Res Pract. 2010;2011:pii: 858262. doi:10.4061/2011/858262.
19. Stewart FA, Seemann I, Hoving S, Russell NS. Understanding radiation-induced cardiovascular damage and strategies for intervention. Clin Oncol. 2013;25(10):617–24. doi:10.1016/j.clon.2013.06.012.

20. Lowe D, Raj K. Premature aging induced by radiation exhibits pro-atherosclerotic effects mediated by epigenetic activation of CD44 expression. Aging Cell. 2014;13(5):900–10. doi:10.1111/acel.12253.

21. Paris F, Fuks Z, Kang A, Capodieci P, Juan G, Ehleiter D, et al. Endothelial apoptosis as the primary lesion initiating intestinal radiation damage in mice. Science. 2001;293(5528):293–7. doi:10.1126/science.1060191.

22. Mendonca MS, Chin-Sinex H, Dhaemers R, Mead LE, Yoder MC, Ingram DA. Differential mechanisms of x-ray-induced cell death in human endothelial progenitor cells isolated from cord blood and adults. Radiat Res. 2011;176(2):208–16.

23. Lee MO, Song SH, Jung S, Hur S, Asahara T, Kim H, et al. Effect of ionizing radiation induced damage of endothelial progenitor cells in vascular regeneration. Arterioscler Thromb Vasc Biol. 2011;32(2):343–52. doi:10.1161/ATVBAHA.111.237651.

24. Dong X, Tong F, Qian C, Zhang R, Dong J, Wu G, et al. NEMO modulates radiation-induced endothelial senescence of human umbilical veins through NF-κB signal pathway. Radiat Res. 2015;183(1):82–93. doi:10.1667/RR13682.1.

25. Chi JT, Chang HY, Haraldsen G, Jahnsen FL, Troyanskaya OG, Chang DS, et al. Endothelial cell diversity revealed by global expression profiling. Proc Natl Acad Sci U S A. 2003;100 (19):10623–8. doi:10.1073/pnas.1434429100.

26. Kirsch DG. Using genetically engineered mice for radiation research. Radiat Res. 2011;176 (3):275–9.

27. Gudkov AV, Komarova EA. The role of p53 in determining sensitivity to radiotherapy. Nat Rev Cancer. 2003;3(2):117–29. doi:10.1038/nrc992.

28. Gudkov AV, Komarova EA. Pathologies associated with the p53 response. Cold Spring Harb Perspect Biol. 2010;2(7):a001180. doi:10.1101/cshperspect.a001180.

29. Lindsay KJ, Coates PJ, Lorimore SA, Wright EG. The genetic basis of tissue responses to ionizing radiation. Br J Radiol. 2007;80(Spec No 1):S2–6. doi:10.1259/bjr/60507340.

30. Schlereth K, Charles JP, Bretz AC, Stiewe T. Life or death: p53-induced apoptosis requires DNA binding cooperativity. Cell Cycle. 2010;9(20):4068–76. doi:10.4161/cc.9.20.13595.

31. Murray-Zmijewski F, Slee EA, Lu X. A complex barcode underlies the heterogeneous response of p53 to stress. Nat Rev Mol Cell Biol. 2008;9(9):702–12. doi:10.1038/nrm2451.

32. Yarom R, Harper IS, Wynchank S, van Schalkwyk D, Madhoo J, Williams K, et al. Effect of captopril on changes in rats' hearts induced by long-term irradiation. Radiat Res. 1993;133 (2):187–97.

33. Boerma M, Zurcher C, Esveldt I, Schutte-Bart CI, Wondergem J. Histopathology of ventricles, coronary arteries and mast cell accumulation in transverse and longitudinal sections of the rat heart after irradiation. Oncol Rep. 2004;12(2):213–9.

34. Khazaie K, Blatner NR, Khan MW, Gounari F, Gounaris E, Dennis K, et al. The significant role of mast cells in cancer. Cancer Metastasis Rev. 2011;30(1):45–60. doi:10.1007/s10555-011-9286-z.

35. Koskinen PK, Kovanen PT, Lindstedt KA, Lemstrom KB. Mast cells in acute and chronic rejection of rat cardiac allografts—a major source of basic fibroblast growth factor. Transplantation. 2001;71(12):1741–7.

36. Li QY, Raza-Ahmad A, MacAulay MA, Lalonde LD, Rowden G, Trethewey E, et al. The relationship of mast cells and their secreted products to the volume of fibrosis in posttransplant hearts. Transplantation. 1992;53(5):1047–51.

37. Boerma M. Experimental radiation-induced heart disease: past, present, and future. Radiat Res. 2012;178(1):1–6.

38. Sridharan V, Tripathi P, Sharma SK, Moros EG, Corry PM, Lieblong BJ, et al. Cardiac inflammation after local irradiation is influenced by the kallikrein-kinin system. Cancer Res. 2012;72(19):4984–92. doi:10.1158/0008-5472.CAN-12-1831.

39. Lee CL, Min H, Befera N, Clark D, Qi Y, Das S, et al. Assessing cardiac injury in mice with dual energy-microCT, 4D-microCT, and microSPECT imaging after partial heart irradiation. Int J Radiat Oncol Biol Phys. 2014;88(3):686–93. doi:10.1016/j.ijrobp.2013.11.238.

40. Giordano SH, Kuo YF, Freeman JL, Buchholz TA, Hortobagyi GN, Goodwin JS. Risk of cardiac death after adjuvant radiotherapy for breast cancer. J Natl Cancer Inst. 2005;97 (6):419–24. doi:10.1093/jnci/dji067.
41. Favourable and unfavourable effects on long-term survival of radiotherapy for early breast cancer: an overview of the randomised trials. Early Breast Cancer Trialists' Collaborative Group. Lancet. 2000;355(9217):1757–70.
42. Darby S, McGale P, Peto R, Granath F, Hall P, Ekbom A. Mortality from cardiovascular disease more than 10 years after radiotherapy for breast cancer: nationwide cohort study of 90 000 Swedish women. BMJ. 2003;326(7383):256–7.
43. Hoskin PJ, Diez P, Williams M, Lucraft H, Bayne M. Recommendations for the use of radiotherapy in nodal lymphoma. Clin Oncol (R Coll Radiol). 2013;25(1):49–58. doi:10.1016/j.clon.2012.07.011.
44. Koh ES, Tran TH, Heydarian M, Sachs RK, Tsang RW, Brenner DJ, et al. A comparison of mantle versus involved-field radiotherapy for Hodgkin's lymphoma: reduction in normal tissue dose and second cancer risk. Radiat Oncol. 2007;2:13. doi:10.1186/1748-717X-2-13.
45. Hoskin PJ, Smith P, Maughan TS, Gilson D, Vernon C, Syndikus I, et al. Long-term results of a randomised trial of involved field radiotherapy vs extended field radiotherapy in stage I and II Hodgkin lymphoma. Clin Oncol (R Coll Radiol). 2005;17(1):47–53.
46. Engert A, Schiller P, Josting A, Herrmann R, Koch P, Sieber M, et al. Involved-field radiotherapy is equally effective and less toxic compared with extended-field radiotherapy after four cycles of chemotherapy in patients with early-stage unfavorable Hodgkin's lymphoma: results of the HD8 trial of the German Hodgkin's Lymphoma Study Group. J Clin Oncol. 2003;21(19):3601–8. doi:10.1200/JCO.2003.03.023.
47. Specht L, Yahalom J, Illidge T, Berthelsen AK, Constine LS, Eich HT, et al. Modern radiation therapy for Hodgkin lymphoma: field and dose guidelines from the international lymphoma radiation oncology group (ILROG). Int J Radiat Oncol Biol Phys. 2014;89(4):854–62. doi:10.1016/j.ijrobp.2013.05.005.
48. Aleman BM, van den Belt-Dusebout AW, De Bruin ML, van't Veer MB, Baaijens MH, de Boer JP, et al. Late cardiotoxicity after treatment for Hodgkin lymphoma. Blood. 2007;109 (5):1878–86. doi:10.1182/blood-2006-07-034405.
49. Hancock SL, Donaldson SS, Hoppe RT. Cardiac disease following treatment of Hodgkin's disease in children and adolescents. J Clin Oncol. 1993;11(7):1208–15.
50. Hancock SL, Tucker MA, Hoppe RT. Factors affecting late mortality from heart disease after treatment of Hodgkin's disease. JAMA. 1993;270(16):1949–55.
51. Hull MC, Morris CG, Pepine CJ, Mendenhall NP. Valvular dysfunction and carotid, subclavian, and coronary artery disease in survivors of Hodgkin lymphoma treated with radiation therapy. JAMA. 2003;290(21):2831–7. doi:10.1001/jama.290.21.2831.
52. Kupeli S, Hazirolan T, Varan A, Akata D, Alehan D, Hayran M, et al. Evaluation of coronary artery disease by computed tomography angiography in patients treated for childhood Hodgkin's lymphoma. J Clin Oncol. 2010;28(6):1025–30. doi:10.1200/JCO.2009.25.2627.
53. Schellong G, Riepenhausen M, Bruch C, Kotthoff S, Vogt J, Bolling T, et al. Late valvular and other cardiac diseases after different doses of mediastinal radiotherapy for Hodgkin disease in children and adolescents: report from the longitudinal GPOH follow-up project of the German-Austrian DAL-HD studies. Pediatr Blood Cancer. 2010;55(6):1145–52. doi:10.1002/pbc.22664.
54. Zittoun R, Audebert A, Hoerni B, Bernadou A, Krulik M, Rojouan J, et al. Extended versus involved fields irradiation combined with MOPP chemotherapy in early clinical stages of Hodgkin's disease. J Clin Oncol. 1985;3(2):207–14.
55. Bonadonna G, Bonfante V, Viviani S, Di Russo A, Villani F, Valagussa P. ABVD plus subtotal nodal versus involved-field radiotherapy in early-stage Hodgkin's disease: long-term results. J Clin Oncol. 2004;22(14):2835–41. doi:10.1200/JCO.2004.12.170.
56. Maraldo MV, Aznar MC, Vogelius IR, Petersen PM, Specht L. Involved node radiation therapy: an effective alternative in early-stage Hodgkin lymphoma. Int J Radiat Oncol Biol Phys. 2013;85(4):1057–65. doi:10.1016/j.ijrobp.2012.08.041.

57. Campbell BA, Voss N, Pickles T, Morris J, Gascoyne RD, Savage KJ, et al. Involved-nodal radiation therapy as a component of combination therapy for limited-stage Hodgkin's lymphoma: a question of field size. J Clin Oncol. 2008;26(32):5170–4. doi:10.1200/JCO.2007.15. 1001.

58. Cuzick J, Stewart H, Rutqvist L, Houghton J, Edwards R, Redmond C, et al. Cause-specific mortality in long-term survivors of breast cancer who participated in trials of radiotherapy. J Clin Oncol. 1994;12(3):447–53.

59. Darby SC, Ewertz M, McGale P, Bennet AM, Blom-Goldman U, Bronnum D, et al. Risk of ischemic heart disease in women after radiotherapy for breast cancer. N Engl J Med. 2013;368 (11):987–98. doi:10.1056/NEJMoa1209825.

60. Marks LB, Yu X, Prosnitz RG, Zhou SM, Hardenbergh PH, Blazing M, et al. The incidence and functional consequences of RT-associated cardiac perfusion defects. Int J Radiat Oncol Biol Phys. 2005;63(1):214–23. doi:10.1016/j.ijrobp.2005.01.029.

61. Nilsson G, Holmberg L, Garmo H, Duvernoy O, Sjogren I, Lagerqvist B, et al. Distribution of coronary artery stenosis after radiation for breast cancer. J Clin Oncol. 2012;30(4):380–6. doi:10.1200/JCO.2011.34.5900.

62. Brenner DJ, Shuryak I, Jozsef G, Dewyngaert KJ, Formenti SC. Risk and risk reduction of major coronary events associated with contemporary breast radiotherapy. JAMA Intern Med. 2014;174(1):158–60. doi:10.1001/jamainternmed.2013.11790.

63. Ling LH, Oh JK, Schaff HV, Danielson GK, Mahoney DW, Seward JB, et al. Constrictive pericarditis in the modern era: evolving clinical spectrum and impact on outcome after pericardiectomy. Circulation. 1999;100(13):1380–6.

64. Saxena P, Joyce LD, Daly RC, Kushwaha SS, Schirger JA, Rosedahl J, et al. Cardiac transplantation for radiation-induced cardiomyopathy: the Mayo Clinic experience. Ann Thorac Surg. 2014;98(6):2115–21. doi:10.1016/j.athoracsur.2014.06.056.

65. Orzan F, Brusca A, Conte MR, Presbitero P, Figliomeni MC. Severe coronary artery disease after radiation therapy of the chest and mediastinum: clinical presentation and treatment. Br Heart J. 1993;69(6):496–500.

66. Katz NM, Hall AW, Cerqueira MD. Radiation induced valvulitis with late leaflet rupture. Heart. 2001;86(6), E20.

67. Siregar S, de Heer F, van Herwerden LA. Cardiac surgery in patients irradiated for Hodgkin's lymphoma. Neth Heart J. 2010;18(2):61–5.

68. Lancellotti P, Nkomo VT, Badano LP, Bergler-Klein J, Bogaert J, Davin L, et al. Expert consensus for multi-modality imaging evaluation of cardiovascular complications of radiotherapy in adults: a report from the European Association of Cardiovascular Imaging and the American Society of Echocardiography. J Am Soc Echocardiogr. 2013;26(9):1013–32. doi:10. 1016/j.echo.2013.07.005.

69. Girinsky T, M'Kacher R, Lessard N, Koscielny S, Elfassy E, Raoux F, et al. Prospective coronary heart disease screening in asymptomatic Hodgkin lymphoma patients using coronary computed tomography angiography: results and risk factor analysis. Int J Radiat Oncol Biol Phys. 2014;89(1):59–66. doi:10.1016/j.ijrobp.2014.01.021.

Chapter 8
Management of Patients with Coronary Disease and Cancer: Interactions Between Cancer, Cancer Treatment, and Ischemia

Ronald J. Krone, Preet Paul Singh, and Chiara Melloni

Introduction

Coronary artery disease (CAD) and cancer share the same demographics and also lifestyle factors to a certain degree. The age groups where cancer is more common are also the age groups where CAD is common. After age 25, cardiac disease, primarily CAD, and malignancy are the two most common causes of death in adults [1, 2] (Fig. 8.1).

Both diseases are more common with advancing age. In addition to age, cancer and coronary disease share risk factors: smoking, diabetes, obesity, and hypertension [3]. The Framingham risk score not only predicts an increased risk of coronary disease but also colorectal cancer [4]. As a result, management of patients with cancer is often complicated by the presence of CAD, and the management of patients with CAD is often complicated by the presence of cancer. In addition, certain cancer therapies, notably radiation therapy and some antimetabolites especially 5-FU (fluorouracil) and its prodrug capecitabine, actively interact with the vascular endothelium leading to activation of atherosclerosis and cardiac events either concurrently with therapy or after a long latent period (radiation)

Electronic supplementary material: The online version of this chapter (doi:10.1007/978-3-319-43096-6_8) contains supplementary material, which is available to authorized users.

R.J. Krone (✉)
Cardiovascular Division, John T Milliken Department of Internal Medicine,
Washington University Medical School, Saint Louis, MO, USA
e-mail: rkrone@wustl.edu

P.P. Singh
Siteman Cancer Center, 4921 Parkview Pl # 7B, Saint Louis, MO 63110, USA
e-mail: psingh@dom.wustl.edu

C. Melloni
Duke Clinical Research Institute, Durham, NC, USA
e-mail: chiara.melloni@dm.duke.edu

© Springer International Publishing Switzerland 2017
G.G. Kimmick et al. (eds.), *Cardio-Oncology*, DOI 10.1007/978-3-319-43096-6_8

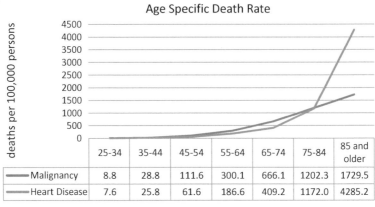

Fig. 8.1 Comparison of age specific death rates for malignancy and cancer, showing that their effects are similar as patients age.

[5–11]. Rarely, as a result of graft versus host disease after bone marrow transplant, the immunologic attack can affect the arteries [12, 13], both coronary and peripheral leading to severe, poorly understood, coronary disease.

The goal of this chapter for the oncologist is to be able to recognize signs that may presage development of manifest coronary ischemia to begin a dialogue with a cardiologist to prevent the development of coronary events which would impact management of the cancer. Once the patient is in the throes of aggressive oncologic therapy, the options for dealing with coronary disease constrict, and management of the coronary disease may be compromised. Early identification of patients at risk for coronary disease may permit the initiation of therapies which may forestall the overt development of coronary events. The oncologist does not need to actually treat the coronary disease, but he/she needs to know when there is a risk of this scenario and start a dialogue.

Pathophysiology of Coronary Atherosclerosis

Atherosclerotic development is a dynamic process which begins early in life, with injury to the endothelium through a variety of interactions and then progresses over time until the vessel lumen is compromised and clinical symptoms are produced. It begins with inactivation of endothelial vasodilation by impairing the production of nitric oxide, the major vasodilator. Endothelial dysfunction is associated with most traditional risk factors: hypercholesterolemia, diabetes, hypertension, cigarette smoking, and especially oxidized low-density lipoprotein (LDL). The oxidized

LDL cholesterol enters the media cell and is taken up by macrophages, forming foam cells. These cells ultimately die leading to the development of a necrotic core in the media. This leads to intimal thickening, fibroatheroma formation with a lesion consisting of a necrotic core with a thin-cap fibroatheroma. This thin-cap fibroatheroma has been called "the vulnerable plaque" as it has a tendency to rupture, leading to acute thrombosis of the vessel [14, 15]. Acute thrombosis can also occur as a result of erosion of the endothelium at the plaque which produces a thrombogenic stress [16]. The rupture of this plaque or the plaque erosion leads to the clinical state of acute coronary syndrome (ACS) which may present as an acute closure of an epicardial artery and subsequent development of ST-segment elevation acute myocardial infarction (STEMI) (type I myocardial infarction) [17] leading to a transmural myocardial infarction [18]. If the resulting thrombus is subtotally occlusive, the ACS can present as a smaller infarction (non-transmural) without elevation of the ST segments: the non-STEMI (NSTEMI) or NSTEMI-ACS [17]. In both events, necrosis of myocardial cells leads to release of cardio-specific proteins and enzymes which constitute cardiac biomarkers such as troponin and CK-MB. Unstable angina is the third manifestation of ACS, and it is also caused by a partial occlusion of the lumen of an epicardial artery, but without myocardial cell death and subsequent elevation in cardiac markers. It has been convincingly opined that as biomarkers become more sensitive, the distinction between NSTEMI-ACS and unstable angina will be lost [19], so in this chapter we will describe ACS as either STEMI or NSTEMI-ACS. ACS is an unstable condition and, if untreated, frequently progresses to a complete occlusion with a transmural infarction.

Chronic stable coronary disease follows different pathway. The plaques can progress into more complicated lesions with fibrosis and calcification, without rupture. There can be hemorrhage into the lipid core which does not expose the necrotic center to the circulating blood, so the lumen may be compromised little by little. ACS does not develop but exercise tolerance or the ability to respond to increased demand is compromised [20]. In situations of extreme demand, such as would occur with surgery, sepsis, hypotension, severe anemia, severe hypertension, and pulmonary embolism with right heart decompensation [17], troponin may be released which defines a NSTEMI type II infarction, a supply/demand imbalance [17]. There can be significant atherosclerosis and lipid accumulation without compromise of the lumen as a result of positive remodeling of the artery where the plaque essentially expands the outer wall of the artery so the lumen may be maintained. This can allow a larger plaque burden to be carried without symptoms [21]. However, these lesions with large plaque burdens may ultimately lead to an ACS infarction at a later date. A goal of therapy, in these cases, is to lower the circulating lipid levels, to permit some stabilization of the plaque interrupting this path to disaster.

Chemotherapy and Promotion of Acute Coronary Syndrome

A number of chemotherapeutic agents have been associated with ischemic events and myocardial infarction [22, 23]. In addition to 5-FU and capecitabine which cause endothelial injury and vasospasm, a wide variety of other agents have been associated with endothelial injury and vasospasm leading to angina, acute coronary syndrome, and myocardial infarction. Paclitaxel and docetaxel-antimicrotubule agents have been associated with these complications [24]. Cisplatin is associated with endothelial damage, platelet activation, and platelet aggregation [25, 26] and has been reported to provoke coronary spasm causing ischemia [27]. When cisplatin is given with bleomycin or vinblastine, endothelial damage can be severe [28]. The vascular endothelial growth factor signaling pathway inhibitors, sunitinib and sorafenib, are associated with marked increase in cardiovascular events [29]. Tyrosine kinase inhibitors including pazopanib, nilotinib, and ponatinib are also associated with progression of coronary disease. Bevacizumab is associated with an increased risk of ischemic heart disease and events [30]. Other drugs which act using hormonal therapy such as aromatase inhibitors, antiandrogens, and others used to treat prostate cancer are associated with myocardial infarctions and angina [31].

Thus, many of the drugs used to treat cancer are known by one mechanism or another to cause or exacerbate cardiac ischemia or even infarction. It has also been shown that a person can harbor a large atherosclerotic burden without overt symptoms. The stresses of cancer treatment, surgery, drug-induced vasospasm, thrombosis, platelet activation, and endothelial damage can "activate" the coronary disease to cause acute coronary syndrome. Alternatively the demands on the heart during non-cardiac surgery or the development of sepsis may stress the coronary reserve and bring coronary disease to the foreground. The similar demographics of cancer and coronary disease suggests that certainly middle-aged and senior patients could harbor an atherosclerotic burden that could set the stage for an acute coronary syndrome. The likelihood of actively developing the coronary complications of chemotherapy is greater in the presence of coronary disease and the injury can be greater. This makes the case to evaluate the patient's risk for coronary disease prior to or simultaneous with treating the cancer so that coronary risk reduction can be performed prophylactically. The major modifiable risk factors are abnormal lipids, hypertension, cigarette smoking, and diabetes (Table 8.1) [32].

Risk Factors and Risk Factor Modification

Standard risk factors such as diabetes, hypertension, hypercholesterolemia, smoking, and obesity need to be addressed in all cases. Smoking cessation, control of diabetes, and control of hypertension all reduce inflammatory stresses on the endothelium and atherosclerotic progression can be controlled in many cases using available risk modification therapy [32–34].

Table 8.1 Risk factors for coronary disease

• Age
• Smoking history (any smoking)
• Family history of coronary disease (coronary interventions, coronary bypass, myocardial infarctions) in relatives <55 years of age
• Diabetes—especially insulin-requiring
• Lipid profile (need not be fasting 2 h after a meal)
• Peripheral vascular disease (carotid and/or femoral bruits)
• Coronary calcifications (can be seen on non-contrast CT examinations of the chest)(Fig. 8.2)
• Risk can be evaluated at http://my.americanheart.org/cvriskcalculator and http://www.cardiosource.org/scienceand-quality/practice-guidelines-and-quality-standards/2013-prevention-guideline-tools.aspx

While hypertension and diabetes need to be controlled, the most effective therapy both for primary and secondary prevention of coronary events is with hydroxymethylglutaryl-CoA reductase inhibitors (statins). Statins have been shown to improve survival in patients with high cholesterol and those who have proven coronary disease [35]. The mechanism of this protection is not clear, since improved survival has been shown by 6 months after the start of the treatment, well before any change in lesion size has occurred [35, 36]. The reduction in clinical events was far greater than what one would expect from the limited lesion regression. This suggests that the statins may cause regression of the lipid-rich lesions which are prone to rupture and or that statins impact atherosclerosis through mechanisms not related to anatomic changes [37, 38].

This concept has been carried further in the most recent guidelines for the use of statins in coronary disease [34] where statin use is indicated over a broad range of LDL values in persons with documented coronary disease and those at high risk of developing it.

The risk for coronary disease has been quantified in several models [39]. A model estimating 10-year and lifetime risk for atherosclerotic cardiovascular disease and calculators are available at http://my.americanheart.org/cvriskcalculator and http://www.cardiosource.org/scienceand-quality/practice-guidelines-and-quality-standards/2013-prevention-guideline-tools.aspx. Coronary calcifications, a marker of coronary disease, may also be seen on staging CT scans in cancer patients (Fig. 8.2).

Because of the results of statin therapy even in patients with cholesterol levels formerly thought to be "normal," the recent guidelines for the use of statin therapy are based more on anticipated risk than on actual levels of LDL cholesterol [34]. The abandonment of targets of LDL has not been without controversy, but identifying populations at risk where statin therapy has been effective may permit protection to persons at risk for developing manifest coronary disease. In addition to the usual risk factors for the development of coronary disease, as established by population studies, the Framingham risk factors, smoking, diabetes, family history with manifest coronary disease in a first-degree relative at age 55 or below, and

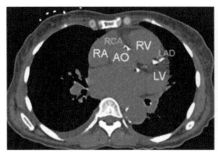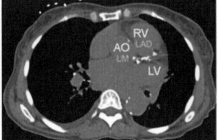

Fig. 8.2 (**a**) Frame from CT of chest showing calcium in LAD and right coronary arteries. (**b**) Frame from CT of chest showing calcification in left main and proximal LAD and circumflex

hypertension, treatment with statins has been recommended for four cohorts of patients [34]:

1. Patients with LDL cholesterol greater than 190 mg%
2. Patients with known coronary or peripheral vascular disease
3. Patients with diabetics and LDL cholesterol levels greater than 70 mg%
4. Patients whose risk calculation is greater than 7.5 % in the next 10 years based on the previously referred model [34]

Assessment before embarking on a course of potentially stressful oncologic therapy is analogous to assessing the coronary risk in a person undergoing non-cardiac surgery. That person, much like the cancer patient, will be undergoing similar stresses, anemia, hypotension, and the potential for sepsis, but the cancer patient also has the potential addition of thrombocytopenia as a result of therapy as well as a potential prothrombotic state [40]. Because of the need for prolonged double antiplatelet therapy (DAPT) after coronary stenting, or the need for hemostasis with coronary artery surgery in the cancer patient, interventions and treatment options may be limited if there is the development of ACS during cancer treatment. Thus an aggressive approach to minimizing coronary risk factors is rational [41]. The mainstay of this "prophylactic" approach, in addition to smoking cessation and control of blood pressure, is aggressive treatment of hyperlipidemia with a statin.

The statins differ in their metabolic pathways. Simvastatin and atorvastatin both are metabolized by the P450 CPY3A4 pathway [42, 43], so that interactions with other drugs, especially drugs used in cancer therapy, some antibiotics and antifungals, are a potential concern in cancer patients (Table 8.2). On the other hand, pravastatin, rosuvastatin, and pitavastatin are excreted largely unchanged and do not interact with the metabolism of other drugs. For that reason many cardio-oncologists prefer to use rosuvastatin or pravastatin as their statin of first choice to avoid interactions. At this time, however, that does pose some real-world problems. Pravastatin is not as effective in lowering the LDL cholesterol as the other statins, while rosuvastatin [34] is perhaps the most efficient in reducing cholesterol.

Table 8.2 Drugs commonly used in cancer patients that are CYP3A4 substrates

Chemotherapeutic agents	Anti-inflammatory agents	Other medications
Etoposide	Cyclosporine	Alprazolam
Doxorubicin	Tacrolimus	Carbamazepine
Ifosfamide	Sirolimus	Macrolide antibiotics
Vincristine	Tamoxifen	Imidazoles
Busulfan		
Everolimus		
Targeted antineoplastic agents		
Imatinib		
Ibrutinib		
Olaparib		
Ruxolitinib		
Sunitinib		
Bosutinib		

A partial list of medications commonly given to cancer patients which are a substrate of the CYP3A4 metabolic pathway. The statins simvastatin and atorvastatin also share this pathway so that serum levels of these drugs change when co-administered and may lead to elevated levels of the statins leading to rhabdomyolysis or unpredictable changes in the levels of the chemotherapeutic drugs [44–47].

ACS Diagnosis and Treatment

Cardiac troponin (cTN) plays a central role in assessing myocardial injury and, especially, the management of coronary artery disease [48]. The cardiac troponin complex has been used for over 15 years as the definitive marker of myocardial necrosis. The troponin complex, consisting of three subunits is located on the actin (thin) filament of striated muscle. Troponin C, the subunit that actually binds calcium is the same in striated and cardiac muscle, but the subunits troponin I which modulates the binding of actin and myosin and troponin T which binds the troponin complex to tropomyosin to complete the actin myosin linkage, have different isoforms in cardiac and skeletal muscle and so are better markers isolating cardiac injury/infarction [49].

Troponin is released when there is myocardial injury or infarction. A number of clinical situations can lead to cardiac injury reflected in low-level elevations in cTN in the absence of coronary disease. These have been enumerated [17, 50] and reflect supply/demand imbalance or underlying myocardial disease. For the patient with cancer, the common scenarios leading to elevated troponin, which may not reflect coronary disease, include atrial tachyarrhythmia, sepsis or septic shock, severe anemia, severe respiratory failure, severe hypertension, coronary spasm, stress cardiomyopathy (takotsubo), or significant pulmonary embolism, among others [17]. Of course, underlying chronic coronary disease, which may not cause symptoms, may lower the threshold for myocardial injury in such situations. Before assuming the limited troponin elevation is due to demand, however, severe underlying coronary disease must be considered. A history of angina, electrocardiographic evidence of infarction, or segmental hypokinesia on an echocardiogram would be clues to a serious underlying coronary stenosis, which may require further evaluation, before dismissing it as the result of increased demand.

Before addressing the specific problems posed by the patients with cancer, it is useful to discuss management of patients with coronary disease in general.

Chronic stable angina in most cases can be handled by reducing demand with beta-blockers; reducing progression of atheroma with aggressive statin administration, control of blood pressure, and excellent management of diabetes; improving cardiac metabolism with ranolazine [51–53]; enhancing coronary vasodilation with nitrates and calcium channel blockers; and reducing thrombogenicity and platelet inhibition with smoking cessation and aspirin in most cases [32, 54–57]. The decision to perform revascularization in patients with chronic stable coronary disease has been a major area of research almost from the development of revascularization procedures [58]. Several studies have shown that in stable patients, in the absence of certain anatomic lesions, such as left main obstruction or large areas of jeopardized myocardium, if symptoms can be controlled medically, there is no survival advantage to revascularization [55, 58–64]. If the symptoms cannot be controlled medically, then revascularization with either coronary artery bypass grafting (CABG) or percutaneous coronary intervention (PCI) is beneficial. The BARI-2D [56] and COURAGE trials compared intervention to medical therapy [65] in patients with stable coronary artery disease. Only 40 % of patients randomized to medical therapy in each trial ultimately required revascularization, primarily to control symptoms which could not be controlled with medical therapy alone [61]. This has been confirmed in other studies [32].

In contrast, acute coronary syndrome requires immediate action [66]. For the acutely occluded artery presenting as a myocardial infarction with ST-segment elevation (STEMI) on the electrocardiogram, success in salvaging myocardium is measured in minutes from the time of occlusion (severe symptoms) until some flow is restored. PCI is the treatment of choice if technically feasible, since surgery in these situations will take longer to institute and results are not necessarily better. In situations with severe multivessel disease, the infarct artery is opened, and then treatment of the other lesions is individualized, with acute multivessel interventions or a staged PCI. If PCI is not technically feasible, then CABG at a later date can complete the revascularization.

In patients presenting with an acute infarction without ST-segment elevation NSTEMI-ACS or "unstable angina," the situation is quite unpredictable, usually a lesion has been unroofed, and a thrombus is forming at the site, which is not yet totally occlusive but certainly has a high likelihood of progressing in a short time [67, 68]. This situation also requires prompt evaluation and treatment. The presence of elevated troponin or ECG changes with symptoms or continuing or recurrent pain identifies patients at high risk [69]. Delay beyond 24 h in high-risk patients is associated with increased 30-day mortality (Table 8.3) [71]. Almost all patients who have suitable anatomy and acceptable procedural risk are revascularized [50]. Medical therapy is usually not adequate to control the situation in the long term, but

Table 8.3 Criteria for high-risk NSTEMI-ACS with indication for invasive management

Primary
Relevant rise or fall in troponin
Dynamic ST- or T-wave changes (symptomatic or silent)
Continuing or recurrent pain
Secondary
Diabetes mellitus
Renal insufficiency (eGFR <60 mL/min/1.73 m^2)
Reduced LV function (ejection fraction <40 %)
Early postinfarction angina
Recent PCI
Prior CABG
Intermediate to high GRACE risk score [70] http://www.outomes.org/grace

anticoagulation and platelet inhibition can usually cool the process down. The decision as to type of definitive therapy can only be made after the coronary anatomy is visualized and is made on an individual basis. An experienced interventionalist can stent most complex anatomies, left main, ostial or proximal LAD, or ostial circumflex lesions or bifurcation lesions, but certain situations are best treated, ideally, with coronary artery bypass graft surgery (CABG). In a substudy by Holvang of the FRISC study of dalteparin in patients with NSTEMI-ACS [49], patients with more ST depression were more likely to undergo bypass surgery because of a higher prevalence of two- and three-vessel disease or left main disease. The choice of therapy requires consideration of the type of cancer, the expected effect of cancer therapy especially on platelets, and the need for cancer surgery in the near future so that in this situation, active consultation with the oncologist is essential.

Revascularization Options for Coronary Disease

Percutaneous coronary intervention (PCI) has been evolving since its introduction by Andreas Gruentzig in 1977 [72, 73]. The initial problems of consistency, stability in the acute setting, and restenosis have been minimized if not solved, and many devices are available to conquer difficult problems such as plaque burden in grafts (filters), thrombotic burden in acute infarction, and heavily calcified lesions (*rotational [74] or orbital athrectomy*) [75]. The introduction of coronary stents in 1985 by Sigwart et al. [76] revolutionized PCI [77], essentially eliminating the need for standby cardiac surgery. Although stents presented many serious problems, most notably thrombosis of the stent and restenosis of the lesion, these problems have been reduced so that the incidence of these complications is low. The problem of immediate and late stent thrombosis has been minimized by emphasis on perfect stent positioning and sizing, out to the medial elastic lamina of the vessel and avoiding stent edge dissections aided by routine use of intravascular ultrasound [78, 79]. In cancer patients where there is a possibility of premature termination of DAPT because of a need for additional cancer surgery or severe thrombocytopenia, perfect stent positioning using ultrasound is essential [41]. The recognition of the role of the platelet in thrombosis and the development of effective antiplatelet agents has minimized the occurrence of stent thrombosis [80–82]. Drug-eluting stents (DESs) using an anti-inflammatory agent bonded to the stent were introduced to reduce the occurrence of restenosis, but these early versions of the drug-eluting stents were susceptible to late thrombosis [83] from hypersensitivity to the polymer [84] or delayed healing or endothelialization [83, 84]. Current stents have been redesigned to limit that problem and have reduced [83] the thrombogenicity, but concern remains [85–87]. A recent study by Valgimigli (ZEUS) [88] and reviewed by Kandzari [89] compared the performance of Endeavor zotarolimus-eluting stent (ZES), designed to improve the rate of endothelialization, with that of bare-metal stents (BMS) in patients thought to be at risk for noncompliance with double antiplatelet therapy (DAPT)-aspirin plus a thienopyridine. In this study, by 30 days 43.6 % of patients had discontinued DAPT (aspirin + a thienopyridine) and by 60 days 62.5 % had done so. The rates of death, myocardial infarction, and stent thrombosis were all lower than the BMS, and the rate of 1-year target vessel revascularization was lower (10.7 % vs 5.9 %) with the ZES.

The original recommendation for duration of DAPT had been to continue the DAPT for 1 year, but the question as to the (minimal) optimal duration with DAPT remains open [90]. Several studies have been reported, and others are in progress to determine if a 6-month DAPT treatment plan would be adequate [91, 92]. Gilard et al. evaluated patients who obtained a Xience V everolimus-eluting stent and who demonstrated responsiveness to aspirin and found non-inferiority in a study, comparing 6 and 12 months of DAPT [93]. On the other hand, Yeh et al. in a review found a lower risk of stent thrombosis and infarction (although a doubling of the risk of bleeding) in patients remaining on DAPT for 30 months [92]. There are no studies comparing optimal duration of DAPT in patients with cancer, so recommendations need to be extrapolated from the available data in patients without cancer, a process that is not necessarily justified [94].

Prasugrel and ticagrelor have since been approved for preventing stent thrombosis. Studies have shown improved results over clopidogrel for stent thrombosis but at a higher risk of bleeding, especially intracranial hemorrhage [95–97]. Patients with cancer were not studied, and there is no experience with these drugs in patients who are thrombocytopenic—for obvious reasons.

Non-cardiac Surgery in Recently Stented Patients: Considerations About Stent Type and Timing of Surgery

Non-cardiac surgery after an artery is stented carries a high risk of stent thrombosis, especially until the stent is incorporated into the vessel wall. This was first reported following surgery within 2 weeks of stenting with BMS with four deaths in patients

Table 8.4 MACE after surgery after percutaneous coronary interventions with stents: the importance of time from procedure [99]

Time from surgery	<30 days	30–90 days	3 months	3–6 months	6-12 months	>12 months
MACE after bare-metal stent	50 %	14 %	4 %			
MACE after drug-eluting stent	35 %	13 %		15 %	6 %	9 %

operated within 1 day of the stenting [98]. The evaluation of the risks following DES placement was based on the first-generation DES which is known to have a higher risk of stent thrombosis than the subsequent generations of stents. Surgery has traditionally been delayed 1 year for elective procedures with semi-elective procedures put off for 6 months [32]. The risk of major adverse cardiac events (MACE) in the experience of the Erasmus Medical Center was reported, and a very high risk of complications was found with both DES and BMS within 30 days, with the complication rate dropping off with delays up to a year [99]. The rate of MACE during non-cardiac surgery for the intervals of <30 days, 30 days to 3 months, and >3 months was 50 %, 14 %, and 4 % in patients getting BMS and for patients getting DES was 35 %, 13 %, 15 %, 6 %, and 9 % for patients undergoing non-cardiac surgery <30 days, 30 days to 3 months, 3–6 months, 6–12 months, and > 12 months, respectively (Table 8.4). This is consistent with other reports [100–108].

Recent guidelines for performing non-cardiac surgery in patients after PCI show a conservative recommendation delaying all elective surgery for 1 year after a drug-eluting stent and 4–12 weeks after a BMS stent [106, 109, 110]. The European guideline permits surgery after a new-generation DES after 6 months [106], but the US guideline recommends delaying elective surgery 1 year for all DESs [111]. The ACC/AHA guidelines do permit surgery after 6 months if the risks of waiting outweigh the risk of the surgery. The recent data on the everolimus-eluting stents, the Endeavor or the Xience V, have not yet been incorporated into these guidelines, but the data are only on spontaneous MACE, not on the MACE following non-cardiac surgery. The prothrombotic state of both surgery and cancer [40] could be expected to increase the occurrence of MACE in the perioperative period.

A careful analysis of the relative advantages of coronary bypass surgery and PCI has been presented in the European Guideline for the Diagnosis and Management of Patients with Stable Ischemic Heart Disease [32, 54] and the American counterpart [54]. The decision as to whether PCI with a drug-eluting stent is the superior treatment when compared with CABG even in patients without cancer is somewhat limited by the paucity of randomized clinical trials [112]. However, it seems reasonable to conclude from SYNTAX which quantified the complexity of the coronary anatomy that outcomes of patients undergoing PCI or CABG in those with relatively uncomplicated and lesser degrees of CAD are comparable, whereas in

Table 8.5 Recommendations for timing of surgery after previous percutaneous coronary intervention

Type of PCI	2014 ESC/ESA guidelines [106]	2014 ACC/AHA guidelines [111]
BMS	4 weeks to 3 months (I, B)	≥30 days (I, B)
DES	≥12 months (IIa, B)	≥12 months (I, B) ≥6 months (IIb, B)
New-generation DES	≥6 months (IIa, B)	
Balloon angioplasty	≥2 weeks (IIa, B)	≥2 weeks (I, C)

PCI percutaneous coronary intervention, *BMS* bare-metal stent, *DES* drug-eluting stent [109]

those with complex and diffuse CAD, CABG appears to be preferable [54]. Most studies have shown that patients with diabetes with three-vessel disease do better in the long run with CABG than with PCI [113]. The long-term results are in part dependent on the complexity of the lesion as well as other factors such as impaired renal function which will be taxed if repeated procedures are required, which is often the case with PCI (Table 8.5).

The circumstance of a cancer patient diagnosed with CAD during active cancer therapy carries a different risk/benefit ratio, and the algorithms that guide ACS management may not apply in the setting of ongoing cancer management. Decision-making needs to consider multiple priorities, both related to the acuity/severity of the cardiac condition, as well as the stage, treatment plan, and goals of care for the cancer. This requires active communication between the oncologist and the cardiologist, The severity and acuity of the coronary disease, the severity and stage of the cancer, the renal function which may be damaged with repeated PCI procedures, the anticipated long-term toxicity of the cancer therapy, the likelihood of developing severe thrombocytopenia on treatment, and the need for cancer surgery within 6 months of the cardiac event all need to be considered by both the oncologist and cardiologist to optimize the overall treatment of the patient. In a patient actively receiving cancer therapy, the primary indication for urgent revascularization is acute coronary syndrome (ACS), where the risks of inaction are high. Additionally, revascularization could be considered in a patient with chronic stable coronary disease where complex cancer surgery is urgently needed and it is felt that the patient would be unable to tolerate the procedure unless some revascularization was done in advance (usually limited to severe left main disease or very proximal anterior descending involving the left main) (Fig. 8.3).

PCI poses several specific problems to the cancer patient but has several important positive aspects. The advantage for PCI is that the procedure is well tolerated and recovery is fast. Frailty and the physical stress of recovery as well as delaying chemotherapy (if thrombocytopenia is not an issue) are not a concern.

However:

1. Bare-metal stents are associated with a high rate of restenosis, possibly as high as 50 % in a year, but only require DAPT for 4–6 weeks at a minimum.
2. Drug-eluting stents reduce the rate of restenosis but require long term, 6–12 months of dual platelet suppression therapy with aspirin and clopidogrel

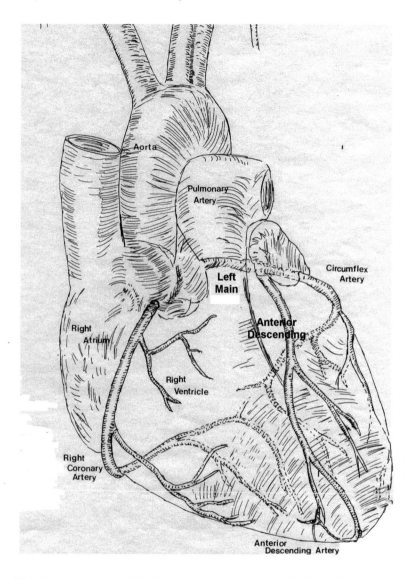

Fig. 8.3 The coronary vessels. The left main divides into the anterior descending and circumflex arteries which supply most of the heart. The anterior descending usually supplies the septum, the apex, and much of the anterolateral wall. The circumflex supplies the lateral wall and a variable amount of the inferior wall. The right coronary supplies the right ventricle and the inferior septum and a variable amount of the inferior–posterior and occasionally lateral wall

[93, 102]. While there is some optimism that the newest generation of stents will endothelialize sooner so that the double platelet therapy can be stopped earlier [88, 89], there are no studies in cancer patients to justify that, and frankly, none are expected.

3. Complex "off-label" stenting (which is used about 50 % of the time [83] and includes long lesions and bifurcation lesions with multiple stents) is associated with delayed endothelialization, which may increase the risk of stent thrombosis under stress. The prothrombotic state found in cancer may be that stress [40, 114].
4. There is some theoretical concern that cancer therapy, designed to inhibit cell growth or inflammation, may impact the endothelialization of the stent [115, 116] which could make it less desirable to reduce the period of DAPT therapy, but there are no data to support this.
5. Non-cardiac surgery in a patient with recent PCI with stent placement carries a high risk of major adverse cardiac events (MACE), death, nonfatal MI, and need for urgent revascularization which is quite high in the 30 days after the stent is placed, and it declines over the first 6 months after the stent is in place. Surgery is commonly employed in the treatment of cancer so this becomes a great concern and can have a major impact on the choice of cancer treatment.

In hematological malignancies, after bone marrow transplant, or as a side effect of gemcitabine, carboplatin, TDM-1 (ado-trastuzumab emtansine), nucleoside inhibitors and others or multi-agent chemotherapy, thrombocytopenia can be severe. The need for DAPT after the stent is placed is a great concern in these patients, although actual data are sparse, but surprisingly encouraging [41, 117]. The development of newer DESs that may not require a year of DAPT [88] has the potential to reduce the risk of this therapy in the future. The limited experience reported suggests that DES may be used, and perhaps ZES, but a prospective study or registry is needed to state this with confidence.

Coronary artery bypass surgery is the alternative method of revascularization. If the therapy for the cancer is expected to lead to severe thrombocytopenia or if non-cardiac surgery is planned in the near future, CABG may be considered as alternative since it poses less of a problem than placing a DES with the need for DAPT, regardless of severe thrombocytopenia. If the patient will require major surgery to remove a cancer, it may be possible to perform both the CABG and the cancer surgery at the same "sitting" or as a two-stage procedure to minimize the delay in the cancer surgery [118, 119]. Frailty adds to CABG risk and may be present in cancer patients [120–123].

1. Recovery from CABG will take at least 2–4 weeks with major impact on quality of life plus draining strength. This is something to consider in the setting of advanced cancer when much time may be spent recovering from CABG.
2. CABG may also delay initiation of chemotherapy to allow for satisfactory wound healing.
3. Immune suppression with chemotherapy and/or the cancer puts patients at risk for non-healing and postoperative infections, most importantly sternal infections.

The cardiologist needs to understand goals of cancer therapy. A sizeable proportion of patients with cancer are treated with curative intent with primary surgery and preoperative or postoperative chemotherapy (generally for fixed duration of

3–6 months). It is important for these patients to receive timely cancer therapy, so interventions for CAD should be chosen to minimize delay or interference with cancer therapy. Definitive treatments like CABG may be delayed till after completion of cancer therapy. Other patients with cancer (typically metastatic cancer or stage IV disease) are seldom cured with anticancer therapy. The patient's non-cardiac prognosis must be a part of the decision-making for selecting the appropriate cardiac intervention, and "the objectives for such patients may be limited to symptom relief and improved quality of life, obtained with the minimum of early hazard and with the shortest duration of functional recovery" [124].

Patients with chronic stable angina usually can be managed in the short run without revascularization. Consider these outcomes of PCI:

- PCI reduces the incidence of angina.
- PCI has not been demonstrated to improve survival in stable patients.
- PCI may increase the short-term risk of MI.
- PCI does not lower the long-term risk of MI [54].

Since the major indication for most patients is a relief of symptoms, there is no imperative to "protect" the patient from cardiac events by performing revascularization. Thus in patients with chronic stable angina or underlying silent ischemia, aggressive medical therapy with the aim of avoiding PCI or surgery during ongoing chemotherapy should be considered until the cancer is stable.

The situation with ACS is quite different. STEMI is a true emergency. The prognosis of a patient with an occluded infarct-related artery is orders of magnitude worse than the prognosis of a patient whose artery is opened promptly and myocardium is protected or salvaged. Myocardium is infarcting and the only way to prevent that or to minimize it is to open the infarct-related artery as promptly as possible. In the case of the active cancer or chemotherapy, this means to develop a technique that permits operating in the setting of possible neutropenia and/or thrombocytopenia.

PCI requires placing a catheter in an artery to access the central circulation, passing the catheter to the ostia of the two coronary arteries, and usually inserting a stent in the "culprit" artery to prevent immediate vessel closure and long-term restenosis. Anticoagulation of the patient with a thrombin inhibitor, usually heparin, is routinely performed to avoid thrombosis in the radial or coronary artery during the procedure.

There are essentially two techniques for access: the femoral artery approach and the radial artery approach. The brachial artery was the original access site, entered with a cut down and suturing the vessel after completion of the procedure, but the simplicity and speed of the percutaneous technique aided by the development of smaller equipment has essentially made the brachial cutdown approach obsolete. Percutaneous brachial access, especially in a thrombocytopenic patient, includes a high risk of brachial hemorrhage with the potential for a compartment syndrome entrapping the median nerve. In thrombocytopenic patients where femoral or radial access is not feasible, brachial artery access utilizing direct entry with direct suture after the procedure remains an option.

With either the femoral or radial approach, care must be taken to avoid uncontrollable bleeding. Although the radial approach takes advantage of the very superficial artery, which simplifies hemostasis after the procedure, there are certain pitfalls that can negate that advantage. The radial approach is a bit more technically challenging so it should not be attempted in thrombocytopenic persons by inexperienced operators. Anatomical variations can lead to failure in 3–7 % of procedures [125], and technical difficulties, mostly with the guide wire, have led to severe bleeding in the arm leading to a compartment syndrome and mediastinal hemorrhage when the right internal thoracic (mammary) artery was entered instead of the ascending aorta and perforated with the wire [126]. Occasionally severe spasm can develop, especially when the radial recurrent artery is inadvertently entered, but hemostasis after the procedure is simpler and more definite using wristband pressure devices.

The femoral approach suffers from the potential to enter the external iliac artery in the retroperitoneum if the entry is too proximal, with the result that hemostasis after the procedure (when the patient is on heparin and antiplatelet agents) is not possible, and thrombosis must be depended upon for hemostasis after the procedure [127]. Entry into the common femoral artery can be assured by entering the artery over the lower half of the femoral head. This approach can be made safer using a "micropuncture set" to establish the safety of the entry prior to enlarging the entry or ultrasound guidance [41, 128]. Closure devices have been devised to plug the hole or suture it, but these devices not infrequently fail, or if arterial entry is in a branch, the closure device cannot be used so that a femoral approach under the best of circumstances carries a risk of uncontrolled bleeding after the procedure [41]. In an obese individual, this becomes more of an issue since pressure on the entry site is not assured and considerable bleeding can be hidden in the obese thigh. In addition, in an immunocompromised thrombocytopenic person, there is concern that the collagen plug of the puncture site can get infected.

Special Considerations in Thrombocytopenic Patients with ACS

Sarkiss et al. showed the importance of aspirin treatment even in patients who were thrombocytopenic [129]. In a group of 27 patients with ACS and with cancer and platelets <100,000 (mean of 32,000), after 7 days, only 6 % were alive if they had not been given aspirin, and 90 % were living at 7 days if they were. There is also experience using double platelet therapy (DAPT) usually with clopidogrel in patients with thrombocytopenia, with good outcomes [41].

Paradoxically, the safest management strategy is to perform a catheterization and then intervene on the culprit artery if possible. Iliescu describes his experience in the first 50 of his over 200 patients with cancer and thrombocytopenia [117, 130]. The results were excellent and several patients were treated with

DAPT for many months with platelet counts less than 25,000. Patients whose thrombocytopenia was due to sepsis, active bleeding, or disseminated intravascular coagulopathy (DIC) were not candidates for the invasive strategy. Most of the patients were thrombocytopenic as a result of their cancer or its treatment. Patients with myeloid dysplastic syndromes (MDS) or leukemias, bone marrow transplant patients, or patients undergoing chemotherapy, most commonly with taxanes or gemcitabine, constituted the majority of patients, and 94 % of patients he intervened on had ACS. All patients were studied using the radial approach. Glycoprotein (GP) IIb/IIIa platelet receptor inhibitors were not used. There are other considerations in these patients which are yet to be tested. What is the role of the newer-generation drug-eluting stents vs the bare-metal stents? The first-generation DES was known to be thrombogenic, and the vascular endothelium covering was delayed often for 1 year or more. Newer stents have been devised to solve that problem with more rapid elution of the drug to avoid delays in endothelialization, metal scaffolds causing less inflammation, and more flexible to distort the artery less. This has raised the question with at least the Endeavor stent that this stent, which was not as efficient in preventing restenosis as other DESs, might be able to compete favorably with a bare-metal stent in terms of thrombogenicity with a limited period of DAPT [88, 89].

The process of stenting itself needs to be optimal. Early in the experience with stents, when there was great concern about thrombosis with the first bare-metal stents, Colombo et al. [79] showed that with careful stent placement using ultrasound to insure optimal interaction with the vessel wall and overstenting edge dissections, they were able to do almost as well with aspirin alone as using DAPT to prevent stent thrombosis. That principle still applies, and it may be critical in this setting, since it may be necessary to prematurely reduce the antiplatelet therapy if the thrombocytopenia becomes extreme [41]. Strut malposition remained important in late stent thrombosis with the first-generation stents [131]. Other questions remain, especially with complex stenting, bifurcation lesions, etc. In the study by Nakazawa et al., stent placement "off label" (bifurcation complex lesions) was associated with poor coverage of the stent by the endothelium [114]. A number of techniques have been devised to simplify the approach to bifurcation lesions, and it is unproven but logical to use the simplest approach possible, minimizing stenting both branches if possible, using a technique of stenting the side branch only if the stenosis remained severe (provisional stenting using the "jailed" wire technique) [132].

Coronary Artery Bypass Grafting for Coronary Stenosis

Coronary insufficiency can also be treated with coronary artery bypass surgery. Coronary bypass often improves the completeness of the revascularization. Studies comparing PCI and bypass often show that while the survival may be similar in most cases, the percutaneous route ends up with more repeat procedures

[133]. However, there may be an increased risk of strokes, and the morbidity is greater with CABG. Importantly for cancer patients, recovery is a problem for a frail person who is dealing with an aggressive cancer. On the other hand, if there is a concern about needing major surgery soon after revascularization, coronary bypass may be safer [134], since even after 6 months there still is concern for stent thrombosis even with continuation of the DAPT [108, 135]. This risk of stent thrombosis needs to be balanced against the morbidity of the CABG surgery. Hawn et al. in a large VA study found a rate of 11.6 % MACE for people operated within 6 weeks of a stent, falling to 6.4 % for operations up to 6 months, 4.2 % if operated within 6–12 months, and 3.5 % after 12 months whether or not DAPT was maintained [136].

Non-cardiac Surgery in the Patient with Stable Coronary Artery Disease

A common role for the cardiologist is "clearing" a patient for major non-cardiac cancer surgery. Recent guidelines from the European Society of Cardiology and the European Society of Anesthesiology [106, 109] have emphasized evaluation in three domains: functional evaluation of the patient, characterization of the patient's risk for coronary disease, and the risk of the surgery itself.

The risk of the surgery itself has been characterized as low, intermediate, and high (Table 8.6). Patients are evaluated by functional capacity and are at low risk if they are able to walk 100 m at 3–6 km/h or climb two flights of stairs, the number of cardiac risk factors based on the Revised Cardiac Risk Index (history of ischemic heart disease, history of congestive heart failure, history of cerebrovascular disease, preoperative treatment with insulin, and preoperative serum creatinine >2.0 mg/ dL), and the risk of the surgery [137]. The preoperative risk of perioperative cardiac arrest or infarction can also be calculated using an interactive risk calculator based

Table 8.6 Risk of surgery: modified from ESC/ESA guidelines on non-cardiac surgery [106, 109]

Low-risk surgery <1 %	Intermediate risk 1–5 %	High risk >5 %
Superficial surgery	Intraperitoneal splenectomy, hiatal hernia repair, cholecystectomy	Major abdominal surgery involving pancreas, liver, etc
Breast surgery	Head and neck surgery	Esophagectomy
Endocrine thyroid	Hip and spine surgery	Repair of perforated bowel
	Major urological surgery	Pulmonary or liver transplant
	Nonmajor intrathoracic	Pneumonectomy
		Total cystectomy
		Adrenal resection

on the American College of Surgeons National Surgical Quality Improvement Program (NSQIP) database (http://www.surgicalriskcalculator.com/miorcardia carrest). The five predictors of perioperative myocardial infarction or cardiac arrest using the NSQIP database were type of surgery, dependent functional status, abnormal creatinine, American Society of Anesthesiologists' class, and increasing age.

Preoperative ECG is recommended only for patients with more than one clinical risk factors and if over age 65. Stress testing can be considered in patients with excellent or good functional status undergoing high-risk surgery if they have risk factors for coronary disease; otherwise it is discouraged. There is a stronger recommendation for stress testing with imaging in patients with poor functional capacity with three or more risk factors undergoing high-risk surgery.

Preoperative coronary revascularization is rarely indicated since there is no convincing evidence that preoperative revascularization is beneficial in the stable patient [138]. Studies have not shown reduction of complications after presurgical revascularization with the non-cardiac surgery, but there may be some long-term benefit. This decision must be individualized bringing together the risk of the surgery and the likelihood of severe coronary disease [111].

Recommendations for Adjunct Medications During Non-Cardiac Surgery [106, 111]

There are three classes of medication which deserve special mention:

1. *Beta-blockers* have been advocated to reduce the cardiac stress on patients undergoing non-cardiac surgery, but the results obtained with randomized studies have been disappointing. The first large randomized trial, the POISE study, testing this concept failed to show benefit, but rather showed increased mortality and stroke with a large (100 mg) dose of metoprolol started just before surgery. The controversy is whether the dose of metoprolol was too high and/or whether metoprolol itself is not the right drug. A large VA study showed a benefit for perioperative beta-blocker with a reduced 30-day mortality [139]. Because of concern that metoprolol might predispose to stroke by attenuating $\beta2$-adrenoceptor-mediated cerebral vasodilation, more cardioselective beta-blockers were studied in this context. Patients getting bisoprolol with a high $\beta1/\beta2$ affinity of 13.5/1 were compared to patients getting atenolol with a $\beta1/\beta2$ affinity of 4.7/1 and to metoprolol, which is a relatively weak cardioselective beta-blocker with a $\beta1/\beta2$ affinity of 2.3/1. In this single-center retrospective cohort study, patients taking bisoprolol had a fivefold reduction in strokes compared to metoprolol [140]. The European guidelines recommend atenolol or bisoprolol may be considered as the first choice beta-blocker in patients

undergoing non-cardiac surgery [106]. The American Guidelines do not mention this distinction [111]. Current recommendations suggest beta-blockers are protective in patients with several cardiac risk factors undergoing non-cardiac surgery [110, 139] and in patients at risk should be started several weeks in advance and up-titrated as tolerated.

2. Aspirin is another drug that may provide benefit to patients at risk for coronary events during non-cardiac surgery. Clearly anyone who has had a previous stent is advised to continue aspirin. If continuation of aspirin is not recommended during surgery (such as spinal cord surgery), then surgery and aspirin interruption should be delayed at least a year after the stent implantation. Patients at low risk for coronary events without previous PCI based on the Lee revised cardiac index [141] can have aspirin stopped if bleeding is a great concern.

3. Statins have been shown to reduce the coronary complications in patients undergoing vascular surgery and are recommended for preoperative treatment [106, 111]. The data for nonvascular surgery is weaker but generally favorable [142], so statin treatment remains in the European and American guidelines [106, 110, 111]. There really are no data for perioperative statins in patients undergoing nonvascular surgery, but the ACC/AHA guidelines, as well as the European guidelines, do recommended it, with the caveat that there are no data to support its use [110].

These recommendations have been independently reviewed, and after deleting the discredited studies that contributed so heavily to the original guidelines [143], the authors found very little in the way of randomized controlled studies to support the use of statins or beta-blockers in the postoperative period. With beta-blockers, the possible increased mortality in some studies does give pause, but there seems to be no downside to pretreating with statins (as long as possible drug interactions are monitored) [110, 142].

We have shown that coronary disease and cancer inhabit the same demographic, so it is not uncommon to have coronary disease in patients with cancer. Treatment of the known disease and aggressive risk factor reduction is hoped to minimize the likelihood of acute coronary disease becoming manifest and influencing the choices for managing the cancer. For that reason, the oncologist would be wise to screen for coronary risk factors in the cancer patient, and if risk is high, referral to a cardiologist to maximally reduce risk factors and hopefully prevent an interruption or alteration of the cancer therapy. The risk factors were enumerated in Table 8.1 and could be incorporated into a simple history form. In a very real sense, embarking on comprehensive cancer therapy is similar to undergoing surgery (although over a much more protracted time). If treatable risk factors are found, smoking, elevated cholesterol, hypertension, and partnering with a cardiologist can reduce the risk of a cardiac event, which has major implications for cancer treatment.

Special Considerations

5-Fluorouracil and Capecitabine: Cardiotoxicity Patterns (Table 8.7)

The pyrimidine analogue 5-flurouracil and its oral prodrug capecitabine are the most common cause of cardiotoxicity after anthracyclines [144], but their toxicity has a special predilection to cause problems with cardiac ischemia. The mechanism of cytotoxicity of 5-FU has been ascribed to the misincorporation of fluoronucleotides into RNA and DNA and to the inhibition of the thymidylate synthase enzyme [145]. While 5-FU has been used in head and neck and breast cancers, its greatest impact has been in gastrointestinal cancers, usually in combination with other agents [146, 147]. While response rates with 5-FU in colorectal cancer are only 10–15 % when used alone, in combination with other agents (e.g., oxaliplatin) response rates of 40–50 % have been reported [145].

Capecitabine is an oral prodrug which through a series of enzymatic steps involving thymidine phosphorylase (TP) in the tumor gets converted to 5-FU [148]. Since TP is at higher concentration in tumors, the capecitabine can develop higher concentrations of 5-FU in the tumor than in the body overall, but it still causes systemic or coronary vascular problems, although at a lower frequency than infusional 5-FU and not necessarily in the same patients [149]. However, its cardiotoxicity is similar to that of 5-FU itself [150–152]. The most common symptom of cardiotoxicity with 5-FU is angina, and the most accepted hypothesis attributes 5-FU cardiotoxicity to coronary vasospasm, which seems to be triggered by 5-FU or its metabolites. The risk of cardiotoxicity is highest with protracted infusions of 5-FU (48 h or 5 days), less common with capecitabine and probably least with bolus administration of 5-FU [153]. As chemotherapeutic drugs are often

Table 8.7 Cardiac toxicities associated with 5-FU and capecitabine

1. Vasospasm
2. Angina pectoris
3. Acute coronary syndrome
4. Myocardial infarction
5. Acute myocarditis
6. Takotsubo stress cardiomyopathy
7. Global cardiomyopathy
8. Sinus bradycardia
9. Ectopic ventricular beats
10. Prolonged QT with torsade de pointes
11. Ventricular tachycardia
12. Cardiogenic shock
13. Sudden death
14. Acute pericarditis

given in combination, cardiotoxicity from other agents should also be considered—especially with agents like trastuzumab, lapatinib, or bevacizumab. The actual frequency of cardiac toxicity is low (2–8 % in various series), but because of the widespread use of 5-FU primarily in gastrointestinal tumors, the cardiologist is frequently called to deal with 5-FU-related cardiotoxicity. In a large randomized clinical trial of patients with colon cancer, approximately 8 % of 2094 patients receiving infusional 5-FU-based chemotherapy reported grade 3 or higher cardio-vascular side effects (http://www.ncbi.nlm.nih.gov/pubmed/19451425). An early study by Akhtar followed 100 patients with no history of cardiac disease and found cardiotoxicity in 8, mostly angina-like pain (5/8) followed by sweating and palpi-tations, ECG changes in 3, and cardiogenic shock in one patient. The symptoms were reversible within 1 h of stopping the infusion and no one died [154]. De Forni in an early study followed 367 patients given first cycle high-dose 5-FU continuous infusion [155]. Almost 90 % were receiving concomitant additional chemotherapy. Cardiac events occurred in 28 patients (7.6 %), nine of whom had a history of cardiac disease. The inaugural symptom was angina in 18 patients (64 %). After 5-FU was stopped, the angina returned to baseline in six, but unstable angina occurred in eight patients. Sudden death occurred in four patients with an overall mortality of 2.2 %. Additionally, 65 % of patients with cardiac events had repolar-ization changes on the ECG and low voltage was found in 22 % of these patients. Wacker et al. followed 102 unselected patients treated with 5-FU for 3 months with ECGs, echocardiograms, and radionuclide ventriculograms [11]. Nineteen percent of patients developed reversible angina symptoms with ECG changes in most, which were severe in six. Coronary angiograms in these six were normal. Two patients demonstrated ejection fractions less than 50 % which did not improve. Bradycardia and PVCs were more common during the infusion than afterwards. Stewart et al. reported a patient developing bradycardia during 5-FU infusion [151]. Kosmas et al. followed 644 patients undergoing therapy with 5-FU and capecitabine-based therapy, and 4.03 % developed symptoms and ECG changes. Those with continuous 5-FU infusion developed these in 6.7 % compared to 2.3 % in the others. Seven of the 20 patients had an acute myocardial infarction. Four patients had ECG changes suggesting coronary vasospasm, and three developed conduction abnormalities, one of which was fatal. Saif et al. reviewed the literature from 1969 to 2007 and were able to evaluate 377 of 448 reported cases of toxicity. Sixty-nine percent of episodes occurred during or within 72 h of the first infusion of 5-FU. Angina occurred in 45 % of the patients with the reported complications, and myocardial infarction occurred in 22 % of patients. ECG changes were seen in 69 % of patients, but abnormal enzymes were seen in only 12 %. On the basis of their analysis, they concluded that preexisting cardiac risk factors were not predictive of cardiotoxicity. They also felt that toxicity may be more commonly related to continuous infusion of 5-FU [156].

Additional case reports describing other toxic effects have been reported. A case of reversible severe stress cardiomyopathy (takotsubo-like) developing 24 h after a FOLFOX treatment was described in a patient who was stabilized using an intra-aortic balloon with an initial total recovery. After 4 months the left ventricular function was normal. (He developed a cardiac arrest at the end of his third course with the development of acute heart failure. His heart function returned to normal several days later [157].) Grunwald et al. described a takotsubo cardiomyopathy in a 60-year-old woman who developed chest pain 26 h into her first infusion which resolved within 8 h. Her ECG was abnormal with 1 mm ST deviations, and an echocardiogram showed an ejection fraction of 15–20 %. Her coronaries were normal on a subsequent coronary angiogram. Four weeks later her LV function returned to normal [158]. Canale et al. reported on a 56-year-old man with no prior heart disease who suffered a myocardial infarction. The troponin peaked at 6.51 and the ECG showed Q waves in $V2$ and $V3$, with akinesis of the apical segments on echocardiogram and an ejection fraction of 45 %. The coronaries were normal on catheterization [159]. Sasson et al. reported two cases of cardiomyopathy developing during 5-FU infusion. One presented with symptoms of angina, but the other developed irreversible cardiogenic shock. Acute myocarditis was found on pathologic examination [160].

The mechanism of the cardiotoxicity of 5-FU is still unknown. Clearly vasospasm plays a central role with the angina. Coronary angiography has been normal in most cases. The effectiveness of vasodilators, nitrates, and calcium channel blockers in some cases is consistent with this hypothesis [161, 162]. It is well established that 5-FU has a very short half-life (10–15 min), and it is catabolized in the liver by dihydropyrimidine dehydrogenase (DPD) into 5,6-dihydrofluorouracil and eventually to α-fluoro-β-alanine (FBAL) [163]. It is hypothesized that the generation and potential accumulation of FBAL is associated with cardiotoxicity, as there are no reports of cardiotoxicity when 5-FU is administered together with the DPD inhibitor eniluracil [164]. In addition, there are reports of patients who experienced 5-FU cardiotoxicity but did not develop any symptoms when treated with the 5-FU derivate S-1, which does not metabolize to FBAL [163]. FBAL may accumulate in patients receiving continuous 5-FU infusion (6.7 % cardiotoxic events) or capecitabine (5.5 % cardiotoxic events), compared with bolus 5-FU therapy (2.3 %; $P < 0.012$) [153].

It is becoming clear that the cardiotoxicity is more than just vasospasm [151]. Cwikiel et al. looked at the endothelium in small arteries in a rabbit ear using scanning and transmission electron microscopy at intervals after in vivo treatment with 5-FU. Severe cell damage with accompanying thrombus formation was found which they interpreted as a thrombogenic effect secondary to direct cytotoxic effect on the endothelium [165]. Eskandari et al. studied the effects of 5-FU and capecitabine on cardiomyocytes freshly isolated from rats and found cytotoxic effects on the mitochondrial membrane leading to mitochondrial dysfunction activating caspase-3 and cell death [148]. Focaccetti et al. provided a comprehensive review of the problem of cardiotoxicity of 5-FU and performed a series of experiments designed to better understand the clinical uncertainties. They examined the effects of 5-FU on primary cell cultures of human cardiomyocytes and endothelial cells and showed autophagic features at the ultrastructural and molecular levels in exposed cardiomyocytes and reactive oxygen species (ROS) elevation in the endothelial cells. Thus they found that 5-FU can affect these cell types which may explain some manifestations of its cardiovascular toxicity. The endothelial response could be prevented with an ROS scavenger [166].

The role of preexisting coronary disease must also be considered. Although many patients who develop coronary symptoms, including vasospasm or myocardial infarction, have no demonstrable coronary disease on catheterization, Meyer et al. reporting on a prospective cohort study in 34 hospitals detailing patients who developed a cardiac event during 5-FU infusion found a relative risk of 6.83 in patients with underlying coronary disease compared to others in developing cardiac toxicity [167]. This was corroborated by Anand [168]. Thymidine phosphorylase is a key enzyme required for the conversion of capecitabine to 5-FU and 5-FU to its active metabolites. Because of higher levels of TP in the tumors 5-FU and capecitabine are more active in tumors than in other tissues. TP expression is upregulated in atherosclerotic plaques and during myocardial infarction, potentially contributing to the higher prevalence of cardiotoxicity in patients with previous cardiovascular disease or 5-FU-induced damage [166]. It is not known whether aggressive treatment of coronary disease with statins will reduce these complications.

Since the mechanism is not clearly known, treatment of 5-FU cardiotoxicity is empirical. The first step should be to discontinue the drug. The second step should be to treat vasospasm with either nitrates or calcium channel blockers. Cases have been reported treating the angina, presumably due to vasospasm, with vasodilators, nitrates, and calcium channel blockers [161, 162, 169]. Others have reported that nitrates and calcium channel blockers are of no or limited value, especially in preventing symptoms upon rechallenge [170, 171]. Patel et al. gave vasodilators on rechallenge and five of six patients had recurrent cardiotoxicity [172]. The cardiomyopathies that have been reported have been generally reversible after stopping administration, so aggressive heart failure management, including devices such as intra-aortic balloons and ECMO, to support these patients until their hearts can recover, would seem appropriate if simpler afterload reduction or even low-dose inotropes are inadequate. There is unpredictable, potentially high risk in rechallenging a patient with documented cardiotoxicity to 5-FU or capecitabine. Patients with previous 5-FU cardiotoxicity other than infarction may be rechallenged. There is no way to predict or avoid potential serious complications. Saif et al. [156] and Sorrentino et al. [144] have recommended the following approach to rechallenging a patient with capecitabine or 5-FU who has documented symptoms. They recommend that a careful evaluation for cardiac or coronary disease should be done prior to the administration of 5-FU or capecitabine. One should be very clear about the need for the 5-FU/capecitabine treatment. Rechallenging should be avoided and consideration given to alternative therapy, if available. The form of treatment should be reevaluated, considering bolus 5-FU, lowering the dose, switching to capecitabine in patients with toxicity from infusional 5-FU or changing to bolus 5-FU in patients with capecitabine therapy. If the patient needs to be rechallenged, close monitoring should be done in the hospital setting with ECG monitoring and cessation of therapy at first signs of cardiotoxicity. Consider coadministration of calcium channel blockers to protect against vasospasm, but recognize that this has not shown consistent benefit in prevention of 5-FU cardiotoxicity.

An alternative to rechallenging is administration of a different fluoropyrimidine [144, 173]. Raltitrexed, was developed as a direct and specific inhibitor of thymidylate synthase, and, although it is not approved by US FDA, is available in Canada, Australia, and some European countries for treatment of colorectal cancer when there is intolerance to 5-FU or capecitabine. In an Australian study, all 42 patients who had experienced cardiac toxicity (most commonly angina) with 5-FU or capecitabine alone or in combination with other chemotherapy did not have further cardiac toxicity after switching to raltitrexed [174]. In another retrospective review of 111 patients who all were given raltitrexed because of high cardiac risk or previous reactions to 5-FU or capecitabine, only 4.5 % patients had cardiotoxicity, all in patients with intolerance to capecitabine [173]. Certainly 5-FU or capecitabine represent the cornerstone component of chemotherapy in patients with multiple cancers. With such widespread use of these two drugs in outpatient settings, this rare but serious side effect of cardiac toxicity should be discussed with patients. Careful patient selection and close monitoring for symptoms are important to minimize the impact of the cardiotoxicity. Vigilance and caution should be used when treating any patient who develops chest pain within hours of an initial infusional dose of 5-FU. Rapid cessation of the drug and appropriate management may prevent serious events, including possible sudden cardiac death.

Radiation Therapy and Coronary Disease

Approximately half of cancer patients receive radiotherapy as part of their treatment, and it is now well recognized that mediastinal radiotherapy is associated with increased risk of cardiovascular disease including myocardial infarction, angina pectoris, heart failure, and valvular disorders [175].

The majority of the evidence for this risk has been abstracted from data obtained from patients treated decades ago for Hodgkin lymphoma (HL), although radiation doses were higher than those that are currently used and techniques are now in place to shield the vital structures, namely, the coronary arteries [176].

Radiotherapy techniques have improved progressively in the past years, but the heart still receives considerable exposure during radiotherapy for several cancers as (left) breast, lung, or HL [177–179].

Modern techniques of radiation therapy allow radiologists to deliver doses with increased accuracy, radiating the target tumors with three-dimensional modeling to minimize direct radiation to the heart and the anterior vessels more effectively than in the past. Patients treated with modern techniques of radiotherapy, however, have had a shorter follow-up so far, so it is not well defined yet as to what degree the theoretical benefits of these methods' reduced dose and volume will obtain. Although radiation doses have decreased significantly in the past few years, recent data have demonstrated that mean heart doses <20 Gy and even <5 Gy can increase the risk of heart damage [178, 180, 181]. A recently developed dose-response relationship seems to suggest that the risk of ischemic heart disease increases by approximately 7 % (95 CI, 3–14 %) for each 1-Gy increase in the mean dose of radiation to the heart. Data from the same analysis found no evidence of a threshold dose below which no risk occurs, but this still needs to be confirmed [177].

All structures of the heart such as the pericardium, myocardium, especially of the right heart, valves especially mitral and aortic valves, and coronary arteries [182] can potentially be damaged by irradiation; therefore, the spectrum of radiation-induced cardiac disease can be very broad, ranging from acute and chronic effusion of the pericardium to constrictive pericarditis, from myocardial fibrosis to restrictive cardiomyopathy, and from accelerated atherosclerosis of the vessels to obstructing lesions that are typically located at the proximal segments or ostium of coronary arteries. The morphology of radiation-related coronary artery disease (CAD) appears to be the same as CAD resulting from atherosclerosis from other causes [182, 183]. Thoracic radiation is therefore now considered as a risk factor for CAD.

Clinical presentation of coronary artery disease in cancer survivors who have received radiotherapy is overall similar to that in general population, although data suggest that silent myocardial infarction may occur more frequently in these patients. Risk of fatal ischemic cardiovascular disease seems also to be higher in patients who have received radiation to the chest, perhaps because of the involvement of the proximal left main [184] and proximal right arteries [185].

Konings et al. showed that in rabbits, radiating the carotid artery allowed increased penetration of the vessel by circulating lipid and allowed atherosclerosis to develop. These data suggest that lipid control may be important to limit the development of atherosclerosis in radiated patients [186].

Patients who receive mediastinal radiotherapy need to be followed for years since radiation-related CAD is usually detected decades after exposure and the risk of cardiotoxicity increases overtime [176]. Those most at risk are survivors treated as children and those with HL treated decades ago with higher doses. Based on this it appears evident that one-time screening of survivors is not enough. Girinsky et al. followed 111 survivors of radiation for HL using coronary CT angiography (CCTA). Five years after treatment, lesions were found in 15 % of patients, but by 10 years the number had grown to 34 %. Ten of the patients underwent revascularization. Most defects were non-ostial (89 %) but ostial lesions were found in 28 %. Appropriate timing and length of follow-up needs to be defined [187].

Unfortunately at present it is not known yet if any type of intervention such as administration of antiplatelet drugs, statins, or ACE inhibitor after exposure can be of any benefit and reduce the subsequent risk of cardiovascular disease.

Percutaneous coronary intervention and coronary artery bypass graft are both valuable options to treat symptomatic coronary obstructions. There is not much evidence but the available data demonstrate that non-ostial, isolated coronary artery lesions can be treated with percutaneous coronary intervention and coronary artery bypass graft can represent a better option in good surgical candidate [188]. However, percutaneous treatment of coronary stenosis may be associated with a higher rate of restenosis than non-radiated arteries [188]. Surgery in these patients must contend with radiation fibrosis frequently of the right ventricle, plus coexistent valve disease which may progress and require a second operation in the future. The vessels may have thinner media and fibrotic adventitia [5] which may influence the anastomoses, and frequently the internal mammary artery is damaged, precluding its use, possibly compromising the long-term results. Stenting of left main lesions in non-radiated persons has been shown to be equivalent to CABG in the short term if the complexity of the disease is low [189]. There are no data at present on the rate of stent restenosis in radiation-induced coronary artery disease.

Treating patients with severe coronary disease and aggressive cancer presents the physician with a true dilemma. The physician must prioritize therapy: can the cancer be treated without revascularizing the coronary disease or does the coronary disease manifest so acutely that it must take priority? This is epitomized in two recent cases where the treating physicians reached out for opinions to experienced cardio-oncologists, surgeons, and oncologists (Parashar S. Patient with severe coronary disease and gastric cancer. Personal communication, 2015).

Patient 1

The patient is a 66-year-old male with a history of diabetes, hypertension, hyperlipidemia, and a previous TIA who presented 2 days earlier with reports of worsening shortness of breath for at least 2 weeks. He noticed some right thigh fullness and swelling and right leg edema starting several weeks ago. Around the same time, he noticed a gradual onset of dyspnea, primarily dyspnea on minimal exertion without chest discomfort. In the emergency room, his troponin was minimally elevated, and chest X-ray showed three masses thought to be metastases. He was noted to have a firm right thigh mass. His ECG showed an anterior MI of unknown age with Q waves $V1$ to $V4$. A biopsy of the mass showed a high-grade malignant spindle cell lesion composed of large pleomorphic spindled cells with myxoid stromal background. He was in intense pain, determined to be due to the tumor encircling the femoral nerve. A diagnostic catheterization on the day after admission showed a 90 % lesion in the proximal right coronary and a 90 % ulcerated lesion in the proximal left anterior descending artery with a second long diffuse lesion in a large diagonal branch. His echocardiogram showed normal left ventricular function.

Thus the situation that presented was a previously active 67-year-old man with multivessel complex coronary disease, with diabetes, in intense pain in his right thigh from the presumed sarcoma with some evidence of pulmonary metastases.

Consultation was obtained with a cardiovascular surgeon and interventional cardiologist. The key features to consider were the impending nature of his coronary disease which, with his severe symptoms of dyspnea, needed to be treated with revascularization, the question whether treatment of the sarcoma would lead to severe thrombocytopenia which would put him at risk for bleeding if kept on double antiplatelet therapy, and the feasibility of a percutaneous approach—it was complex but all major lesions could be treated. After discussion which considered his poor prognosis, the convalescent time required for CABG, the intense pain in his thigh which required immediate treatment with radiation, and the anticipated lack of thrombocytopenia, it was elected to proceed with the PCI which successfully treated all three lesions.

His postoperative course was marred by a fall with small intracerebral bleed leading to some confusion. Platelet function both for aspirin and Plavix was normal, i.e., unresponsive to the antiplatelet agents which were increased.

Two and one-half months later, he presented dyspneic and septic with marked increase in the metastatic lesions and elected to discontinue chemotherapy. Post-mortem was not performed.

This patient demonstrates several important points. First there is the presentation with two severe problems needing immediate attention, acute coronary syndrome with an unstable plaque in a large coronary artery and intense pain from the tumor which would seriously compromise surgical recovery, but a poor overall prognosis so that the recovery period from cardiac surgery might well encompass his remaining functional life. In addition, the lack of platelet response to standard DAPT in this patient with metastatic sarcoma was unexpected. PCI was able to deal with the unstable coronary situation, permitting prompt treatment of the severe pain with radiation, and the treatment of the sarcoma could proceed without interruption. Unfortunately in this man, the tumor did not respond.

Patient 2

The patient's oncologist reached out to a wide group of cardio-oncologists and oncologists by internet so their comments could all be recorded.

A 75-year-old man was admitted to the hospital with chest pain. Cardiac catheterization showed a 60 % ostial left main lesion, a 90 % proximal LAD lesion, 80 % sequential left circumflex lesions, and an occluded proximal RCA. His ejection fraction was 35–40 %. He was being considered for CABG when the workup for a concomitant anemia led to a diagnosis of stage IV metastatic gastric adenocarcinoma. The tumor was shown to overexpress HER2. The chemotherapies considered were trastuzumab which could have a spectacular result but risks worsening CHF and 5-FU which risks angina/MI in the face of this severe CAD.

The Responses

Cardiologist 1

What is the prognosis and do they see any gastric surgery in the future? Trastuzumab is off the table since he is bordering on serious decompensated heart failure already. But what about PCI with bare-metal stents (to limit the duration of double platelet therapy to 1 month)? This approach would of course increase the long-term risk of restenosis. If he is in good shape, the better approach may be CABG so there would be less concern about thrombocytopenia and less concern with the use of 5-FU in a patient with such severe underlying cardiac disease. It may also be that the revascularized LV would improve its contractility which could open the door to trastuzumab.

Cardiologist 2

Try to optimize the hematological problems and put him on appropriate cardiac meds. Then PCI of the LAD lesion (our preference would be DES—not BMS—new data indicates less stent thrombosis with modern DES) likely that LVEF will improve after revascularization. Then 5-FU (bolus may be better than continuous—less coronary spasms)—coronary vasodilators if needed. I would not categorically deny this patient this sometimes incredibly effective therapy (Trastuzumab).

Oncologist 1

Any role for radiating his stomach if he's bleeding to control ongoing blood loss? Also early palliative care involvement might be helpful.

Oncologist 2

He is not a surgical candidate nor can he currently receive trastuzumab. I would recommend optimizing his cardiac function and plan on 5-FU. If cardiac function improves, then trastuzumab can be added.

Cardiologist 3

The goal here is palliation. I would not go down the CABG route, which is far more likely to cause downside/discomfort than upside. I agree with the recommendation of a sequential plan of transfusion/medical therapy with beta-blockers/nitrates to see if he still has angina; depending on what his baseline Hgb and hemodynamics were, it is very conceivable option that he will be angina-free at that point. In addition, his systolic function could be significantly be improved by medical therapy alone. I would not rush to do PCI in this patient unless he had refractory angina despite maximal medical therapy.

Oncologist 3

1. From an oncology standpoint, prognosis is not good
2. If the tumor is HER2 positive, would try trastuzumab. The cardiac effects seem to be mild and reversible. This is probably the best palliative option

3. Coronary spasm from fluorouracil is rare and reversible. If 5-FU is deemed appropriate, consider giving small IV test dose, probably preferable to oral capecitabine which could theoretically cause coronary vasospasm too, but it takes longer to clear from the system. (I have an elderly lady with terrible CAD who has done marvelously on Xeloda (capecitabine) for a couple of years.)
4. It will be important to carefully maintain Hgb with transfusions, with diuretics to avoid fluid overload.

Result

He had a pyloric stent placement for the obstructing pyloric mass. Oncology proceeded with mFOLFOX (5-FU-based chemotherapy). His repeat echo during the admission showed normalized EF. He was discharged home after he finished his first cycle.

Comment

This case demonstrates the problems posed by patients with both coronary disease and severe cancer. The treatment for the coronary disease was clearly compromised. On its own, with the severe three-vessel disease (left main, 90 % LAD, 80 % circumflex, and complete RCA), CABG would ordinarily be recommended, but the morbidity in this man with such a poor prognosis was unacceptable. PCI would potentially open the culprit artery, but if he could be controlled medically, that would be just as good. The chemotherapy was similarly impacted by the cardiac situation. Trastuzumab, which was the choice of several of the oncologists, was a major concern based on the potential for further cardiac dysfunction, with a high potential for developing clinical failure. The 5-FU-based therapy had its unknown risks but was ultimately chosen as the best of the available options. Obviously, the cardiac situation can deteriorate at any time which would force another crisis, but hopefully by then, the prognosis based on response to therapy could be better defined.

A major aspect to this "virtual conference" as it is presented is the importance of the collaboration of the players; the oncologist, the cardiologist, and the gastroenterologist all contributed important insight from their unique points of view. This then developed a strategy which could provide the patient the best quality of life, while avoiding unnecessary treatment-related morbidity.

References

1. Murphy SL, Xu J, Kochanek KD. Deaths: final data for 2010. Natl Vital Stat Rep. 2013;61:1–117.

2. Driver JA, Djousse L, Logroscino G, Gaziano JM, Kurth T. Incidence of cardiovascular disease and cancer in advanced age: prospective cohort study. BMJ. 2008;337:a2467.
3. Koene RJ, Prizment AE, Blaes A, Konety SH. Shared risk factors in cardiovascular disease and cancer. Circulation. 2016;133:1104–14.
4. Basyigit S, Ozkan S, Uzman M, et al. Should screening for colorectal neoplasm be recommended in patients at high risk for coronary heart disease: a cross-sectional study. Medicine (Baltimore). 2015;94, e793.
5. Virmani R, Farb A, Carter AJ, Jones RM. Pathology of radiation-induced coronary artery disease in human and pig. Cardiovasc Radiat Med. 1999;1:98–101.
6. Mulrooney DA, Ness KK, Huang S, et al. Pilot study of vascular health in survivors of osteosarcoma. Pediatr Blood Cancer. 2013;60:1703–8.
7. Tzonevska A, Chakarova A, Tzvetkov K. GSPECT-CT myocardial scintigraphy plus calcium scores as screening tool for prevention of cardiac side effects in left-sided breast cancer radiotherapy. J BUON. 2014;19:667–72.
8. Takahashi I, Ohishi W, Mettler Jr FA, et al. A report from the 2013 international workshop: radiation and cardiovascular disease, Hiroshima, Japan. J Radiol Prot. 2013;33:869–80.
9. Plummer C, Henderson RD, O'Sullivan JD, Read SJ. Ischemic stroke and transient ischemic attack after head and neck radiotherapy: a review. Stroke. 2011;42:2410–8.
10. Hicks Jr GL. Coronary artery operation in radiation-associated atherosclerosis: long-term follow-up. Ann Thorac Surg. 1992;53:670–4.
11. Wacker A, Lersch C, Scherpinski U, Reindl L, Seyfarth M. High incidence of angina pectoris in patients treated with 5-fluorouracil. A planned surveillance study with 102 patients. Oncology. 2003;65:108–12.
12. Rackley C, Schultz KR, Goldman FD, et al. Cardiac manifestations of graft-versus-host disease. Biol Blood Marrow Transplant. 2005;11:773–80.
13. Prevost D, Taylor G, Sanatani S, Schultz KR. Coronary vessel involvement by chronic graft-versus-host disease presenting as sudden cardiac death. Bone Marrow Transplant. 2004;34:655–6.
14. Virmani R, Kolodgie FD, Burke AP, Farb A, Schwartz SM. Lessons from sudden coronary death: a comprehensive morphological classification scheme for atherosclerotic lesions. Arterioscler Thromb Vasc Biol. 2000;20:1262–75.
15. Vancraeynest D, Pasquet A, Roelants V, Gerber BL, Vanoverschelde JL. Imaging the vulnerable plaque. J Am Coll Cardiol. 2011;57:1961–79.
16. Niccoli G, Montone RA, Di Vito L, et al. Plaque rupture and intact fibrous cap assessed by optical coherence tomography portend different outcomes in patients with acute coronary syndrome. Eur Heart J. 2015;36:1377–84.
17. Thygesen K, Alpert JS, Jaffe AS, et al. Third universal definition of myocardial infarction. Circulation. 2012;126:2020–35.
18. Lind PA, Pagnanelli R, Marks LB, et al. Myocardial perfusion changes in patients irradiated for left-sided breast cancer and correlation with coronary artery distribution. Int J Radiat Oncol Biol Phys. 2003;55:914–20.
19. Braunwald E, Morrow DA. Unstable angina: is it time for a requiem? Circulation. 2013;127:2452–7.
20. Fuster V, Moreno PR, Fayad ZA, Corti R, Badimon JJ. Atherothrombosis and high-risk plaque: Part I: evolving concepts. J Am Coll Cardiol. 2005;46:937–54.
21. Glagov S, Weisenberg E, Zarins CK, Stankunavicius R, Kolettis GJ. Compensatory enlargement of human atherosclerotic coronary arteries. N Engl J Med. 1987;316(22):1371–5.
22. Yeh ETH, Bickford CL. Cardiovascular complications of cancer therapy: incidence, pathogenesis, diagnosis, and management. J Am Coll Cardiol. 2009;53:2231–47.
23. Curigliano G, Mayer EL, Burstein HJ, Winer EP, Goldhirsch A. Cardiac toxicity from systemic cancer therapy: a comprehensive review. Prog Cardiovasc Dis. 2010;53:94–104.
24. Shah K, Gupta S, Ghosh J, Bajpai J, Maheshwari A. Acute non-ST elevation myocardial infarction following paclitaxel administration for ovarian carcinoma: a case report and review of literature. J Cancer Res Ther. 2012;8:442–4.

25. Jafri M, Protheroe A. Cisplatin-associated thrombosis. Anticancer Drugs. 2008;19:927–9.
26. Togna GI, Togna AR, Franconi M, Caprino L. Cisplatin triggers platelet activation. Thromb Res. 2000;99:503–9.
27. Berliner S, Rahima M, Sidi Y, et al. Acute coronary events following cisplatin-based chemotherapy. Cancer Investig. 1990;8:583–6.
28. Samuels BL, Vogelzang NJ, Kennedy BJ. Severe vascular toxicity associated with vinblastine, bleomycin, and cisplatin chemotherapy. Cancer Chemother Pharmacol. 1987;19:253–6.
29. Choueiri TK, Schutz FA, Je Y, Rosenberg JE, Bellmunt J. Risk of arterial thromboembolic events with sunitinib and sorafenib: a systematic review and meta-analysis of clinical trials. J Clin Oncol. 2010;28:2280–5.
30. Chen XL, Lei YH, Liu CF, et al. Angiogenesis inhibitor bevacizumab increases the risk of ischemic heart disease associated with chemotherapy: a meta-analysis. PLoS One. 2013;8, e66721.
31. Cuppone F, Bria E, Verma S, et al. Do adjuvant aromatase inhibitors increase the cardiovascular risk in postmenopausal women with early breast cancer? Meta-analysis of randomized trials. Cancer. 2008;112:260–7.
32. Montalescot G, Sechtem U, Achenbach S, et al. 2013 ESC guidelines on the management of stable coronary artery disease: the Task Force on the management of stable coronary artery disease of the European Society of Cardiology. Eur Heart J. 2013;34:2949–3003.
33. Goff Jr DC, Lloyd-Jones DM, Bennett G, et al. 2013 ACC/AHA guideline on the assessment of cardiovascular risk: a report of the American College of Cardiology/American Heart Association Task Force on Practice Guidelines. J Am Coll Cardiol. 2014;63:2935–59.
34. Stone NJ, Robinson JG, Lichtenstein AH, et al. 2013 ACC/AHA guideline on the treatment of blood cholesterol to reduce atherosclerotic cardiovascular risk in adults: a report of the American College of Cardiology/American Heart Association Task Force on Practice Guidelines. J Am Coll Cardiol. 2014;63:2889–934.
35. Vaughan CJ, Gotto Jr AM, Basson CT. The evolving role of statins in the management of atherosclerosis. J Am Coll Cardiol. 2000;35:1–10.
36. Furberg CD, Byington RP, Crouse JR, Espeland MA. Pravastatin, lipids, and major coronary events. Am J Cardiol. 1994;73:1133–4.
37. Brown BG, Zhao XQ, Chait A, et al. Simvastatin and niacin, antioxidant vitamins, or the combination for the prevention of coronary disease. N Engl J Med. 2001;345:1583–92.
38. Go AS, Iribarren C, Chandra M, et al. Statin and beta-blocker therapy and the initial presentation of coronary heart disease. Ann Intern Med. 2006;144:229–38.
39. DeFilippis AP, Young R, Carrubba CJ, et al. An analysis of calibration and discrimination among multiple cardiovascular risk scores in a modern multiethnic cohort. Ann Intern Med. 2015;162:266–75.
40. Lip GY, Chin BS, Blann AD. Cancer and the prothrombotic state. Lancet Oncol. 2002;3:27–34.
41. Iliescu CA, Grines CL, Herrmann J, et al. SCAI Expert consensus statement: evaluation, management, and special considerations of cardio-oncology patients in the cardiac catheterization laboratory (endorsed by the Cardiological Society of India, and Sociedad Latino Americana de Cardiologia Intervencionista). Catheter Cardiovasc Interv. 2016;87(5): E202–23.
42. Shitara Y, Sugiyama Y. Pharmacokinetic and pharmacodynamic alterations of 3-hydroxy-3-methylglutaryl coenzyme A (HMG-CoA) reductase inhibitors: drug-drug interactions and interindividual differences in transporter and metabolic enzyme functions. Pharmacol Ther. 2006;112:71–105.
43. Neuvonen PJ, Niemi M, Backman JT. Drug interactions with lipid-lowering drugs: mechanisms and clinical relevance. Clin Pharmacol Ther. 2006;80:565–81.
44. Neuvonen PJ, Kantola T, Kivisto KT. Simvastatin but not pravastatin is very susceptible to interaction with the CYP3A4 inhibitor itraconazole. Clin Pharmacol Ther. 1998;63:332–41.

45. Zhou SF, Xue CC, Yu XQ, Li C, Wang G. Clinically important drug interactions potentially involving mechanism-based inhibition of cytochrome P450 3A4 and the role of therapeutic drug monitoring. Ther Drug Monit. 2007;29:687–710.
46. Ogu CC, Maxa JL. Drug interactions due to cytochrome P450. Proc (Bayl Univ Med Cent). 2000;13:421–3.
47. Guengerich FP. Cytochrome p450 and chemical toxicology. Chem Res Toxicol. 2008;21:70–83.
48. Christenson RH, Assay HME. Biomarkers of myocardial necrosis. Totowa, NJ: Humana Press; 2006.
49. Christenson RH, Azzazy HM. Biochemical markers of the acute coronary syndromes. Clin Chem. 1998;44:1855–64.
50. Hamm CW, Bassand JP, Agewall S, et al. ESC Guidelines for the management of acute coronary syndromes in patients presenting without persistent ST-segment elevation: the Task Force for the management of acute coronary syndromes (ACS) in patients presenting without persistent ST-segment elevation of the European Society of Cardiology (ESC). Eur Heart J. 2011;32:2999–3054.
51. Wilson SR, Scirica BM, Braunwald E, et al. Efficacy of ranolazine in patients with chronic angina observations from the randomized, double-blind, placebo-controlled MERLIN-TIMI (Metabolic Efficiency with Ranolazine for Less Ischemia in Non-ST-Segment Elevation Acute Coronary Syndromes) 36 Trial. J Am Coll Cardiol. 2009;53:1510–6.
52. Stone PH, Chaitman BR, Stocke K, Sano J, DeVault A, Koch GG. The anti-ischemic mechanism of action of ranolazine in stable ischemic heart disease. J Am Coll Cardiol. 2010;56:934–42.
53. Chaitman BR. Ranolazine for the treatment of chronic angina and potential use in other cardiovascular conditions. Circulation. 2006;113:2462–72.
54. Fihn SD, Gardin JM, Abrams J, et al. ACCF/AHA/ACP/AATS/PCNA/SCAI/STS Guideline for the diagnosis and management of patients with stable ischemic heart disease: a report of the American College of Cardiology Foundation/American Heart Association Task Force on Practice Guidelines, and the American College of Physicians, American Association for Thoracic Surgery, Preventive Cardiovascular Nurses Association, Society for Cardiovascular Angiography and Interventions, and Society of Thoracic Surgeons. J Am Coll Cardiol. 2012;60:e44–164.
55. Boden WE. Interpreting the COURAGE trial. It takes COURAGE to alter our belief system. Cleve Clin J Med. 2007;74:623–5. 9–33.
56. The BARI 2D Study Group. A randomized trial of therapies for type 2 diabetes and coronary artery disease. N Engl J Med. 2009;360:2503–15.
57. Chow CK, Jolly S, Rao-Melacini P, Fox KA, Anand SS, Yusuf S. Association of diet, exercise, and smoking modification with risk of early cardiovascular events after acute coronary syndromes. Circulation. 2010;121:750–8.
58. CASS Principal Investigators and Their Associates. Myocardial infarction and mortality in the coronary artery surgery study (CASS) randomized trial. N Engl J Med. 1984;310:750–8.
59. Chaitman BR, Hardison RM, Adler D, et al. The Bypass Angioplasty Revascularization Investigation 2 Diabetes randomized trial of different treatment strategies in type 2 diabetes mellitus with stable ischemic heart disease: impact of treatment strategy on cardiac mortality and myocardial infarction. Circulation. 2009;120:2529–40.
60. Fuster V, Farkouh ME. General cardiology perspective: decision making regarding revascularization of patients with type 2 diabetes mellitus and cardiovascular disease in the Bypass Angioplasty Revascularization Investigation 2 Diabetes (BARI 2D) trial. Circulation. 2010;121:2450–2.
61. Krone RJ, Althouse AD, Tamis-Holland J, et al. Appropriate revascularization in stable angina: lessons from the BARI 2D trial. Can J Cardiol. 2014;30:1595–601.
62. Stergiopoulos K, Brown DL. Initial coronary stent implantation with medical therapy vs medical therapy alone for stable coronary artery disease: meta-analysis of randomized controlled trials. Arch Intern Med. 2012;172:312–9.

63. Kottke TE. The lessons of COURAGE for the management of stable coronary artery disease. J Am Coll Cardiol. 2011;58:138–9.

64. Coronary artery surgery study (CASS): a randomized trial of coronary artery bypass surgery. Comparability of entry characteristics and survival in randomized patients and nonrandomized patients meeting randomization criteria. J Am Coll Cardiol. 1984;3:114–28.

65. Boden WE, O'Rourke RA, Teo KK, et al. Optimal medical therapy with or without PCI for stable coronary disease. N Engl J Med. 2007;356:1503–16.

66. Anderson JL, Adams CD, Antman EM, et al. 2011 ACCF/AHA Focused Update Incorporated into the ACC/AHA 2007 Guidelines for the Management of Patients with Unstable Angina/Non-ST-Elevation Myocardial Infarction: a report of the American College of Cardiology Foundation/American Heart Association Task Force on Practice Guidelines. Circulation. 2011;123:e426–579.

67. Amsterdam EA, Wenger NK, Brindis RG, et al. 2014 AHA/ACC Guideline for the Management of Patients with Non–ST-Elevation Acute Coronary Syndromes: a report of the American College of Cardiology/American Heart Association Task Force on Practice Guidelines. J Am Coll Cardiol. 2014;64:e139–228.

68. Thanavaro S, Krone RJ, Kleiger RE, et al. In-hospital prognosis of patients with first nontransmural and transmural infarctions. Circulation. 1980;61:29–33.

69. Wright RS, Anderson JL, Adams CD, et al. ACCF/AHA focused update of the Guidelines for the Management of Patients with Unstable Angina/Non-ST-Elevation Myocardial Infarction (updating the 2007 guideline): a report of the American College of Cardiology Foundation/American Heart Association Task Force on Practice Guidelines developed in collaboration with the American College of Emergency Physicians, Society for Cardiovascular Angiography and Interventions, and Society of Thoracic Surgeons. J Am Coll Cardiol. 2011;57:1920–59.

70. Fox KA, Dabbous OH, Goldberg RJ, et al. Prediction of risk of death and myocardial infarction in the six months after presentation with acute coronary syndrome: prospective multinational observational study (GRACE). BMJ. 2006;333:1091.

71. Sorajja P, Gersh BJ, Cox DA, et al. Impact of delay to angioplasty in patients with acute coronary syndromes undergoing invasive management: analysis from the ACUITY (Acute Catheterization and Urgent Intervention Triage strategY) trial. J Am Coll Cardiol. 2010;55:1416–24.

72. Gruntzig AR, Senning A, Siegenthaler WE. Nonoperative dilatation of coronary-artery stenosis: percutaneous transluminal coronary angioplasty. N Engl J Med. 1979;301:61.

73. Krone R. Thirty years of coronary angioplasty. Cardiol J. 2008;15:201–2.

74. Tomey MI, Kini AS, Sharma SK. Current status of rotational atherectomy. JACC Cardiovasc Interv. 2014;7:345–53.

75. Chambers JW, Feldman RL, Himmelstein SI, et al. Pivotal trial to evaluate the safety and efficacy of the orbital atherectomy system in treating de novo, severely calcified coronary lesions (ORBIT II). JACC Cardiovasc Interv. 2014;7:510–8.

76. Sigwart U, Puel J, Mirkovitch V, Joffre F, Kappenberger L. Intravascular stents to prevent occlusion and restenosis after transluminal angioplasty. N Engl J Med. 1987;316:701–6.

77. Topol EJ. The stentor and the sea change. Am J Cardiol. 1995;76:307–8.

78. Hall P, Nakamura S, Maiello L, et al. A randomized comparison of combined ticlopidine and aspirin therapy versus aspirin therapy alone after successful intravascular ultrasound-guided stent implantation. Circulation. 1996;93:215–22.

79. Colombo A, Hall P, Nakamura S, et al. Intracoronary stenting without anticoagulation accomplished with intravascular ultrasound guidance. Circulation. 1995;91:1676–88.

80. Karrillon GJ, Morice MC, Benveniste E, et al. Intracoronary stent implantation without ultrasound guidance and with replacement of conventional anticoagulation by antiplatelet therapy: 30-day clinical outcome of the French Multicenter Registry. Circulation. 1996;94:1519–27.

81. Morice MC, Zemour G, Benveniste E, et al. Intracoronary stenting without coumadin: one month results of a French multicenter study. Cathet Cardiovasc Diagn. 1995;35:1–7.
82. Albiero R, Hall P, Itoh A, et al. Results of a consecutive series of patients receiving only antiplatelet therapy after optimized stent implantation. Comparison of aspirin alone versus combined ticlopidine and aspirin therapy. Circulation. 1997;95:1145–56.
83. Krone RJ, Rao SV, Dai D, et al. Acceptance, panic, and partial recovery the pattern of usage of drug-eluting stents after introduction in the U.S. (a report from the American College of Cardiology/National Cardiovascular Data Registry). JACC Cardiovasc Interv. 2010;3:902–10.
84. Virmani R, Farb A, Guagliumi G, Kolodgie FD. Drug-eluting stents: caution and concerns for long-term outcome. Coron Artery Dis. 2004;15:313–8.
85. McFadden EP, Stabile E, Regar E, et al. Late thrombosis in drug-eluting coronary stents after discontinuation of antiplatelet therapy. Lancet. 2004;364:1519–21.
86. Grines CL, Bonow RO, Casey Jr DE, et al. Prevention of premature discontinuation of dual antiplatelet therapy in patients with coronary artery stents: a science advisory from the American Heart Association, American College of Cardiology, Society for Cardiovascular Angiography and Interventions, American College of Surgeons, and American Dental Association, with representation from the American College of Physicians. Circulation. 2007;115:813–8.
87. Chieffo A, Park SJ, Meliga E, et al. Late and very late stent thrombosis following drug-eluting stent implantation in unprotected left main coronary artery: a multicentre registry. Eur Heart J. 2008;29:2108–15.
88. Valgimigli M, Patialiakas A, Thury A, et al. Zotarolimus-eluting versus bare-metal stents in uncertain drug-eluting stent candidates. J Am Coll Cardiol. 2015;65:805–15.
89. Kandzari DE. Stent selection and antiplatelet therapy duration: one size does not fit all. J Am Coll Cardiol. 2015;65:816–9.
90. Montalescot G, Brieger D, Dalby AJ, Park SJ, Mehran R. Duration of dual antiplatelet therapy after coronary stenting: a review of the evidence. J Am Coll Cardiol. 2015;66:832–47.
91. Colombo A, Chieffo A, Frasheri A, et al. Second-generation drug-eluting stent implantation followed by 6- versus 12-month dual antiplatelet therapy: the SECURITY randomized clinical trial. J Am Coll Cardiol. 2014;64:2086–97.
92. Yeh RW, Mauri L, Kereiakes DJ. Dual antiplatelet platelet therapy duration following coronary stenting. J Am Coll Cardiol. 2015;65:787–90.
93. Gilard M, Barragan P, Noryani AA, et al. 6- versus 24-month dual antiplatelet therapy after implantation of drug-eluting stents in patients nonresistant to aspirin: the randomized, multicenter italic trial. J Am Coll Cardiol. 2015;65:777–86.
94. Kahneman D. Thinking, fast and slow. New York, NY: Farrar, Straus and Giroux; 2011.
95. Wallentin L, Becker RC, Cannon CP, et al. Review of the accumulated PLATO documentation supports reliable and consistent superiority of ticagrelor over clopidogrel in patients with acute coronary syndrome: commentary on: DiNicolantonio JJ, Tomek A, Inactivations, deletions, non-adjudications, and downgrades of clinical endpoints on ticagrelor: serious concerns over the reliability of the PLATO trial, International Journal of Cardiology, 2013. Int J Cardiol. 2014;170:e59–62.
96. Lindholm D, Varenhorst C, Cannon CP, et al. Ticagrelor vs. clopidogrel in patients with non-ST-elevation acute coronary syndrome with or without revascularization: results from the PLATO trial. Eur Heart J. 2014;35:2083–93.
97. Udell JA, Braunwald E, Antman EM, Murphy SA, Montalescot G, Wiviott SD. Prasugrel versus clopidogrel in patients with ST-segment elevation myocardial infarction according to timing of percutaneous coronary intervention: a TRITON-TIMI 38 subgroup analysis (Trial to Assess Improvement in Therapeutic Outcomes by Optimizing Platelet Inhibition with Prasugrel-Thrombolysis In Myocardial Infarction 38). JACC Cardiovasc Interv. 2014;7:604–12.

98. Kaluza GL, Joseph J, Lee JR, Raizner ME, Raizner AE. Catastrophic outcomes of noncardiac surgery soon after coronary stenting. J Am Coll Cardiol. 2000;35:1288–94.

99. van Kuijk JP, Flu WJ, Schouten O, et al. Timing of noncardiac surgery after coronary artery stenting with bare metal or drug-eluting stents. Am J Cardiol. 2009;104:1229–34.

100. Alshawabkeh LI, Banerjee S, Brilakis ES. Systematic review of the frequency and outcomes of non-cardiac surgery after drug-eluting stent implantation. Hellenic J Cardiol. 2011;52:141–8.

101. Botto F, Alonso-Coello P, Chan MT, et al. Myocardial injury after noncardiac surgery: a large, international, prospective cohort study establishing diagnostic criteria, characteristics, predictors, and 30-day outcomes. Anesthesiology. 2014;120:564–78.

102. Brilakis ES, Patel VG, Banerjee S. Medical management after coronary stent implantation: a review. JAMA. 2013;310:189–98.

103. Devereaux PJ, Goldman L, Cook DJ, Gilbert K, Leslie K, Guyatt GH. Perioperative cardiac events in patients undergoing noncardiac surgery: a review of the magnitude of the problem, the pathophysiology of the events and methods to estimate and communicate risk. CMAJ. 2005;173:627–34.

104. Gandhi NK, Abdel-Karim AR, Banerjee S, Brilakis ES. Frequency and risk of noncardiac surgery after drug-eluting stent implantation. Catheter Cardiovasc Interv. 2011;77:972–6.

105. Khan J, Alonso-Coello P, Devereaux PJ. Myocardial injury after noncardiac surgery. Curr Opin Cardiol. 2014;29:307–11.

106. Kristensen SD, Knuuti J, Saraste A, et al. 2014 ESC/ESA Guidelines on non-cardiac surgery: cardiovascular assessment and management: the Joint Task Force on non-cardiac surgery: cardiovascular assessment and management of the European Society of Cardiology (ESC) and the European Society of Anaesthesiology (ESA). Eur Heart J. 2014;35:2383–431.

107. Luckie M, Khattar RS, Fraser D. Non-cardiac surgery and antiplatelet therapy following coronary artery stenting. Heart. 2009;95:1303–8.

108. Sanon S, Rihal CS. Non-cardiac surgery after percutaneous coronary intervention. Am J Cardiol. 2014;114:1613–20.

109. Guarracino F, Baldassarri R, Priebe HJ. Revised ESC/ESA guidelines on non-cardiac surgery: cardiovascular assessment and management. Implications for preoperative clinical evaluation. Minerva Anestesiol. 2015;81:226–33.

110. Patel AY, Eagle KA, Vaishnava P. Cardiac risk of noncardiac surgery. J Am Coll Cardiol. 2015;66:2140–8.

111. Fleisher LA, Fleischmann KE, Auerbach AD, et al. 2014 ACC/AHA guideline on perioperative cardiovascular evaluation and management of patients undergoing noncardiac surgery: a report of the American College of Cardiology/American Heart Association Task Force on Practice Guidelines. J Am Coll Cardiol. 2014;64:e77–137.

112. Serruys PW, Morice MC, Kappetein AP, et al. Percutaneous coronary intervention versus coronary-artery bypass grafting for severe coronary artery disease. N Engl J Med. 2009;360:961–72.

113. The BARI Investigators. Seven-year outcome in the Bypass Angioplasty Revascularization Investigation (BARI) by treatment and diabetic status. J Am Coll Cardiol. 2000;35:1122–9.

114. Nakazawa G, Otsuka F, Nakano M, et al. The pathology of neoatherosclerosis in human coronary implants bare-metal and drug-eluting stents. J Am Coll Cardiol. 2011;57:1314–22.

115. Smith SC, Winters KJ, Lasala JM. Stent thrombosis in a patient receiving chemotherapy. Cathet Cardiovasc Diagn. 1997;40:383–6.

116. Lee JM, Yoon CH. Acute coronary stent thrombosis in cancer patients: a case series report. Korean Circ J. 2012;42:487–91.

117. Iliescu C, Durand JB, Kroll M. Cardiovascular interventions in thrombocytopenic cancer patients. Tex Heart Inst J. 2011;38:259–60.

118. Saxena P, Tam RK. Combined off-pump coronary artery bypass surgery and pulmonary resection. Ann Thorac Surg. 2004;78:498–501.

119. Tsuji Y, Morimoto N, Tanaka H, et al. Surgery for gastric cancer combined with cardiac and aortic surgery. Arch Surg. 2005;140:1109–14.
120. Soong J, Poots AJ, Scott S, Donald K, Bell D. Developing and validating a risk prediction model for acute care based on frailty syndromes. BMJ Open. 2015;5, e008457.
121. Herman CR, Buth KJ, Legare JF, Levy AR, Baskett R. Development of a predictive model for major adverse cardiac events in a coronary artery bypass and valve population. J Cardiothorac Surg. 2013;8:177.
122. Cervera R, Bakaeen FG, Cornwell LD, et al. Impact of functional status on survival after coronary artery bypass grafting in a veteran population. Ann Thorac Surg. 2012;93:1950–4. Discussion 4–5.
123. Sundermann S, Dademasch A, Praetorius J, et al. Comprehensive assessment of frailty for elderly high-risk patients undergoing cardiac surgery. Eur J Cardiothorac Surg. 2011;39:33–7.
124. Teo KK, Cohen E, Buller C, et al. Canadian Cardiovascular Society/Canadian Association of Interventional Cardiology/Canadian Society of Cardiac Surgery position statement on revascularization-multivessel coronary artery disease. Can J Cardiol. 2014;30:1482–91.
125. Vorobcsuk A, Konyi A, Aradi D, et al. Transradial versus transfemoral percutaneous coronary intervention in acute myocardial infarction Systematic overview and meta-analysis. Am Heart J. 2009;158:814–21.
126. Tatli E, Gunduz Y, Buturak A. Hematoma of the breast: a rare complication of transradial angiography and its treatment with handmade stent graft. J Invasive Cardiol. 2014;26:E24–6.
127. Pitta SR, Prasad A, Kumar G, Lennon R, Rihal CS, Holmes DR. Location of femoral artery access and correlation with vascular complications. Catheter Cardiovasc Interv. 2011;78:294–9.
128. Seto AH, Abu-Fadel MS, Sparling JM, et al. Real-time ultrasound guidance facilitates femoral arterial access and reduces vascular complications: FAUST (Femoral Arterial Access with Ultrasound Trial). JACC Cardiovasc Interv. 2010;3:751–8.
129. Sarkiss MG, Yusuf SW, Warneke CL, et al. Impact of aspirin therapy in cancer patients with thrombocytopenia and acute coronary syndromes. Cancer. 2007;109:621–7.
130. Iliescu C. Cardiovascular procedures in patients with cancer and thrombocytopenia. MD Anderson Practices (MAP) in Onco-Cardiology. 2014.
131. Nakazawa G, Finn AV, Vorpahl M, Ladich ER, Kolodgie FD, Virmani R. Coronary responses and differential mechanisms of late stent thrombosis attributed to first-generation sirolimus- and paclitaxel-eluting stents. J Am Coll Cardiol. 2011;57:390–8.
132. Singh J, Patel Y, Depta JP, et al. A modified provisional stenting approach to coronary bifurcation lesions: clinical application of the "jailed-balloon technique". J Interv Cardiol. 2012;25:289–96.
133. Al Ali J, Franck C, Filion KB, Eisenberg MJ. Coronary artery bypass graft surgery versus percutaneous coronary intervention with first-generation drug-eluting stents: a meta-analysis of randomized controlled trials. JACC Cardiovasc Interv. 2014;7:497–506.
134. Albaladejo P, Marret E, Samama CM, et al. Non-cardiac surgery in patients with coronary stents: the RECO study. Heart. 2011;97:1566–72.
135. Assali A, Vaknin-Assa H, Lev E, et al. The risk of cardiac complications following noncardiac surgery in patients with drug eluting stents implanted at least six months before surgery. Catheter Cardiovasc Interv. 2009;74:837–43.
136. Hawn MT, Graham LA, Richman JS, Itani KF, Henderson WG, Maddox TM. Risk of major adverse cardiac events following noncardiac surgery in patients with coronary stents. JAMA. 2013;310(14):1462–72.
137. Gupta PK, Gupta H, Sundaram A, et al. Development and validation of a risk calculator for prediction of cardiac risk after surgery. Circulation. 2011;124:381–7.
138. McFalls EO, Ward HB, Moritz TE, et al. Coronary-artery revascularization before elective major vascular surgery. N Engl J Med. 2004;351:2795–804.
139. London MJ, Hur K, Schwartz GG, Henderson WG. Association of perioperative beta-blockade with mortality and cardiovascular morbidity following major noncardiac surgery. JAMA. 2013;309:1704–13.

140. Ashes C, Judelman S, Wijeysundera DN, et al. Selective beta1-antagonism with bisoprolol is associated with fewer postoperative strokes than atenolol or metoprolol: a single-center cohort study of 44,092 consecutive patients. Anesthesiology. 2013;119:777–87.
141. Lim W, Qushmaq I, Cook DJ, et al. Elevated troponin and myocardial infarction in the intensive care unit: a prospective study. Crit Care. 2005;9:R636–44.
142. Nowbar AN, Cole GD, Shun-Shin MJ, Finegold JA, Francis DP. International RCT-based guidelines for use of preoperative stress testing and perioperative beta-blockers and statins in non-cardiac surgery. Int J Cardiol. 2014;172:138–43.
143. Poldermans D, Boersma E, Bax JJ, et al. The effect of bisoprolol on perioperative mortality and myocardial infarction in high-risk patients undergoing vascular surgery. Dutch Echocardiographic Cardiac Risk Evaluation Applying Stress Echocardiography Study Group. N Engl J Med. 1999;341:1789–94.
144. Sorrentino MF, Kim J, Foderaro AE, Truesdell AG. 5-fluorouracil induced cardiotoxicity: review of the literature. Cardiol J. 2012;19:453–8.
145. Longley DB, Harkin DP, Johnston PG. 5-fluorouracil: mechanisms of action and clinical strategies. Nat Rev Cancer. 2003;3:330–8.
146. Shields AF, Zalupski MM, Marshall JL, Meropol NJ. Treatment of advanced colorectal carcinoma with oxaliplatin and capecitabine: a phase II trial. Cancer. 2004;100:531–7.
147. Hoff PM, Ansari R, Batist G, et al. Comparison of oral capecitabine versus intravenous fluorouracil plus leucovorin as first-line treatment in 605 patients with metastatic colorectal cancer: results of a randomized phase III study. J Clin Oncol. 2001;19:2282–92.
148. Eskandari MR, Moghaddam F, Shahraki J, Pourahmad J. A comparison of cardiomyocyte cytotoxic mechanisms for 5-fluorouracil and its pro-drug capecitabine. Xenobiotica. 2015;45:79–87.
149. Fernandez-Martos C, Nogue M, Cejas P, Moreno-Garcia V, Machancoses AH, Feliu J. The role of capecitabine in locally advanced rectal cancer treatment: an update. Drugs. 2012;72:1057–73.
150. Ng M, Cunningham D, Norman AR. The frequency and pattern of cardiotoxicity observed with capecitabine used in conjunction with oxaliplatin in patients treated for advanced colorectal cancer (CRC). Eur J Cancer. 2005;41:1542–6.
151. Stewart T, Pavlakis N, Ward M. Cardiotoxicity with 5-fluorouracil and capecitabine: more than just vasospastic angina. Intern Med J. 2010;40:303–7.
152. Frickhofen N, Beck FJ, Jung B, Fuhr HG, Andrasch H, Sigmund M. Capecitabine can induce acute coronary syndrome similar to 5-fluorouracil. Ann Oncol. 2002;13:797–801.
153. Kosmas C, Kallistratos MS, Kopterides P, et al. Cardiotoxicity of fluoropyrimidines in different schedules of administration: a prospective study. J Cancer Res Clin Oncol. 2008;134:75–82.
154. Akhtar SS, Salim KP, Bano ZA. Symptomatic cardiotoxicity with high-dose 5-fluorouracil infusion: a prospective study. Oncology. 1993;50:441–4.
155. de Forni M, Malet-Martino MC, Jaillais P, et al. Cardiotoxicity of high-dose continuous infusion fluorouracil: a prospective clinical study. J Clin Oncol. 1992;10:1795–801.
156. Saif MW, Shah MM, Shah AR. Fluoropyrimidine-associated cardiotoxicity: revisited. Expert Opin Drug Saf. 2009;8:191–202.
157. Basselin C, Fontanges T, Descotes J, et al. 5-Fluorouracil-induced Tako-Tsubo-like syndrome. Pharmacotherapy. 2011;31:226.
158. Grunwald MR, Howie L, Diaz Jr LA. Takotsubo cardiomyopathy and Fluorouracil: case report and review of the literature. J Clin Oncol. 2012;30:e11–4.
159. Canale ML, Camerini A, Stroppa S, et al. A case of acute myocardial infarction during 5-fluorouracil infusion. J Cardiovasc Med (Hagerstown). 2006;7:835–7.
160. Sasson Z, Morgan CD, Wang B, Thomas G, MacKenzie B, Platts ME. 5-Fluorouracil related toxic myocarditis: case reports and pathological confirmation. Can J Cardiol. 1994;10:861–4.
161. Farina A, Malafronte C, Valsecchi MA, Achilli F. Capecitabine-induced cardiotoxicity: when to suspect? How to manage? A case report. J Cardiovasc Med (Hagerstown). 2009;10:722–6.

162. Senturk T, Kanat O, Evrensel T, Aydinlar A. Capecitabine-induced cardiotoxicity mimicking myocardial infarction. Neth Heart J. 2009;17:277–80.
163. McDermott BJ, van den Berg HW, Murphy RF. Nonlinear pharmacokinetics for the elimination of 5-fluorouracil after intravenous administration in cancer patients. Cancer Chemother Pharmacol. 1982;9:173–8.
164. Jensen SA, Sorensen JB. Risk factors and prevention of cardiotoxicity induced by 5-fluorouracil or capecitabine. Cancer Chemother Pharmacol. 2006;58:487–93.
165. Cwikiel M, Eskilsson J, Wieslander JB, Stjernquist U, Albertsson M. The appearance of endothelium in small arteries after treatment with 5-fluorouracil. An electron microscopic study of late effects in rabbits. Scanning Microsc. 1996;10:805–18. Discussion 19.
166. Focaccetti C, Bruno A, Magnani E, et al. Effects of 5-fluorouracil on morphology, cell cycle, proliferation, apoptosis, autophagy and ROS production in endothelial cells and cardiomyocytes. PLoS One. 2015;10, e0115686.
167. Meyer CC, Calis KA, Burke LB, Walawander CA, Grasela TH. Symptomatic cardiotoxicity associated with 5-fluorouracil. Pharmacotherapy. 1997;17:729–36.
168. Anand AJ. Fluorouracil cardiotoxicity. Ann Pharmacother. 1994;28:374–8.
169. Kleiman NS, Lehane DE, Geyer Jr CE, Pratt CM, Young JB. Prinzmetal's angina during 5-fluorouracil chemotherapy. Am J Med. 1987;82:566–8.
170. Akpek G, Hartshorn KL. Failure of oral nitrate and calcium channel blocker therapy to prevent 5-fluorouracil-related myocardial ischemia: a case report. Cancer Chemother Pharmacol. 1999;43:157–61.
171. Eskilsson J, Albertsson M. Failure of preventing 5-fluorouracil cardiotoxicity by prophylactic treatment with verapamil. Acta Oncol. 1990;29:1001–3.
172. Patel B, Kloner RA, Ensley J, Al-Sarraf M, Kish J, Wynne J. 5-Fluorouracil cardiotoxicity: left ventricular dysfunction and effect of coronary vasodilators. Am J Med Sci. 1987;294:238–43.
173. Kelly C, Bhuva N, Harrison M, Buckley A, Saunders M. Use of raltitrexed as an alternative to 5-fluorouracil and capecitabine in cancer patients with cardiac history. Eur J Cancer. 2013;49:2303–10.
174. Ransom D, Wilson K, Fournier M, et al. Final results of Australasian Gastrointestinal Trials Group ARCTIC study: an audit of raltitrexed for patients with cardiac toxicity induced by fluoropyrimidines. Ann Oncol. 2014;25:117–21.
175. Darby SC, Cutter DJ, Boerma M, et al. Radiation-related heart disease: current knowledge and future prospects. Int J Radiat Oncol Biol Phys. 2010;76:656–65.
176. Hancock SL, Donaldson SS, Hoppe RT. Cardiac disease following treatment of Hodgkin's disease in children and adolescents. J Clin Oncol. 1993;11:1208–15.
177. Darby SC, Ewertz M, McGale P, et al. Risk of ischemic heart disease in women after radiotherapy for breast cancer. N Engl J Med. 2013;368:987–98.
178. Clarke M, Collins R, Darby S, Davies C, Elphinstone P, Evans V, Godwin J, Gray R, Hicks C, James S, MacKinnon E, McGale P, McHugh T, Peto R, Taylor C, Wang Y, Early Breast Cancer Trialists' Collaborative Group (EBCTCG). Effects of radiotherapy and of differences in the extent of surgery for early breast cancer on local recurrence and 15-year survival: an overview of the randomised trials. Lancet. 2005;366:2087–106.
179. Brenner DJ, Shuryak I, Jozsef G, Dewyngaert KJ, Formenti SC. Risk and risk reduction of major coronary events associated with contemporary breast radiotherapy. JAMA Intern Med. 2014;174:158–60.
180. Carr ZA, Land CE, Kleinerman RA, et al. Coronary heart disease after radiotherapy for peptic ulcer disease. Int J Radiat Oncol Biol Phys. 2005;61:842–50.
181. Taylor CW, Nisbet A, McGale P, Darby SC. Cardiac exposures in breast cancer radiotherapy: 1950s–1990s. Int J Radiat Oncol Biol Phys. 2007;69:1484–95.
182. Orzan F, Brusca A, Conte MR, Presbitero P, Figliomeni MC. Severe coronary artery disease after radiation therapy of the chest and mediastinum: clinical presentation and treatment. Br Heart J. 1993;69:496–500.

183. Veinot JP, Edwards WD. Pathology of radiation-induced heart disease: a surgical and autopsy study of 27 cases. Hum Pathol. 1996;27:766–73.

184. Chinnasami BR, Schwartz RC, Pink SB, Skotnicki RA. Isolated left main coronary stenosis and mediastinal irradiation. Clin Cardiol. 1992;15:459–61.

185. Gyenes G, Rutqvist LE, Liedberg A, Fornander T. Long-term cardiac morbidity and mortality in a randomized trial of pre- and postoperative radiation therapy versus surgery alone in primary breast cancer. Radiother Oncol. 1998;48:185–90.

186. Konings AW, Smit Sibinga CT, Aarnoudse MW, de Wit SS, Lamberts HB. Initial events in radiation-induced atheromatosis. II Damage to intimal cells. Strahlentherapie. 1978;154:795–800.

187. Girinsky T, M'Kacher R, Lessard N, et al. Prospective coronary heart disease screening in asymptomatic Hodgkin lymphoma patients using coronary computed tomography angiography: results and risk factor analysis. Int J Radiat Oncol Biol Phys. 2014;89:59–66.

188. Veeragandham RS, Goldin MD. Surgical management of radiation-induced heart disease. Ann Thorac Surg. 1998;65:1014–9.

189. Morice MC, Serruys PW, Kappetein AP, et al. Outcomes in patients with de novo left main disease treated with either percutaneous coronary intervention using paclitaxel-eluting stents or coronary artery bypass graft treatment in the Synergy between Percutaneous Coronary Intervention with TAXUS and Cardiac Surgery (SYNTAX) trial. Circulation. 2010;121:2645–53.

Chapter 9
Vascular Complications of Cancer and Cancer Therapy

Gary H. Lyman, Anna Catino, and Bonnie Ky

The Risk of Venous Thromboembolism in Patients with Cancer

The risk of venous thromboembolism (VTE) is increased considerably in patients with cancer, most notably hospitalized patients, the elderly, and those with major medical comorbidities [1–4]. Of particular importance is the primary site of cancer with the highest rates observed in those with cancers of the brain, pancreas, stomach, kidney, ovary, and lung as well as in those with hematologic malignancies [4–6]. Additional risk factors for VTE include comorbid conditions such as infection, pulmonary or renal disease, and obesity, elevations in leukocyte and platelet counts, and reductions in hemoglobin.

As discussed later in this chapter, the risk of VTE is further increased in patients receiving systemic therapies including chemotherapy, hormonal therapy, and

Electronic supplementary material: The online version of this chapter (doi:10.1007/978-3-319-43096-6_9) contains supplementary material, which is available to authorized users.

G.H. Lyman (✉)
Hutchinson Institute for Cancer Outcomes Research, Fred Hutchinson Cancer Research Center, Seattle, WA, USA

University of Washington, Seattle, WA, USA
e-mail: glyman@fredhutch.org

A. Catino
Division of Cardiovascular Medicine, Department of Medicine, University of Utah, Salt Lake City, UT, USA
e-mail: anna.catino@hsc.utah.edu

B. Ky
Division of Cardiology, Department of Medicine, University of Pennsylvania, Philadelphia, PA, USA
e-mail: bonnie.ky@uphs.upenn.edu

G.G. Kimmick et al. (eds.), *Cardio-Oncology*, DOI 10.1007/978-3-319-43096-6_9

Table 9.1 Risk score for predicting outpatient VTE in cancer patients [16]

Patient characteristics	Risk score
Site of cancer	2
Very high risk (stomach, pancreas)	1
High risk (lung, lymphoma, gynecologic, bladder, testicular)	
Prechemotherapy platelet count 350,000/mm^3 or more	1
Hemoglobin level less than 10 g/dL or use of red cell growth factors	1
Prechemotherapy leukocyte count more than 11,000/mm^3	1
Body mass index 35 kg/m^2 or more	1

High-risk score ≥ 3
Intermediate-risk score $= 1$–2
Low-risk score $= 0$

certain targeted agents, especially the anti-angiogenesis agents which appear to be associated with an increased risk of arterial and potentially venous thrombosis [7–12]. While the risk of arterial thrombotic events is increased with bevacizumab, it remains unclear whether the risk of VTE is increased after adjustment for treatment duration [13]. The use of the erythropoiesis-stimulating agents, epoetin alfa and darbepoetin alfa, as well as blood transfusions has also been associated with an increased risk of VTE [3, 14, 15]. Due to the multiple disease, treatment, and patient-specific risk factors associated with VTE, a predictive risk model for VTE in ambulatory cancer patients receiving systemic chemotherapy based on clinical and laboratory measures has been developed [16, 17]. The risk score has now been validated in multiple retrospective and prospective studies [16, 18–20] (Table 9.1). Retrospective evaluations of randomized controlled trials have also shown that the risk of VTE in high-risk patients identified on the basis of the risk score is significantly reduced in those receiving thromboprophylaxis [21, 22].

Consequences of Venous Thromboembolism in Patients with Cancer

VTE in patients with cancer is associated with several adverse consequences including early mortality [2, 23–26]. Additional serious clinical complications include recurrent VTE, major bleeding associated with anticoagulation, and interruption of optimal cancer treatment along with an impact on quality of life and healthcare costs [27, 28]. Importantly, the risk of recurrence, bleeding, and mortality in cancer patients with incidental or unsuspected VTE appears to be similar to those with symptomatic VTE [29]. The majority of patients with unsuspected pulmonary embolism (PE) identified on staging computerized tomography scans are symptomatic with similar clinical consequences [20, 30–32]. Clinical symptoms of chest pain, shortness of breath, and fatigue are often attributed to the underlying malignancy [20, 31, 32].

Prevention and Treatment of Cancer-Associated Venous Thromboembolism

There is experimental evidence that the heparins may interfere with cancer cell proliferation, angiogenesis, and the formation of metastases [33]. Several RCTs in patients with cancer but without VTE have evaluated whether anticoagulants improve overall survival with varied results [34–40]. In a meta-analysis of 11 RCTs of patients with cancer receiving anticoagulants or no anticoagulants, a significant reduction in 1-year mortality with LMWHs but not with warfarin was observed with relative risks for all-cause mortality of 0.88 [95 % CI, 0.79–0.98; $P = 0.015$] and 0.94 [95 % CI, 0.85–1.04; $P = 0.239$], respectively [41]. Greater risk of major bleeding was reported in patients receiving anticoagulation reaching statistical significance in warfarin studies [41]. Therefore, while anticoagulation is not recommended in this situation due to the recognized limitations of these trials and the increased risk for bleeding, a number of clinical practice guidelines address the appropriate role of thromboprophylaxis in the treatment and preventions of VTE in patients with cancer [42–46]. As summarized in Table 9.2, recommendations cover treatment and prevention of VTE in hospitalized medical and surgical cancer patients, the current limited role of prophylaxis in the ambulatory setting, and secondary prophylaxis of patients with established VTE. These guidelines also recommend that patients with cancer be educated about the symptoms and signs of VTE and that VTE risk be assessed at the time of chemotherapy initiation and periodically over the course of treatment.

Treatment of VTE in Patients with Cancer

The initial treatment of established VTE in cancer patients is generally patterned after therapeutic approaches in other non-cancer settings. However, the duration of therapy to prevent early recurrence is often extended in cancer patients with persistent disease or continuing on cancer treatment [47]. Current recommendations call for low molecular weight heparin (LMWH) for the initial 5–10 days of anticoagulation in cancer patients with established VTE, as well as for secondary prevention of recurrence for at least 6 months. Patients with unsuspected or incidental VTE should be treated the same as symptomatic VTE. High-risk patients on systemic therapy for persistent malignancy should be considered for extended anticoagulation to prevent VTE recurrence. The development of a number of new oral and parenteral antithrombotic agents is likely to have future application to patients with cancer [48, 49].

Table 9.2 VTE treatment and prophylaxis recommendations [46, 124]

ASCO recommendations

Inpatient

    1.1 Hospitalized patients who have active malignancy with acute medical illness or reduced mobility should receive pharmacologic thromboprophylaxis in the absence of bleeding or other contraindications

    1.2 Hospitalized patients who have active malignancy without additional risk factors may be considered for pharmacologic thromboprophylaxis in the absence of bleeding or other contraindications

    1.3 Data are inadequate to support routine thromboprophylaxis in patients admitted for minor procedures or brief infusional chemotherapy or in patients undergoing stem cell/ bone marrow transplantation

Outpatient

    2.1 Routine pharmacologic thromboprophylaxis is not recommended in cancer outpatients

    2.2 Based on limited RCT data, clinicians may consider LMWH prophylaxis on a case-by-case basis in highly selected outpatients with solid tumors receiving chemotherapy. Consideration of such therapy should be accompanied by a discussion with the patient about the uncertainty concerning benefits and harms, as well as dose and duration of prophylaxis in this setting

    2.3 Patients with multiple myeloma receiving thalidomide- or lenalidomide-based regimens with chemotherapy and/or dexamethasone should receive pharmacologic thromboprophylaxis with either aspirin or LMWH for low-risk patients and LMWH for high-risk patients

Perioperative

    3.1 All patients with malignant disease undergoing major surgical intervention should be considered for pharmacologic thromboprophylaxis with either UFH or LMWH unless contraindicated because of active bleeding or a high risk of bleeding with the procedure

    3.2 Prophylaxis should be commenced preoperatively

    3.3 Mechanical methods may be added to pharmacologic thromboprophylaxis, but should not be used as monotherapy for VTE prevention unless pharmacologic methods are contraindicated because of active bleeding or high bleeding risk

    3.4 A combined regimen of pharmacologic and mechanical prophylaxis may improve efficacy, especially in the highest-risk patients

    3.5 Pharmacologic thromboprophylaxis should be continued for at least 7–10 days in all patients. Extended prophylaxis with LMWH for up to 4 weeks postoperatively should be considered for patients undergoing major abdominal or pelvic surgery for cancer who have high-risk features such as restricted mobility, obesity, history of VTE, or with additional risk factors

Treatment and secondary prophylaxis

    4.1 LMWH is preferred over UFH for the initial 5–10 days of anticoagulation for the cancer patient with newly diagnosed VTE who does not have severe renal impairment (defined as creatinine clearance <30 mL/min)

    4.2 For long-term anticoagulation, LMWH for at least 6 months is preferred due to improved efficacy over vitamin K antagonists. Vitamin K antagonists are an acceptable alternative for long-term therapy if LMWH is not available

    4.3 Anticoagulation with LMWH or vitamin K antagonist beyond the initial 6 months may be considered for select patients with active cancer, such as those with metastatic disease or those receiving chemotherapy

    4.4 The insertion of a vena cava filter is only indicated for patients with contraindications to anticoagulant therapy. It may be considered as an adjunct to anticoagulation in patients with progression of thrombosis (recurrent VTE or extension of existing thrombus) despite maximal therapy with LMWH

(continued)

Table 9.2 (continued)

4.5 For patients with central nervous system malignancies, anticoagulation is recommended for established VTE as described for other patients with cancer. Careful monitoring is necessary to limit the risk of hemorrhagic complications
4.6 Use of novel oral anticoagulants for either prevention or treatment of VTE in cancer patients is not recommended at this time
4.7 Incidental PE and DVT should be treated in the same manner as symptomatic VTE. Treatment of splanchnic or visceral vein thrombi diagnosed incidentally should be considered on a case-by-case basis, considering potential benefits and risks of anticoagulation
Anticoagulation and survival
5.1 Anticoagulants are not recommended to improve survival in patients with cancer without VTE
5.2 Patients with cancer should be encouraged to participate in clinical trials designed to evaluate anticoagulant therapy as an adjunct to standard anticancer therapies
Risk assessment
6.1 Cancer patients should be assessed for VTE risk at the time of chemotherapy initiation and periodically thereafter
6.1a In the outpatient setting, risk assessment can be conducted based on a validated risk assessment tool
6.1b Solitary risk factors, including biomarkers or cancer site, do not reliably identify cancer patients at high risk of VTE
6.2 Oncologists should educate patients regarding VTE, particularly in settings that increase risk such as major surgery, hospitalization, and while receiving systemic antineoplastic therapy. Patient education should at least include a discussion of the warning signs and symptoms of VTE, including leg swelling or pain, sudden-onset chest pain, and shortness of breath

Thromboprophylaxis of Hospitalized Medical or Surgical Patients with Cancer

Although reported rates vary considerably, VTE is a common cause of death in hospitalized cancer patients [2, 4, 50–53]. Although three large randomized controlled trials (RCTs) have demonstrated that thromboprophylaxis reduces VTE risk in hospitalized patients with acute medical illness, cancer represented only a small proportion of the study populations [54–57]. Nevertheless, due to the increased risk of VTE associated with malignancy, prophylactic anticoagulation of most hospitalized patients with major medical illnesses including cancer or reduced mobility is recommended in the absence of a serious bleeding risk with anticoagulation.

Likewise, patients undergoing major cancer surgery are at an increased risk for VTE as well as for bleeding complications [58]. Patients undergoing major surgical procedures for cancer should receive thromboprophylaxis unless contraindicated, while combined mechanical prophylaxis and anticoagulation may be considered in high-risk patients [59]. Prophylactic anticoagulation should be initiated preoperatively when possible and continued for at least 7–10 days. Extended prophylaxis for up to 4 weeks postoperatively should also be considered in high-risk patients including those with restricted mobility, obesity, or a history of VTE. Of note, there remain inadequate data to support routine thromboprophylaxis in those with short admissions for chemotherapy or for minor procedures [46, 60].

Thromboprophylaxis of Ambulatory Patients with Cancer

The risk of VTE in ambulatory cancer patients varies widely with the type of cancer and treatment and associated comorbid conditions. As discussed further in this chapter, the emergence of more aggressive interventions and a number of new cancer therapies and supportive care agents with an increased risk of VTE has resulted in increased interest in the potential value of VTE prophylaxis in this setting [8, 61–72]. Several RCTs of thromboprophylaxis in ambulatory cancer patients have been reported including nine with LMWHs. The greatest impact on the absolute risk of VTE has been observed in patients with advanced pancreatic cancer receiving specified chemotherapy [73, 74]. A meta-analysis has estimated a relative risk for symptomatic VTE across studies of 0.47 (0.36–0.61; $P < 0.001$) but with only an absolute reduction in VTE risk of 2.8 % (1.8–3.7 %; $P < 0.001$) [75]. Due to the small incremental benefit observed in most trials of ambulatory cancer patients, routine thromboprophylaxis is not recommended with the exception of patients with multiple myeloma receiving thalidomide or lenalidomide with chemotherapy and dexamethasone where the risk of VTE is very high. However, real-world studies in unselected ambulatory cancer patients receiving cancer chemotherapy have suggested rates of VTE twofold to threefold greater than those reported in selected patients in reported RCTs (Fig. 9.1) [76]. Therefore, thromboprophylaxis may be considered on an individual basis in selected high-risk patients with solid tumors receiving chemotherapy balancing the potential benefits and harms [46, 77].

Vascular Complications of Endocrine Cancer Therapies

VTE is a recognized adverse event associated with estrogens as well as certain estrogen-like agents such as tamoxifen and other selective estrogen receptor modulating agents (SERMS) [78–81]. Increased risk of VTE with these agents has been observed both in patients receiving endocrine treatment for cancer but also in those receiving SERMs as chemoprevention to reduce cancer risk [82]. Despite an apparent lower risk, an increased risk of VTE has also been associated with endocrine treatment with the aromatase inhibitors [83].

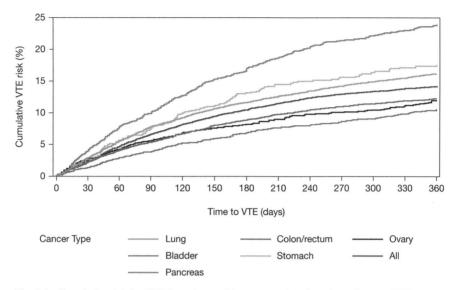

Fig. 9.1 Cumulative risk for VTE in patients with cancer undergoing chemotherapy. *VTE* venous thromboembolism [76]

Vascular Complications Associated with Targeted Cancer Therapeutics

While several traditional cytotoxic chemotherapeutic agents including 5-fluorouracil and cisplatin have been associated with vascular toxicities such as coronary vasospasm and arterial thrombotic events [84, 85], newer targeted biological agents, including monoclonal antibodies and tyrosine kinase inhibitors, are also associated with a significant risk of vascular complications. In the following sections, we will provide an overview of these cardiovascular toxicities and specifically focus on the vascular complications of newer anti-VEGF (vascular endothelial growth factor) therapies, tyrosine kinase inhibitors, and immunomodulatory therapies.

Monoclonal Antibodies: VEGF Inhibitors

The relationship between vascular endothelial growth factor and tumor angiogenesis was first introduced in the 1970s by Dr. Judah Folkman, when an association between solid tumor growth and vascular supply was observed. He identified a soluble factor released from tumors ("tumor angiogenesis factor"), which promoted neovascularization, and he proposed that inhibition of this factor could halt tumor neo-angiogenesis [86]. Dr. Napoleone Ferrara's group subsequently sequenced this factor, now known as VEGF, and since then this signaling pathway has been the target of multiple pharmacotherapies for the treatment of various malignancies [86]. Bevacizumab (Avastin™), a humanized monoclonal antibody that binds and neutralizes VEGF, was the first VEGF inhibitor approved by the FDA in 2004 after a landmark study demonstrated that the addition of bevacizumab to fluorouracil-based combination chemotherapy resulted in improved survival among patients with metastatic colorectal cancer [87]. It has since been approved as monotherapy for the treatment of advanced non-squamous non-small cell lung cancer, metastatic renal cell carcinoma, and recurrent glioblastoma [86–88]. VEGF, while crucial to tumor angiogenesis, is also fundamental for endothelial cell function and proliferation and thus the formation of new vessels. As might be expected, VEGF inhibition has been associated with a significant increase in vascular complications, in particular arterial thrombotic events and bleeding [86, 87].

Mechanism of Action and Toxicity

VEGF is essential for tumor angiogenesis and increased VEGF expression is associated with increased tumor invasiveness, metastatic ability, and recurrence [87, 88]. There are three receptors (VEGFR-1/Flt-1, VEGFR-2/Flk-1/KDR, VEGFR-3/Flt-4). The ligand VEGF-A, generally referred to as VEGF, binds to VEGFR-2 on endothelial cells leading to pro-angiogenic effects [89]. By binding to the VEGF receptor, bevacizumab disrupts downstream VEGF signaling, preventing tumor angiogenesis and increasing the delivery of cancer therapy to tumor cells [90]. It is hypothesized that the vascular toxicities of bevacizumab, which include both thrombosis and bleeding, occur through similar mechanisms and are the result of an imbalance in the tightly regulated hemostatic system. This system includes a balance of pro- and anticoagulant proteins, platelet-activating and platelet-inhibiting factors, and pro- and antifibrinolytic products [12, 90]. Inhibition of VEGF results in decreased endothelial cell survival, platelet aggregation and thrombosis, increased platelet reactivity, and downregulation of several factors. The vasculature is susceptible to damage induced by trauma [12, 90], and disruption of the endothelial barrier results in exposure of the subendothelial von Willebrand factor and tissue factor, platelet aggregation, and thrombus formation [86, 91]. The increase in platelet-endothelial interactions may further precipitate thrombosis [92]. Finally, downregulation of several factors that are modulated by VEGF including nitric oxide, prostacyclin, and thrombolytic serine proteases (u-PA and t-PA) contributes to increased vascular toxicity such as vasoconstriction, endothelial cell apoptosis, and increased arterial stiffness [86, 90]. Several other mechanisms have been proposed as contributing to VEGF inhibitor-induced vascular toxicity. Drug-induced hypertension generating high shear stress at plaque sites may accelerate atherothrombosis [88, 91]. Associated inflammation and cell lysis have also been shown to increase thrombogenicity, and apoptotic cell blebs may sustain vascular inflammation and activate the complement cascade [88, 91]. Anti-angiogenic drugs are known to hinder the recognized insulin anti-atherogenic actions, including glucose uptake, lipogenesis, and antilipolysis, ultimately producing a thrombophilic hyperglycemic, atherogenic lipoprotein prone to thrombosis [9]. Finally, VEGF inhibition may result in lack of protective growth factors, potentially resulting in plaque instability and thrombosis [93]. Figure 9.2 illustrates the proposed mechanisms for the vascular toxic effects of bevacizumab.

Clinical Presentation and Epidemiology

The major cardiovascular toxicities of bevacizumab are hypertension, hemorrhage, perforation, and thrombosis [90]. Thrombotic events include thrombosis and thromboembolism, generally in the form of acute coronary syndrome, stroke, and peripheral vascular disease, although coronary ischemia is the most frequent arterial thrombotic event (ATE) [94]. While initial trials of bevacizumab only reported an insignificant increase in thrombotic or bleeding events, multiple subsequent larger clinical studies have demonstrated an elevated risk of vascular events [87]. A meta-analysis of 1745 patients from five randomized trials showed combination treatment with bevacizumab and chemotherapy, compared with chemotherapy alone, was associated with an increased risk of ATE (HR 2.0, 95 % CI 1.05–3.75, $P = 0.031$), but not venous thromboembolism [10]. A meta-analysis published in 2010 to evaluate the incidence of arterial thromboembolic events associated with bevacizumab included over 12,500 patients with various advanced solid tumors and found a 3.3 % incidence of ATE (95 % CI 2.0–5.6) and a 2.0 % incidence of high-grade arterial thrombotic events (95 % CI 1.7–2.5), defined as acute coronary syndrome, transient ischemic attack, stroke, life-threatening peripheral arterial thrombosis or requiring surgery, and death [94]. Compared to controls, bevacizumab was associated with a relative risk of ATE of 1.44 (95 % CI 1.08–1.91, $p < 0.013$). In particular, this meta-analysis found that bevacizumab was associated with a significantly increased risk of cardiac ischemia (RR 2.14, 95 % CI 1.12–4.08, $p < 0.021$) [94]. Vascular events have been noted early after starting VEGF inhibitor therapy, with a median time of event occurrence after drug initiation of 7 months (1–12 months is general range) [88, 95]. Moreover, the risk of ATE associated with bevacizumab may differ by tumor type. One meta-analysis found a significantly higher risk of high-grade ATE in patients with renal cell carcinoma (RR 5.14 95 % CI 1.35–19.64) [94]. Patients with pre-existing cardiovascular disease are at an increased high risk for thrombotic complications [96, 97]. Specifically, patients older than 65 years of age, with diabetes, with known atherosclerosis, or with a history of a prior cardiovascular event, appear to be at a higher risk for bevacizumab-associated ATE [97].

Management

Traditionally arterial thrombotic events have been associated with grave prognosis in cancer patients [98]. Once an arterial thrombotic event develops in a patient receiving VEGF inhibitor therapy, it is generally recommended therapy be permanently stopped and the ATE treated as per guidelines for the particular event, such as the American College of Cardiology/American Heart Association (ACC/AHA) recommendations for acute coronary events [99, 100]. Some clinicians advocate for avoiding anti-VEGF therapies in patients with a history of coronary or peripheral vascular disease. Others recommend prophylactic antiplatelet therapy such as aspirin or clopidogrel [86]. Aspirin therapy has been shown to be associated with a significant improvement in short-term cardiovascular outcomes [10, 88]. Theoretically, statins and angiotensin-converting-enzyme inhibitors (ACE-inhibitors) may also exert antioxidant and anti-inflammatory effects resulting in a decrease in atherothrombotic risk [10]. However, the use of anticoagulants and antiplatelet agents in patients receiving VEGF inhibitors remains controversial, especially in the setting of thromboembolic events given their association with bleeding.

Despite the increased frequency of thromboembolic events in cancer patients, there are limited data on the use of bevacizumab concurrently in patients being treated with therapeutic anticoagulation. A post hoc analysis of three phase III clinical trials of bevacizumab compared to control evaluated the incidence of thrombotic and bleeding in patients receiving therapeutic anticoagulation (warfarin and low molecular weight heparin) [95]. The incidence of thrombotic adverse events for patients receiving bevacizumab compared to the placebo group was primarily venous and on the order of 9.6–17.3 %. The overall rates of severe bleeding for all patients in the control group were 2.5 % versus 3.3 % in the bevacizumab group. The authors concluded that combining bevacizumab with therapeutic anticoagulation did not substantially increase the risk of bleeding beyond the risk of bleeding expected from therapeutic anticoagulation alone [95]. Similarly, a prospective observational cohort study including 1953 patients to assess the safety of bevacizumab for treatment of metastatic colorectal cancer (BRiTE study) showed serious bleeding events were comparable among patients on prophylactic anticoagulation therapy versus not [101]. In the absence of formal guidelines, it is generally recommended that patients be treated for thrombotic events with anticoagulation albeit cautiously with close monitoring for adverse bleeding events. There are insufficient data and therefore no standard recommendations to use prophylactic anticoagulation in this setting. Of course, an individual approach for patients should be conducted based on comorbidities and prior thrombotic and bleeding events. Furthermore, a cardiovascular risk assessment is recommended in all patients undergoing such therapy, with consideration for additional testing in certain patient populations.

Small Molecule Tyrosine Kinase Inhibitors: VEGF Inhibitors

Tyrosine kinase inhibitors (TKIs) are a growing and widely used group of therapies for various malignancies, and many TKIs have anti-angiogenic properties. Examples include, but are not limited to, sunitinib (Sutent™), sorafenib (Nexavar™), and pazopanib (Votrient™). These agents, used widely in metastatic renal cell cancer, as well as for the treatment of other malignancies, have been associated with coronary ischemia and small vessel disease [12, 86].

Mechanisms of Action and Toxicity

Similar to bevacizumab, these small molecule TKIs work by blocking the intracellular domain of the VEGF receptor leading to inhibition of the VEGF pathway. Moreover, these TKIs affect multiple additional pathways. Sunitinib has activity against all three VEGFRs, platelet-derived growth factor receptor (PDGF) α and β, stem cell factor receptor (KIT), and fms-like kinase receptor 3 (FLT3). It is approved for treatment of advanced renal cell carcinoma, gastrointestinal stromal tumors (GIST), and advanced pancreatic neuroendocrine tumors [86, 88, 97]. Sorafenib has activity against all VEGFRs, PDGF-β, KIT, FLT3, and RET, as well as the intracellular kinases CRAF, BRAF, and mutant BRAF. It has been approved for the treatment of advanced hepatocellular carcinoma, thyroid cancer, and advanced renal cell carcinoma [86, 88, 97]. Pazopanib also has activity against VEGFRs, PDGFRs, fibroblast growth factor receptors (FGFRs) 1 and 3. It has been approved for the treatment of metastatic renal cell carcinoma and advanced soft tissue sarcomas that have received prior chemotherapy [86, 88, 97].

The mechanisms for vascular toxicity in these TKIs with VEGF pathway inhibiting characteristics may be similar to those proposed for bevacizumab. Individual response to VEGF inhibition and variation in response to the growth factor pathway blocking lends to variation in vascular complications and individual vulnerability to off-target effects [12, 86, 88, 97]. Figure 9.2 illustrates proposed mechanisms for vascular toxic effects of VEGF signaling pathway inhibitors.

Clinical Presentation and Epidemiology

The major cardiac vascular toxicities of small molecule tyrosine kinase inhibitors with VEGF-inhibiting properties include hypertension, hemorrhage, perforation, and thrombosis [90]. As it relates to thrombosis, there is an increased incidence of acute coronary syndrome, cerebrovascular accidents, peripheral vascular disease, and bleeding observed with these anti-angiogenic TKIs.

Cardiac ischemia and related coronary artery disease has been a common manifestation of ATE associated with TKIs (Fig. 9.3). One observational study showed that among patients treated with sorafenib or sunitinib, there was an extremely high rate of cardiac events (33.8 %) leading to interruption or discontinuation of TKI therapy in 60 % of those patients [102]. Of the patients who experienced cardiac events, 52 % were symptomatic with angina, dyspnea, and dizziness while 48 % of the patients were asymptomatic with cardiac biomarker

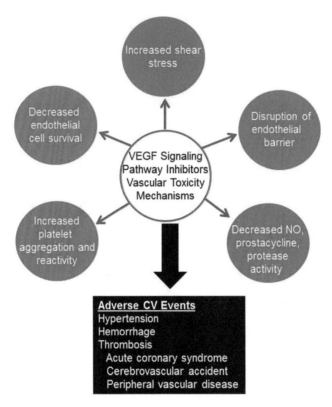

Fig. 9.2 Proposed mechanisms for the "off-target" vascular toxicities from VEGF signaling pathway inhibitors [12, 86, 88, 90–92, 97]

elevation or ECG changes [102]. In a large meta-analyses of over 38,000 patients evaluating the vascular complications of VEGF inhibitors, including both TKIs and bevacizumab, there was an increased risk of myocardial infarction, hypertension, and arterial thromboembolism [103]. Compared to the control group, recipients of VEGF inhibitors had significantly higher risk of myocardial infarction (RR 3.54, 95 % CI 1.61–7.80, $I^2 = 0$ %, tau2 = 0), arterial thrombotic events (RR 1.80, 95 % CI 1.24–2.59, $I^2 = 0$ %, tau2 = 0), and hypertension (RR 3.46, 95 % CI 2.89–4.15, $I^2 = 58$ %, tau2 = 0.16) [103]. In 2010, Choueiri et al. published a meta-analysis of clinical trials with sorafenib or sunitinib that included over 10,000 patients [91]. The rate of arterial thrombotic events was increased threefold (2 % absolute risk) with these drugs, and this finding was independent of type of malignancy or TKI [91]. Again, the most common type of ATE was coronary ischemia, followed by stroke [91].

Interestingly, a newer agent under investigation semaxanib, a potent and selective inhibitor of VEGFR-2/Flk-1/KDR, with activity against VEGFR-1, KIT, and FLT3, was aborted because of a remarkably high thrombosis rate of 42 % during a phase I trial [12, 88, 104]. The authors concluded that semaxanib likely causes

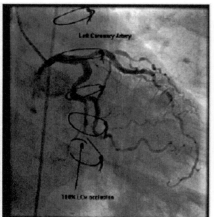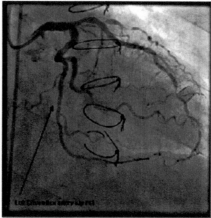

Fig. 9.3 Coronary angiogram of a 60-year-old male with metastatic renal cell cancer treated with multiple angiogenic inhibitors over a 9-year period. (**a**) Shows pre-percutaneous coronary intervention with occlusion of the left circumflex. (**b**) Shows post-percutaneous coronary intervention with restoration of flow in the left circumflex

endothelial cell activation, and in the setting of chemotherapy-induced triggered coagulation cascade, high thrombosis rates can occur. However, it is speculated that this high rate of thrombosis (both arterial and venous) is most likely related to the combination of semaxanib with cisplatin and gemcitabine, which are also associated with vascular events independently [104, 105].

Management

As with bevacizumab, there are no standardized recommendations on specifically how to manage these patients within the realm of cardio-oncology. Withdrawal of TKI therapy and treatment of arterial thrombosis as per oncology and cardiology guidelines is currently advised [99, 100]. The role of screening and prophylactic anticoagulation is not defined. Furthermore, large studies assessing the role of various risk stratification tools to evaluate patients vulnerable to the atherothrombotic effects of TKIs are lacking [12, 86].

Small Molecule Tyrosine Kinase Inhibitors: Bcr-Abl Inhibitors

Bcr-Abl tyrosine kinase inhibitors are also small molecule TKIs that appear to have anti-angiogenic activity, although they do not directly inhibit the VEGF pathway. Bcr-Abl TKIs are first-line therapy for treatment of chronic myelogenous leukemia

(CML). More than 90 % of CMLs are caused by a chromosomal abnormality with formation of a "Philadelphia chromosome" which is essentially the fusion between the Abelson (Abl) tyrosine kinase gene on chromosome 9 and the breakpoint cluster (Bcr) gene at chromosome 22 [106]. Therapy targeting this specific mutation has been developed and the first approved therapy was imatinib (Gleevec™) by the FDA in 2001 [107]. The therapeutic benefits from this targeted therapy have been astounding and truly revolutionized CML therapy. However, resistance has since emerged to imatinib in more than 20 % of patients. Therefore, second- and third-generation Bcr-Abl inhibitors (dasatinib (Sprycel™), nilotinib (Tasigna™), bosutinib (Bosulif™), and ponatinib (Iclusig™)) have been developed to overcome imatinib resistance. These are promising therapies from an oncologic standpoint, but they have been associated with significant vascular complications. Specifically these agents have been associated with acute coronary syndromes, stroke, and acute limb ischemia [96, 107].

Mechanisms of Action and Toxicity

The mutated fusion protein, Bcr-Abl, is expressed only on malignant cells, and thus Bcr-Abl-inhibiting TKIs are theoretically specific to leukemic cells. The TKIs bind to the amino acids of the Bcr-Abl tyrosine kinase ATP-binding site and stabilize the inactive form of the protein, preventing tyrosine autophosphorylation and downstream phosphorylation of its substrates [108]. Second- and third-generation Bcr-Abl-inhibiting TKIs target the genetic mutations leading to imatinib resistance. Ponatinib is an example and has activity against the specific T3151 mutation in Bcr-Abl implicated in many imatinib-resistant cases [107]. The mechanisms underlying the association between the second- and third-generation Bcr-Abl-inhibiting TKIs and vascular complications are largely unknown. Unlike other anti-angiogenic therapies, these small molecule TKIs do not have established VEGF receptor or pathway inhibiting properties. However, they are often referred to as "accidental" angiogenesis inhibitors as they likely still affect the angiogenesis pathway [88, 96, 109]. There is some speculation that the vascular toxicity associated with these agents may be related to unrecognized kinase targets being inhibited or at least preferentially blocked by the second- and third-generation TKIs which have demonstrated acute atherothrombosis and accelerated atherosclerosis [110]. These TKIs have been demonstrated to have effects on the discoidin domain receptor 1 (DDR1), which has been implicated in plaque formation in atherosclerosis [110]. Additional targets of these TKIs, KIT and PDGFR, appear to be involved in regulation of various vascular and perivascular cells, and thus disruption may lead to vascular events [110]. Some small prospective trials show evidence that nilotinib may also result in metabolic derangements including glucose intolerance and even diabetes, altered lipid profiles, and atherogenesis [110–112].

Clinical Presentation and Epidemiology

Clinically the adverse vascular events attributed to Bcr-Abl-inhibiting TKIs appear to be dose related and have manifested as acute thrombotic events and accelerated atherosclerosis [88]. Ponatinib has been associated with acute myocardial infarction, cerebral vascular accidents, and severe peripheral vascular disease (PAD) including acute limb ischemia [96, 113]. Rapid development and progression of atherosclerosis has been observed in the absence of significant cardiovascular risk factors, underlying atherosclerosis, or other vascular trauma [96]. The phase II Ponatinib for CML Evaluation and Philadelphia Chromosome-Positive Acute Lymphoblastic Leukemia (PACE) trial [34], evaluating ponatinib in patients with resistant forms of CML, showed an 11.8 % incidence of serious arterial thrombotic events (cardiovascular 6.2 %, cerebrovascular 4.0 %, and peripheral vascular 3.6 %,) and 17.1 % incidence of all arterial thrombotic events at 24 months. The majority of these events occurred within the first 11 months of therapy. These adverse vascular events were seen across all age groups and in patients with and without cardiovascular risk factors [113]. However, 55 % of these patients had a history of ischemic vascular disease prior to initiation of ponatinib, and 95 % had one or more cardiovascular risk factors including hypertension, diabetes, hypercholesterolemia, or obesity [113]. Since then, the FDA has placed a black box warning and announced an investigation into the frequency of "serious and life-threatening blood clots and severe narrowing of blood vessels" among patients taking ponatinib [107, 110, 114, 115]. Nilotinib is also associated with high rate of arterial thrombotic events and accelerated atherosclerosis [96, 107]. In the initial studies evaluating nilotinib, the therapy was associated with rapidly progressive peripheral artery disease, acute myocardial infarction, spinal infarction, and even sudden death in 25 % of the 24 patients [110]. Moreover, renovascular hypertension and thrombotic events including ischemic nephropathy and mesenteric ischemia have also been observed [19, 96]. A study of nilotinib in 129 CML patients treated with imatinib or nilotinib showed the development of PAD occurred quickly in the nilotinib group compared to imatinib (median 30 versus 102 months, respectively), despite similar cardiovascular risk factors [116]. Pathological peripheral artery disease (using ankle-brachial index (ABI) of <0.9 for screening in asymptomatic patients being treated with TKI therapy) was seen in 6.3 % of patients receiving first-line imatinib and up to 26–35.7 % receiving nilotinib as first- or second-line therapy [116]. Interestingly the original Bcr-Abl inhibitor, imatinib, with less potent activity has not been associated with the same rate of arterial vascular complications despite similar underlying patient characteristics [96, 117]. Levato et al. evaluated 82 CML patients at their institution treated with imatinib or nilotinib. While none of the patients treated with imatinib developed peripheral vascular disease, 14.8 % treated with nilotinib developed peripheral vascular disease [117].

Management

There is little guidance regarding treatment of patients who suffer from such adverse vascular events, and very little is known about the progression/regression of disease once discontinuation of these more potent Bcr-Abl TKIs. However there are data that suggest limiting dose and avoiding use of successive TKIs may lessen the risk [112]. Similar to the thrombotic events that occur with other cancer therapies, it is generally recommended that therapy be permanently discontinued [110, 112]. As noted above, a black box warning has now been issued outlining a risk of arterial vascular events of up to 27 % of patients with ponatinib [96, 107, 114, 115]. Nilotinib is still in clinical use however. As these highly potent therapies remain an essential treatment to certain patients with resistance to other TKIs, the significant vascular events associated with the second- and third-generation TKIs raise the importance of considering the risk/benefit ratio for individual patients. Accordingly, some oncologists are now proposing first-line therapy with imatinib and turning to the second- and third-line agents in the presence of less than complete hematological or molecular remission [111]. There are no formal recommendations addressing screening patients for cardiovascular events prior to initiating second- and third-line Bcr-Abl TKIs. Accelerated atherosclerosis and acute arterial thrombosis occurred in the absence of pre-existing vascular disease. There is a general consensus in the literature that caution must be taken in patients with underlying cardiovascular disease [86] and comorbidities that increase the risk of CV disease such as hypertension, hyperlipidemia, diabetes, and obesity should be aggressively controlled [88, 97].

Immunomodulatory Therapies: Thalidomide and Lenalidomide

Immunomodulatory therapies including thalidomide (Thalomid™) and its derivatives such as lenalidomide (Revlimid™) and pomalidomide (Pomalyst™) alter the immune response against cancer cells. Thalidomide was first of this class to be used for patients with multiple myeloma refractory to other chemotherapy. Used alone, there has been no significant increase in vascular complications associated with thalidomide or with lenalidomide beyond those associated with multiple myeloma [71, 118]. However, there is a more potent anti-angiogenic and antitumor effect when these agents are used in combination with other therapies, and a significant rate of venous thromboembolic (VTE) emerged when used in combination with other agents in the treatment of multiple myeloma and solid tumors [118].

Mechanism of Action and Toxicity

The anticancer activity of immunomodulatory agents is not well understood. However in myeloma, it appears that these drugs cause direct downregulation of critical tumor cell survival functions such as cell adhesion and cytokine production [119]. The mechanism for venous thrombotic events associated with thalidomide and its derivatives is likely multifactorial. Studies on the teratogenic effects of thalidomide indicate an anti-angiogenic effect possibly associated with the generation of reactive oxygen species [12, 85]. Architectural alterations in endothelial cells treated with thalidomide and dexamethasone have been noted, and bone marrow-derived endothelial cells have shown a dose-dependent downregulation of important angiogenic genes when exposed to thalidomide [12, 85]. Additionally, serum levels of the anticoagulant thrombomodulin have been shown to decrease in response to thalidomide [120], and von Willebrand factor antigen and factor VIII have been noted to be upregulated during thalidomide treatment [121]. In the setting of thalidomide and doxorubicin, upregulation of endothelial expression of PAR-1 has been observed, potentially leading to increased vascular endothelial thrombin binding and subsequent clot formation [97, 122].

Clinical Presentation and Epidemiology

Thrombotic events in patients treated with thalidomide or its derivatives tend to be venous thrombosis, although arterial thrombotic events have also been reported. Immunomodulatory therapy-related venous thrombosis occurs in the form of deep or superficial vein thrombosis and embolic events such as pulmonary embolism [12]. The risk of VTE with thalidomide and its derivatives appears to be variable and as previously noted is primarily observed when used in combination with other therapies. Thalidomide alone is associated with an incidence of VTE of 3–4 % in newly diagnosed multiple myeloma and 2–4 % in relapsed or refractory multiple myeloma [118]. Similar rates of VTE exist for lenalidomide as single therapy. It is estimated that the rate of thalidomide associated VTE when used in combination with dexamethasone is 14–26 % in newly diagnosed multiple myeloma patient and approximately 2–8 % in patients with recurrent disease [118]. The highest incidence of venous thromboembolism observed in multiple myeloma were in patients treated with thalidomide and doxorubicin-containing chemotherapy with a VTE rate of up to 34 and 43 % in renal cell carcinoma [12, 85, 123]. VTE also occurs with greater frequency when thalidomide derivatives (lenalidomide and pomalidomide) are used in combination with dexamethasone or standard chemotherapy. Lenalidomide with dexamethasone or chemotherapy has been associated with an 11 % risk of thrombotic events [12]. However, some reports suggest up to a 75 % incidence in newly diagnosed patients [118]. Interestingly, when used in combination with bortezomib, the increase in VTE is not observed as it is with other therapies, and the etiology for this remains unclear [12, 72, 118]. Zangari et al. analyzed risk factors associated with the development of VTE in a large group of myeloma patients treated either with thalidomide in combination with multi-agent chemotherapy or with dexamethasone. They found an overall incidence of VTE of 15 %. Multivariable analysis suggests that regimens with doxorubicin were associated with a 4.3-fold increase in VTE and newly diagnosed disease was associated with a 2.5-fold increase of VTE compared to relapsed/refractory disease [120]. Newly diagnosed myeloma and combination of thalidomide with anthracycline are the two strongest predictors of VTE [12, 72]. Obesity, stasis, prior VTE, indwelling catheters, hormone therapy, and inherited thrombophilias are also important risk factors [118].

Management

Observational studies using aspirin in the setting of immunomodulating therapy with dexamethasone or chemotherapy have reduced cardiovascular complications, but there are no randomized trial data. Aspirin, low-dose LMWH, and fixed low-dose warfarin have all been shown to decrease risk of thrombotic events in patients treated with thalidomide and high-dose dexamethasone or chemotherapy in observational studies [12]. A prospective randomized study of enoxaparin versus aspirin or low fixed-dose warfarin in patients with myeloma treated with thalidomide, corticosteroids, and bortezomib was performed and showed no significant difference in cardiovascular episodes between the three arms of the study, but the prophylaxis was instituted only during the induction phase of the trial [12]. Larger experiences with aspirin are available for lenalidomide, and aspirin seems to be effective in reducing the VTE risk in some studies [12, 118]. In 2007, the International Myeloma Working Group devised a set of recommendations to address venous thromboembolism in the setting of myeloma and immunomodulatory therapy [118]. They recommended tailoring therapy according to the individual patient based upon risk factors (age, obesity, previous VTE, central catheter, immobility, comorbidities, myeloma risk factors such as diagnosis and viscosity, as well as other treatment-related risk factors) [118]. No specific prophylaxis in patients being treated with single-agent thalidomide or lenalidomide was advised. However, they did suggest the use of aspirin for none or one risk factor if patients are treated with combination therapy (thalidomide/lenalidomide with dexamethasone or doxorubicin). They also recommended low molecular weight heparin or full-dose warfarin for two or more risk factors or on concomitant high-dose dexamethasone or doxorubicin [118].

Conclusions

Patients with cancer are at an increased risk for thrombosis. Due to the complex interaction of the coagulation system with cancer growth, angiogenesis, and metastases, the potential role of anticoagulants in improving cancer patient survival represents an intriguing but unrealized possibility requiring the results of additional clinical trials. At the same time, current evidence-based clinical practice guidelines recommend that hospitalized cancer patients including those undergoing major surgery should be considered for routine thromboprophylaxis. Additional studies are needed to better define the appropriate role of thromboprophylaxis in ambulatory patients receiving systemic cancer therapies. Clinical practice guidelines based on rigorous systematic reviews and evidence summaries can provide clinicians with a balanced resource for the use of anticoagulants in the specific management of patients with cancer. While the use of clinical risk models for VTE among ambulatory cancer patients is promising, identification and validation of new clinical and molecular biomarkers for VTE are awaited to further improve the selection of high-risk patients for more personalized prophylactic strategies. Through optimal application of current strategies along with increased investment into basic and translational clinical research, further reductions in the morbidity and mortality associated with thromboembolic complications in patients with cancer can be realized. At the same time, many newer therapies, ranging from anti-angiogenic antibodies, to tyrosine kinase inhibitors, to immunomodulatory therapies, have significant cardiotoxic effects involving the vasculature. Arterial thrombotic events are primarily observed with bevacizumab and the anti-angiogenic TKIs. The Bcr-Abl TKIs are also associated with a surprising incidence of acute thrombotic events and accelerated atherosclerosis. Finally, the immunomodulating agents have an increased incidence of venous thromboembolism, particularly when used in conjunction with additional agents. Additional translational and epidemiologic studies are needed to understand these complications and guide clinical management strategies.

Conflict of Interest   The authors have no financial or personal conflicts of interest related to the subject matter of this review.

References

1. Heit JA, Silverstein MD, Mohr DN, Petterson TM, O'Fallon WM, Melton 3rd LJ. Risk factors for deep vein thrombosis and pulmonary embolism: a population-based case–control study. Arch Intern Med. 2000;160(6):809–15.
2. Chew HK, Wun T, Harvey D, Zhou H, White RH. Incidence of venous thromboembolism and its effect on survival among patients with common cancers. Arch Intern Med. 2006;166 (4):458–64.

3. Khorana AA, Francis CW, Culakova E, Lyman GH. Risk factors for chemotherapy-associated venous thromboembolism in a prospective observational study. Cancer. 2005;104(12):2822–9.

4. Khorana AA, Francis CW, Culakova E, Fisher RI, Kuderer NM, Lyman GH. Thromboembolism in hospitalized neutropenic cancer patients. J Clin Oncol. 2006;24 (3):484–90.

5. Komrokji RS, Uppal NP, Khorana AA, Lyman GH, Kaplan KL, Fisher RI, et al. Venous thromboembolism in patients with diffuse large B-cell lymphoma. Leuk Lymphoma. 2006;47 (6):1029–33.

6. Falanga A, Marchetti M. Venous thromboembolism in the hematologic malignancies. J Clin Oncol. 2009;27(29):4848–57.

7. Cavo M, Zamagni E, Cellini C, Tosi P, Cangini D, Cini M, et al. Deep-vein thrombosis in patients with multiple myeloma receiving first-line thalidomide-dexamethasone therapy. Blood. 2002;100(6):2272–3.

8. Kabbinavar F, Hurwitz HI, Fehrenbacher L, Meropol NJ, Novotny WF, Lieberman G, et al. Phase II, randomized trial comparing bevacizumab plus fluorouracil (FU)/leucovorin (LV) with FU/LV alone in patients with metastatic colorectal cancer. J Clin Oncol. 2003;21(1):60–5.

9. Kuenen BC, Levi M, Meijers JC, van Hinsbergh VW, Berkhof J, Kakkar AK, et al. Potential role of platelets in endothelial damage observed during treatment with cisplatin, gemcitabine, and the angiogenesis inhibitor SU5416. J Clin Oncol. 2003;21(11):2192–8.

10. Scappaticci FA, Skillings JR, Holden SN, Gerber HP, Miller K, Kabbinavar F, et al. Arterial thromboembolic events in patients with metastatic carcinoma treated with chemotherapy and bevacizumab. J Natl Cancer Inst. 2007;99(16):1232–9.

11. Nalluri SR, Chu D, Keresztes R, Zhu X, Wu S. Risk of venous thromboembolism with the angiogenesis inhibitor bevacizumab in cancer patients: a meta-analysis. JAMA. 2008;300 (19):2277–85.

12. Zangari M, Fink LM, Elice F, Zhan F, Adcock DM, Tricot GJ. Thrombotic events in patients with cancer receiving antiangiogenesis agents. J Clin Oncol. 2009;27(29):4865–73.

13. Hurwitz HI, Saltz LB, Van Cutsem E, Cassidy J, Wiedemann J, Sirzen F, et al. Venous thromboembolic events with chemotherapy plus bevacizumab: a pooled analysis of patients in randomized phase II and III studies. J Clin Oncol. 2011;29(13):1757–64.

14. Bohlius J, Wilson J, Seidenfeld J, Piper M, Schwarzer G, Sandercock J, et al. Recombinant human erythropoietins and cancer patients: updated meta-analysis of 57 studies including 9353 patients. J Natl Cancer Inst. 2006;98(10):708–14.

15. Khorana AA, Francis CW, Blumberg N, Culakova E, Refaai MA, Lyman GH. Blood transfusions, thrombosis, and mortality in hospitalized patients with cancer. Arch Intern Med. 2008;168(21):2377–81.

16. Khorana AA, Kuderer NM, Culakova E, Lyman GH, Francis CW. Development and validation of a predictive model for chemotherapy-associated thrombosis. Blood. 2008;111 (10):4902–7.

17. Khorana AA, Connolly GC. Assessing risk of venous thromboembolism in the patient with cancer. J Clin Oncol. 2009;27(29):4839–47.

18. American Cancer Society. Cancer facts and figures for African Americans 2011–2012. Atlanta: American Cancer Society; 2011.

19. Ay C, Dunkler D, Marosi C, Chiriac AL, Vormittag R, Simanek R, et al. Prediction of venous thromboembolism in cancer patients. Blood. 2010;116(24):5377–82.

20. Khorana AA, O'Connell C, Agnelli G, Liebman HA, Lee AY, Subcommittee on Hemostasis and Malignancy of the SSC of the ISTH. Incidental venous thromboembolism in oncology patients. J Thromb Haemost. 2012;10(12):2602–4.

21. George DJ, Agnelli G, Fisher W, AK K, Lassen MR, Mismetti P, et al. Venous thromboembolism (VTE) prevention with semuloparin in cancer patients initiating chemotherapy:

benefit-risk assessment by VTE risk in SAVE-ONCO. Blood. 2011;ASH Annual Meeting Program and Proceedings (206).

22. Verso M, Agnelli G, Barni S, Gasparini G, LaBianca R. A modified Khorana risk assessment score for venous thromboembolism in cancer patients receiving chemotherapy: the Protecht score. Intern Emerg Med. 2012;7(3):291–2.

23. Alcalay A, Wun T, Khatri V, Chew HK, Harvey D, Zhou H, et al. Venous thromboembolism in patients with colorectal cancer: incidence and effect on survival. J Clin Oncol. 2006;24 (7):1112–8.

24. Chew HK, Wun T, Harvey DJ, Zhou H, White RH. Incidence of venous thromboembolism and the impact on survival in breast cancer patients. J Clin Oncol. 2007;25(1):70–6.

25. Kuderer NM, Ortel TL, Francis CW. Impact of venous thromboembolism and anticoagulation on cancer and cancer survival. J Clin Oncol. 2009;27(29):4902–11.

26. Sorensen HT, Mellemkjaer L, Olsen JH, Baron JA. Prognosis of cancers associated with venous thromboembolism. N Engl J Med. 2000;343(25):1846–50.

27. Prandoni P, Lensing AW, Piccioli A, Bernardi E, Simioni P, Girolami B, et al. Recurrent venous thromboembolism and bleeding complications during anticoagulant treatment in patients with cancer and venous thrombosis. Blood. 2002;100(10):3484–8.

28. Elting LS, Escalante CP, Cooksley C, Avritscher EB, Kurtin D, Hamblin L, et al. Outcomes and cost of deep venous thrombosis among patients with cancer. Arch Intern Med. 2004;164 (15):1653–61.

29. den Exter PL, Hooijer J, Dekkers OM, Huisman MV. Risk of recurrent venous thromboembolism and mortality in patients with cancer incidentally diagnosed with pulmonary embolism: a comparison with symptomatic patients. J Clin Oncol. 2011;29(17):2405–9.

30. O'Connell CL, Boswell WD, Duddalwar V, Caton A, Mark LS, Vigen C, et al. Unsuspected pulmonary emboli in cancer patients: clinical correlates and relevance. J Clin Oncol. 2006;24 (30):4928–32.

31. O'Connell C, Razavi P, Ghalichi M, Boyle S, Vasan S, Mark L, et al. Unsuspected pulmonary emboli adversely impact survival in patients with cancer undergoing routine staging multirow detector computed tomography scanning. J Thromb Haemost. 2011;9(2):305–11.

32. O'Connell CL, Razavi PA, Liebman HA. Symptoms adversely impact survival among patients with cancer and unsuspected pulmonary embolism. J Clin Oncol. 2011;29 (31):4208–9. Author reply 9–10.

33. Castelli R, Porro F, Tarsia P. The heparins and cancer: review of clinical trials and biological properties. Vasc Med. 2004;9(3):205–13.

34. Zacharski LR, Henderson WG, Rickles FR, Forman WB, Cornell Jr CJ, Forcier RJ, et al. Effect of warfarin anticoagulation on survival in carcinoma of the lung, colon, head and neck, and prostate. Final report of VA Cooperative Study #75. Cancer. 1984;53(10):2046–52.

35. Chahinian AP, Propert KJ, Ware JH, Zimmer B, Perry MC, Hirsh V, et al. A randomized trial of anticoagulation with warfarin and of alternating chemotherapy in extensive small-cell lung cancer by the Cancer and Leukemia Group B. J Clin Oncol. 1989;7(8):993–1002.

36. Maurer LH, Herndon 2nd JE, Hollis DR, Aisner J, Carey RW, Skarin AT, et al. Randomized trial of chemotherapy and radiation therapy with or without warfarin for limited-stage small-cell lung cancer: a Cancer and Leukemia Group B study. J Clin Oncol. 1997;15(11):3378–87.

37. Lebeau B, Chastang C, Brechot JM, Capron F, Dautzenberg B, Delaisements C, et al. Subcutaneous heparin treatment increases survival in small cell lung cancer. "Petites Cellules" Group. Cancer. 1994;74(1):38–45.

38. Altinbas M, Coskun HS, Er O, Ozkan M, Eser B, Unal A, et al. A randomized clinical trial of combination chemotherapy with and without low-molecular-weight heparin in small cell lung cancer. J Thromb Haemost. 2004;2(8):1266–71.

39. Klerk CP, Smorenburg SM, Otten HM, Lensing AW, Prins MH, Piovella F, et al. The effect of low molecular weight heparin on survival in patients with advanced malignancy. J Clin Oncol. 2005;23(10):2130–5.

40. Sideras K, Schaefer PL, Okuno SH, Sloan JA, Kutteh L, Fitch TR, et al. Low-molecular-weight heparin in patients with advanced cancer: a phase 3 clinical trial. Mayo Clin Proc. 2006;81(6):758–67.

41. Kuderer NM, Khorana AA, Lyman GH, Francis CW. A meta-analysis and systematic review of the efficacy and safety of anticoagulants as cancer treatment: impact on survival and bleeding complications. Cancer. 2007;110(5):1149–61.

42. Streiff MB, Bockenstedt PL, Cataland SR, Chesney C, Eby C, Fanikos J, et al. Venous thromboembolic disease. J Natl Compr Canc Netw. 2013;11(11):1402–29.

43. Mandala M, Falanga A, Roila F. Management of venous thromboembolism (VTE) in cancer patients: ESMO clinical practice guidelines. Ann Oncol. 2011;22 Suppl 6:vi85–92.

44. Siragusa S, Armani U, Carpenedo M, Falanga A, Fulfaro F, Imberti D, et al. Prevention of venous thromboembolism in patients with cancer: guidelines of the Italian Society for Haemostasis and Thrombosis (SISET)(1). Thromb Res. 2012;129(5):e171–6.

45. Farge D, Debourdeau P, Beckers M, Baglin C, Bauersachs RM, Brenner B, et al. International clinical practice guidelines for the treatment and prophylaxis of venous thromboembolism in patients with cancer. J Thromb Haemost. 2013;11(1):56–70.

46. Lyman GH, Bohlke K, Khorana AA, Kuderer NM, Lee AY, Arcelus JI, et al. Venous thromboembolism prophylaxis and treatment in patients with cancer: American Society of Clinical Oncology Clinical Practice Guideline Update 2014. J Clin Oncol. 2015;33(6):654–6.

47. Lee AY. Anticoagulation in the treatment of established venous thromboembolism in patients with cancer. J Clin Oncol. 2009;27(29):4895–901.

48. Lyman GH. Thromboprophylaxis with low-molecular-weight heparin in medical patients with cancer. Cancer. 2009;115(24):5637–50.

49. Levine MN. New antithrombotic drugs: potential for use in oncology. J Clin Oncol. 2009;27 (29):4912–8.

50. Ambrus JL, Ambrus CM, Mink IB, Pickren JW. Causes of death in cancer patients. J Med. 1975;6(1):61–4.

51. Sallah S, Wan JY, Nguyen NP. Venous thrombosis in patients with solid tumors: determination of frequency and characteristics. Thromb Haemost. 2002;87(4):575–9.

52. Stein PD, Beemath A, Meyers FA, Skaf E, Sanchez J, Olson RE. Incidence of venous thromboembolism in patients hospitalized with cancer. Am J Med. 2006;119(1):60–8.

53. Levitan N, Dowlati A, Remick SC, Tahsildar HI, Sivinski LD, Beyth R, et al. Rates of initial and recurrent thromboembolic disease among patients with malignancy versus those without malignancy. Risk analysis using Medicare claims data. Medicine (Baltimore). 1999;78 (5):285–91.

54. Cohen AT, Davidson BL, Gallus AS, Lassen MR, Prins MH, Tomkowski W, et al. Efficacy and safety of fondaparinux for the prevention of venous thromboembolism in older acute medical patients: randomised placebo controlled trial. BMJ. 2006;332(7537):325–9.

55. Leizorovicz A, Cohen AT, Turpie AG, Olsson CG, Vaitkus PT, Goldhaber SZ. Randomized, placebo-controlled trial of dalteparin for the prevention of venous thromboembolism in acutely ill medical patients. Circulation. 2004;110(7):874–9.

56. Samama MM, Cohen AT, Darmon JY, Desjardins L, Eldor A, Janbon C, et al. A comparison of enoxaparin with placebo for the prevention of venous thromboembolism in acutely ill medical patients. Prophylaxis in Medical Patients with Enoxaparin Study Group. N Engl J Med. 1999;341(11):793–800.

57. Francis CW. Prevention of venous thromboembolism in hospitalized patients with cancer. J Clin Oncol. 2009;27(29):4874–80.

58. Kakkar AK, Haas S, Wolf H, Encke A. Evaluation of perioperative fatal pulmonary embolism and death in cancer surgical patients: the MC-4 cancer substudy. Thromb Haemost. 2005;94 (4):867–71.

59. Geerts WH, Pineo GF, Heit JA, Bergqvist D, Lassen MR, Colwell CW, et al. Prevention of venous thromboembolism: the Seventh ACCP Conference on Antithrombotic and Thrombolytic Therapy. Chest. 2004;126(3 Suppl):338S–400.

60. Carrier M, Khorana AA, Moretto P, Le Gal G, Karp R, Zwicker JI. Lack of evidence to support thromboprophylaxis in hospitalized medical patients with cancer. Am J Med. 2014;127(1):82–6. e1.
61. Wun T, Law L, Harvey D, Sieracki B, Scudder SA, Ryu JK. Increased incidence of symptomatic venous thrombosis in patients with cervical carcinoma treated with concurrent chemotherapy, radiation, and erythropoietin. Cancer. 2003;98(7):1514–20.
62. Rosenzweig MQ, Bender CM, Lucke JP, Yasko JM, Brufsky AM. The decision to prematurely terminate a trial of R-HuEPO due to thrombotic events. J Pain Symptom Manage. 2004;27(2):185–90.
63. Barlogie B, Tricot G, Anaissie E, Shaughnessy J, Rasmussen E, van Rhee F, et al. Thalidomide and hematopoietic-cell transplantation for multiple myeloma. N Engl J Med. 2006;354 (10):1021–30.
64. Rajkumar SV, Blood E, Vesole D, Fonseca R, Greipp PR. Phase III clinical trial of thalidomide plus dexamethasone compared with dexamethasone alone in newly diagnosed multiple myeloma: a clinical trial coordinated by the Eastern Cooperative Oncology Group. J Clin Oncol. 2006;24(3):431–6.
65. Zonder JA, Durie BGM, McCoy J, Crowley J, Zeldis JB, Ghannam L, et al. High Incidence of Thrombotic Events Observed in Patients Receiving Lenalidomide (L) + Dexamethasone (D) (LD) as First-Line Therapy for Multiple Myeloma (MM) without Aspirin (ASA) Prophylaxis. Blood. 2005;106:3455.
66. Zangari M, Anaissie E, Barlogie B, Badros A, Desikan R, Gopal AV, et al. Increased risk of deep-vein thrombosis in patients with multiple myeloma receiving thalidomide and chemotherapy. Blood. 2001;98(5):1614–5.
67. Zangari M, Barlogie B, Anaissie E, Saghafifar F, Eddlemon P, Jacobson J, et al. Deep vein thrombosis in patients with multiple myeloma treated with thalidomide and chemotherapy: effects of prophylactic and therapeutic anticoagulation. Br J Haematol. 2004;126(5):715–21.
68. Rus C, Bazzan M, Palumbo A, Bringhen S, Boccadoro M. Thalidomide in front line treatment in multiple myeloma: serious risk of venous thromboembolism and evidence for thromboprophylaxis. J Thromb Haemost. 2004;2(11):2063–5.
69. Rajkumar SV. Thalidomide therapy and deep venous thrombosis in multiple myeloma. Mayo Clin Proc. 2005;80(12):1549–51.
70. Barlogie B, Jagannath S, Desikan KR, Mattox S, Vesole D, Siegel D, et al. Total therapy with tandem transplants for newly diagnosed multiple myeloma. Blood. 1999;93(1):55–65.
71. Weber D, Rankin K, Gavino M, Delasalle K, Alexanian R. Thalidomide alone or with dexamethasone for previously untreated multiple myeloma. J Clin Oncol. 2003;21(1):16–9.
72. Zangari M, Barlogie B, Thertulien R, Jacobson J, Eddleman P, Fink L, et al. Thalidomide and deep vein thrombosis in multiple myeloma: risk factors and effect on survival. Clin Lymphoma. 2003;4(1):32–5.
73. Maraveyas A, Waters J, Roy R, Fyfe D, Propper D, Lofts F, et al. Gemcitabine versus gemcitabine plus dalteparin thromboprophylaxis in pancreatic cancer. Eur J Cancer. 2012;48(9):1283–92.
74. Riess H, Pelzer U, Opitz B, et al. A prospective, randomized trial of simultaneous pancreatic cancer treatment with enoxaparin and chemotherapy. Final Results of the CONKO-004 trial. American Society of Clinical Oncology (ASCO) Annual Meeting, June 2010. 2010.
75. Kuderer NM, Ortel TL, Khorana AA, et al. Low-molecular-weight heparin for venous thromboprophylaxis in ambulatory cancer patients: A systematic review meta-analysis of randomized controlled trials. American Society of Hematology (ASH) Annual Meeting, December 2009. 2009.
76. Lyman GH, Eckert L, Wang Y, Wang H, Cohen A. Venous thromboembolism risk in patients with cancer receiving chemotherapy: a real-world analysis. Oncologist. 2013;18(12):1321–9.
77. Lyman GH. The incidence of venous thromboembolism in cancer patients: a real-world analysis. Clin Adv Hematol Oncol. 2012;10(1):40–2.

78. Blom JW, Doggen CJ, Osanto S, Rosendaal FR. Malignancies, prothrombotic mutations, and the risk of venous thrombosis. JAMA. 2005;293(6):715–22.

79. Fisher B, Costantino JP, Wickerham DL, Redmond CK, Kavanah M, Cronin WM, et al. Tamoxifen for prevention of breast cancer: report of the National Surgical Adjuvant Breast and Bowel Project P-1 Study. J Natl Cancer Inst. 1998;90(18):1371–88.

80. Pritchard KI, Paterson AH, Paul NA, Zee B, Fine S, Pater J. Increased thromboembolic complications with concurrent tamoxifen and chemotherapy in a randomized trial of adjuvant therapy for women with breast cancer. National Cancer Institute of Canada Clinical Trials Group Breast Cancer Site Group. J Clin Oncol. 1996;14(10):2731–7.

81. Saphner T, Tormey DC, Gray R. Venous and arterial thrombosis in patients who received adjuvant therapy for breast cancer. J Clin Oncol. 1991;9(2):286–94.

82. Nelson HD, Smith ME, Griffin JC, Fu R. Use of medications to reduce risk for primary breast cancer: a systematic review for the U.S. Preventive Services Task Force. Ann Intern Med. 2013;158(8):604–14.

83. Deitcher SR, Gomes MP. The risk of venous thromboembolic disease associated with adjuvant hormone therapy for breast carcinoma: a systematic review. Cancer. 2004;101 (3):439–49.

84. Sanon S, Lenihan DJ, Mouhayar E. Peripheral arterial ischemic events in cancer patients. Vasc Med. 2011;16(2):119–30.

85. Yeh ET, Bickford CL. Cardiovascular complications of cancer therapy: incidence, pathogenesis, diagnosis, and management. J Am Coll Cardiol. 2009;53(24):2231–47.

86. Bair SM, Choueiri TK, Moslehi J. Cardiovascular complications associated with novel angiogenesis inhibitors: emerging evidence and evolving perspectives. Trends Cardiovasc Med. 2013;23(4):104–13.

87. Hurwitz H, Fehrenbacher L, Novotny W, Cartwright T, Hainsworth J, Heim W, et al. Bevacizumab plus irinotecan, fluorouracil, and leucovorin for metastatic colorectal cancer. N Engl J Med. 2004;350(23):2335–42.

88. Conti E, Romiti A, Musumeci MB, Passerini J, Zezza L, Mastromarino V, et al. Arterial thrombotic events and acute coronary syndromes with cancer drugs: are growth factors the missed link?: what both cardiologist and oncologist should know about novel angiogenesis inhibitors. Int J Cardiol. 2013;167(6):2421–9.

89. Ferrara N, Gerber HP, LeCouter J. The biology of VEGF and its receptors. Nat Med. 2003;9 (6):669–76.

90. Keefe D, Bowen J, Gibson R, Tan T, Okera M, Stringer A. Noncardiac vascular toxicities of vascular endothelial growth factor inhibitors in advanced cancer: a review. Oncologist. 2011;16(4):432–44.

91. Choueiri TK, Schutz FA, Je Y, Rosenberg JE, Bellmunt J. Risk of arterial thromboembolic events with sunitinib and sorafenib: a systematic review and meta-analysis of clinical trials. J Clin Oncol. 2010;28(13):2280–5.

92. Verheul HM, Pinedo HM. Possible molecular mechanisms involved in the toxicity of angiogenesis inhibition. Nat Rev Cancer. 2007;7(6):475–85.

93. Dunmore BJ, McCarthy MJ, Naylor AR, Brindle NP. Carotid plaque instability and ischemic symptoms are linked to immaturity of microvessels within plaques. J Vasc Surg. 2007;45 (1):155–9.

94. Ranpura V, Hapani S, Chuang J, Wu S. Risk of cardiac ischemia and arterial thromboembolic events with the angiogenesis inhibitor bevacizumab in cancer patients: a meta-analysis of randomized controlled trials. Acta Oncol. 2010;49(3):287–97.

95. Leighl NB, Bennouna J, Yi J, Moore N, Hambleton J, Hurwitz H. Bleeding events in bevacizumab-treated cancer patients who received full-dose anticoagulation and remained on study. Br J Cancer. 2011;104(3):413–8.

96. Herrmann J, Lerman A. An update on cardio-oncology. Trends Cardiovasc Med. 2014;24 (7):285–95.

97. Passerini J, Romiti A, D'Antonio C, Mastromarino V, Marchetti P, Volpe M, et al. Tailored angiogenesis inhibition in cancer therapy: respecting the heart to improve the net outcome. Curr Signal Transduct Ther. 2012;7(3):265–88.

98. Javid M, Magee TR, Galland RB. Arterial thrombosis associated with malignant disease. Eur J Vasc Endovasc Surg. 2008;35(1):84–7.

99. Amsterdam EA, Wenger NK, Brindis RG, Casey Jr DE, Ganiats TG, Holmes Jr DR, et al. 2014 AHA/ACC guideline for the management of patients with non-ST-elevation acute coronary syndromes: a report of the American College of Cardiology/American Heart Association Task Force on Practice Guidelines. J Am Coll Cardiol. 2014;64(24):e139–228.

100. O'Gara PT, Kushner FG, Ascheim DD, Casey Jr DE, Chung MK, de Lemos JA, et al. 2013 ACCF/AHA guideline for the management of ST-elevation myocardial infarction: executive summary: a report of the American College of Cardiology Foundation/American Heart Association Task Force on Practice Guidelines: developed in collaboration with the American College of Emergency Physicians and Society for Cardiovascular Angiography and Interventions. Catheter Cardiovasc Interv. 2013;82(1):E1–27.

101. Flynn P, Sugrue M, Feng S, et al. Incidence of serious bleeding events (sBE) in patients (pts) with metastatic colorectal cancer (mCRC) receiving bevacizumab (BV) as part of a first-line regimen: results from the BRiTE observational cohort study (OCS). J Clin Oncol. 2008;26 (15 Suppl):4104.

102. Schmidinger M, Zielinski CC, Vogl UM, Bojic A, Bojic M, Schukro C, et al. Cardiac toxicity of sunitinib and sorafenib in patients with metastatic renal cell carcinoma. J Clin Oncol. 2008;26(32):5204–12.

103. Faruque LI, Lin M, Battistella M, Wiebe N, Reiman T, Hemmelgarn B, et al. Systematic review of the risk of adverse outcomes associated with vascular endothelial growth factor inhibitors for the treatment of cancer. PLoS One. 2014;9(7), e101145.

104. Kuenen BC, Rosen L, Smit EF, Parson MR, Levi M, Ruijter R, et al. Dose-finding and pharmacokinetic study of cisplatin, gemcitabine, and SU5416 in patients with solid tumors. J Clin Oncol. 2002;20(6):1657–67.

105. Marx GM, Steer CB, Harper P, Pavlakis N, Rixe O, Khayat D. Unexpected serious toxicity with chemotherapy and antiangiogenic combinations: time to take stock! J Clin Oncol. 2002;20(6):1446–8.

106. Deininger M, Buchdunger E, Druker BJ. The development of imatinib as a therapeutic agent for chronic myeloid leukemia. Blood. 2005;105(7):2640–53.

107. Groarke JD, Cheng S, Moslehi J. Cancer-drug discovery and cardiovascular surveillance. N Engl J Med. 2013;369(19):1779–81.

108. Marcucci G, Perrotti D, Caligiuri MA. Understanding the molecular basis of imatinib mesylate therapy in chronic myelogenous leukemia and the related mechanisms of resistance. Commentary re: A. N. Mohamed et al., The effect of imatinib mesylate on patients with Philadelphia chromosome-positive chronic myeloid leukemia with secondary chromosomal aberrations. Clin. Cancer Res., 9: 1333–1337, 2003. Clin Cancer Res. 2003;9(4):1248–52.

109. Kerbel RS, Viloria-Petit A, Klement G, Rak J. 'Accidental' anti-angiogenic drugs. anti-oncogene directed signal transduction inhibitors and conventional chemotherapeutic agents as examples. Eur J Cancer. 2000;36(10):1248–57.

110. Aichberger KJ, Herndlhofer S, Schernthaner GH, Schillinger M, Mitterbauer-Hohendanner G, Sillaber C, et al. Progressive peripheral arterial occlusive disease and other vascular events during nilotinib therapy in CML. Am J Hematol. 2011;86(7):533–9.

111. Tefferi A. Nilotinib treatment-associated accelerated atherosclerosis: when is the risk justified? Leukemia. 2013;27(9):1939–40.

112. Valent P, Hadzijusufovic E, Schernthaner GH, Wolf D, Rea D, le Coutre P. Vascular safety issues in CML patients treated with BCR/ABL1 kinase inhibitors. Blood. 2015;125(6):901–6.

113. Cortes JE, Kim DW, Pinilla-Ibarz J, le Coutre P, Paquette R, Chuah C, et al. A phase 2 trial of ponatinib in Philadelphia chromosome-positive leukemias. N Engl J Med. 2013;369 (19):1783–96.

114. Food and Drug Administration. FDA drug safety communication: FDA investigating leukemia drug Iclusig (ponatinib) after increased reports of serious blood clots in arteries and veins. 2013.
115. ARIAD announces changes in the clinical development program of Iclusig. Press release of ARIAD Pharmaceuticals. 2013.
116. Kim TD, Rea D, Schwarz M, Grille P, Nicolini FE, Rosti G, et al. Peripheral artery occlusive disease in chronic phase chronic myeloid leukemia patients treated with nilotinib or imatinib. Leukemia. 2013;27(6):1316–21.
117. Levato L, Cantaffa R, Kropp MG, Magro D, Piro E, Molica S. Progressive peripheral arterial occlusive disease and other vascular events during nilotinib therapy in chronic myeloid leukemia: a single institution study. Eur J Haematol. 2013;90(6):531–2.
118. Palumbo A, Rajkumar SV, Dimopoulos MA, Richardson PG, San Miguel J, Barlogie B, et al. Prevention of thalidomide- and lenalidomide-associated thrombosis in myeloma. Leukemia. 2008;22(2):414–23.
119. Latif T, Chauhan N, Khan R, Moran A, Usmani SZ. Thalidomide and its analogues in the treatment of Multiple Myeloma. Exp Hematol Oncol. 2012;1(1):27.
120. Corso A, Lorenzi A, Terulla V, Airo F, Varettoni M, Mangiacavalli S, et al. Modification of thrombomodulin plasma levels in refractory myeloma patients during treatment with thalidomide and dexamethasone. Ann Hematol. 2004;83(9):588–91.
121. Minnema MC, Fijnheer R, De Groot PG, Lokhorst HM. Extremely high levels of von Willebrand factor antigen and of procoagulant factor VIII found in multiple myeloma patients are associated with activity status but not with thalidomide treatment. J Thromb Haemost. 2003;1(3):445–9.
122. Kaushal V, Kaushal GP, Melkaveri SN, Mehta P. Thalidomide protects endothelial cells from doxorubicin-induced apoptosis but alters cell morphology. J Thromb Haemost. 2004;2(2):327–34.
123. Farge D, Parfrey PS, Forbes RD, Dandavino R, Guttmann RD. Reduction of azathioprine in renal transplant patients with chronic hepatitis. Transplantation. 1986;41(1):55–9.
124. Lyman GH, Khorana AA, Kuderer NM, Lee AY, Arcelus JI, Balaban EP, et al. Venous thromboembolism prophylaxis and treatment in patients with cancer: American Society of Clinical Oncology clinical practice guideline update. J Clin Oncol. 2013;31(17):2189–204.

Chapter 10
Breast Cancer Cardio-Oncology

Angela Esposito, Carmen Criscitiello, Douglas B. Sawyer, and Giuseppe Curigliano

Introduction

Cardiovascular toxicity is a potential short- or long-term complication of breast cancer therapy, involving direct effects on the cardiovascular system, as well as potential exacerbation and/or unmasking of preexisting heart disease. In recent years, the awareness of cardiac toxicity related to anticancer treatment has increased, likely related to improvements in patient survival, the aging of cancer patients, and the introduction of new anticancer drugs with unique effects on the cardiovascular system. The advent of novel biologic agents, including monoclonal antibodies and tyrosine kinase inhibitors, has led to substantial improvement in the treatment of breast cancers. Although targeted therapies in general are considered less toxic and better tolerated by patients compared with classic chemotherapy agents, rare serious complications have been observed, and longer-term follow-up is needed to determine the exact cardiovascular side-effect profile.

Many breast cancer patients have multiple risk factors for both cardiac and coronary disease, such as cigarette smoking, diabetes, dyslipidemia, alcohol consumption, and obesity, that may increase risk for the detrimental effects of cardiotoxic drugs used in conventional breast cancer treatment. Preexisting

Electronic supplementary material: The online version of this chapter (doi:10.1007/978-3-319-43096-6_10) contains supplementary material, which is available to authorized users.

A. Esposito • C. Criscitiello • G. Curigliano (✉)
Division of Early Drug Development for Innovative Therapies, Istituto Europeo di Oncologia, Via Ripamonti 435, 20133 Milano, Italy
e-mail: angela.esposito@ieo.it; Carmen.Criscitiello@ieo.it; giuseppe.curigliano@ieo.it

D.B. Sawyer
Maine Medical Center, Cardiovascular Institute, Portland, ME, USA
e-mail: DSawyer@mmc.org

cardiovascular disease may significantly limit the diagnosis, staging, and choice of therapy for the breast cancer patient. In patients with either breast cancer or cardiovascular disease such as heart failure or ischemia, a wealth of evidence helps guide choices of therapies that maximize an individual's likelihood of successful treatment. However in a patient with both breast cancer and cardiovascular disease, known adverse cardiovascular effects and lack of clear evidence create uncertainty and complexity for patients and providers. This is a particularly common problem in the older patient because of the strong age-associated risk for both breast cancer and cardiovascular disease.

Cardiac toxicity associated with breast cancer therapies can range from asymptomatic subclinical abnormalities, including electrocardiographic changes and temporary left ventricular ejection fraction decline, to life-threatening events such as congestive heart failure or acute coronary syndromes. Assessment of the prevalence, type, and severity of cardiac toxicity caused by various cancer treatments is a critical topic for patient management and specifically for new drug development. The purpose of this chapter is to attempt to summarize the current state of knowledge of common cardiovascular complications, such as left ventricular dysfunction (LVD), cardiac ischemia, hypertension (HTN), venous thromboembolism (VTE), and QT prolongation associated with frequently used breast anticancer medications.

Anticancer Drugs and Cardiovascular Toxicity

The use of specific chemotherapeutic agents and molecular targeted therapies can affect the cardiovascular system, either through a direct effect on the myocardium or coronary circulation or peripherally through hemodynamic flow alteration (hypertension and/or thrombotic events). The literature describes several kinds of cardiotoxicities induced by anticancer chemotherapeutic agents (Table 10.1). Ewer et al. [1] proposed a system distinguishing therapeutics that have the potential to cause irreversible damage (type 1) versus those that with reversible effects (type

Table 10.1 Potential cardiac toxicity induced by anticancer chemotherapeutic agents

DRUG	Toxic dose range	Cardiac toxicity	%
Doxorubicin	>450 mg/m^2	Left venticular dysfunction	3–12%
Epirubicin	>900 mg/m^2		0.9–3.3%
Paclitaxel	Conventional dose	Left venticular dysfunction	5–15%
Docetaxel			2.3–8%
Cyclophosphamide	>100–120 mg/kg	Left venticular dysfunction	3–5%
Capecitabine	Conventional dose	Cardiac ischemia	3–9%
Fluorouracil			1–68%
Paclitaxel	Conventional dose	Cardiac ischemia	<1–5%
Docetaxel			1.7%
Paclitaxel	Conventional dose	QTc prolongation	0.1–31%

II). In type I cardiac toxicity, exemplified by anthracyclines, permanent cellular and tissue damage occurs via loss of cardiac myocytes by one or more mechanisms (described further below). Given the limited regenerative capacity of the heart, the number of cardiomyocytes progressively falls, leading to ventricular dysfunction and progressive remodeling [2]. On the other hand, type II cardiac dysfunction is exemplified by trastuzumab. The mechanisms of trastuzumab-induced cardiotoxicity are not fully understood, but some evidence suggests disruption of the ErbB2-neurgulin 1 (NRG1) signaling cascade may play a central role [3, 4].

However, this classification system has some limitations and should be used with caution. For example, trastuzumab can trigger irreversible cardiac damage in patients with severe preexisting cardiac disease or potentiate anthracycline type I cardiotoxicity. In type I cardiotoxicity, typical pathophysiology is related to cell loss; in type II cellular dysfunction, mitochondrial and protein alterations underlie the reversible damage. Type I toxicity may appear after considerable delay from exposure, thus could be missed during early phase clinical trials. Moreover, modern therapy for cardiovascular disease can normalize function in a way that makes it difficult to distinguish permanent from reversible effects. For example, in the setting of left ventricular dysfunction during cancer treatment, standard of care includes introduction of neurohormonal antagonists such as beta-adrenergic receptor blockers, a therapy associated with improvement in ventricular function regardless of the mechanism for cardiac injury. Does normalization of cardiac function in this setting suggest that this type of cardiotoxicity is type II? This is an important concept that can impact decisions related to selection of therapies. Perhaps "type II toxicity" should be reserved for effects that have no associated marker of cardiac injury and do not require other therapy for normalization of cardiovascular function.

Left Ventricular Dysfunction

One of the most common manifestations of cardiotoxicity associated with exposure to anticancer therapies is the development of left ventricular dysfunction (LVD) and overt heart failure. According to the Cardiac Review and Evaluation Committee [5], LVD is characterized by [1] decrease in cardiac left ventricular ejection fraction (LVEF) that was either global or more severe in the septum; [6] symptoms of congestive heart failure (CHF); [7] associated signs of CHF, including but not limited to S3 gallop, tachycardia, or both; and [2] decline in LVEF of at least 5% to less than 55% with accompanying signs or symptoms of CHF or a decline in LVEF of at least 10% to below 55% without accompanying signs or symptoms. Several chemotherapeutic agents may cause LVD such as antimetabolites, alkylating agents, antitumor antibiotics, and anthracyclines.

Anthracyclines, including doxorubicin and epirubicin, are a class of chemotherapeutics widely used in the management of breast cancer. Risk factors for anthracycline toxicity include cumulative dose; intravenous bolus administration;

higher single doses; history of prior mediastinal irradiation; the use of other concomitant agents known to have cardiotoxic effects including cyclophosphamide, trastuzumab, and paclitaxel; female gender; underlying cardiovascular disease; age (young and elderly); increased length of time since completion of chemotherapy; and increase in cardiac biomarkers during or after administration [8–11]. Anthracycline-induced LVD occurs in part from direct myocyte damage that has been ascribed to the production of oxygen free radicals and subsequent rise in oxidative stress [6], either directly through redox cycling of the quinone moiety or indirectly through inhibition of topoisomerase IIb, leading to mitochondrial dysfunction. Iron homeostasis might also have a role in the myocardial injury as anthracyclines inhibit the iron metabolism pathways and induce iron accumulation in the cardiomyocytes [7]. A consequence is cardiac cell death by apoptosis or necrosis after exposure to anthracyclines. Genetic studies have identified several loci associated with sensitivity to anthracycline-induced cardiac damage including polymorphisms of multidrug resistance proteins (MDR) 1 and 2, carbonyl reductase, subunits of NADPH oxidase, and phase II detoxification enzymes such as glutathione-S-transferase P and most recently retinoic acid receptor gamma [12].

Cardiotoxicity induced by anthracyclines can be categorized into acute, early-onset chronic progressive, and late-onset chronic progressive. Acute cardiotoxicity occurs in 1% of patients, and it is usually observed within 14 days from the beginning of the treatment. It manifests as an acute, transient decline in myocardial contractility, which is usually reversible. The early-onset chronic progressive form occurs in 1.6–2.1% of patients, during therapy or within the first year after treatment. Late-onset chronic progressive occurs at least 1 year after completion of therapy in 1.6–5% of patients. Early- and late-onset chronic progressive cardiotoxicity typically present as a dilated cardiomyopathy in adults, which can be progressive. The risk of cardiac complications is relatively lower with the use of liposome-encapsulated doxorubicin, which is associated with lower myocardial accumulation. Some clinical data suggest that patients who previously received conventional anthracyclines can still receive liposomal preparations even if they have received the maximum cumulative dose of the drug [13, 14].

LVD has also been described for two other classes of cytotoxic agents: alkylating agents and inhibitors of microtubule polymerization. In the first case the risk of cardiotoxicity appears to be dose related ($\geq$150 mg/kg and 1.5 g/m^2/day) [15]. Cyclophosphamide cardiotoxicity is not well understood. Extravasation of blood, interstitial edema, and myocardial necrosis associated with fibrin microthrombi could have a role in this process [16]. The incidence of heart failure associated with the inhibitors of microtubule polymerization is relatively low. In the Breast Cancer International Research Group trial 001, the overall incidence of congestive HF (including that during follow-up) was 1.6% among patients treated with TAC regimen (docetaxel, doxorubicin, cyclophosphamide) and 0.7% for those treated with FAC regimen (5-fluorouracil, doxorubicin, cyclophosphamide) (P50.09) [17].

Within the past decade, the advent of biologic targeted agents has brought into the clinic additional therapies with cardiotoxic concerns. Trastuzumab, a humanized monoclonal antibody against the HER2 receptor, has revolutionized the treatment for HER2-positive breast cancer, with landmark adjuvant phase 3 trials demonstrating a 50% reduction in recurrence of disease and a 33% improvement in survival [18–21]. Rates of cardiac toxicity reported in the adjuvant trials of trastuzumab are variable and reflect differences in trial design, chemotherapy administration, and definitions of cardiac events. In the trastuzumab adjuvant trials [18–20, 22] (Table 10.2), the highest reported incidence of symptomatic or severe cardiac heart failure (CHF) with trastuzumab was 4%, which occurred when trastuzumab was administered with paclitaxel after anthracycline exposure. A low rate of 0.4% CHF was reported in the BCIRG 006 adjuvant trial examining the trastuzumab/docetaxel/carboplatin combination regimen without prior anthracycline therapy [18]. The exact pathogenesis of trastuzumab-induced cardiac damage remains unclear. Trastuzumab is thought to cause cardiac dysfunction through the interruption of the HER2/ErbB2 signaling pathway in myocardium, thus interfering with normal growth, repair, and survival of cardiomyocytes [24]. Another suggested mechanism of trastuzumab cardiotoxicity is linked to the effect on cardiomyocytes of cytotoxic immune reactions triggered by the IgG1 domain of trastuzumab [25]

Table 10.2 Cardiac toxicity induced by trastuzumab

Trial	Design	Asymptomatic drop in LVEF ($\geq$10 percentage points to <55%)	Severe CHF/cardiac events (NYHA class III/IV CHF or death)	Discontinued for cardiac reasons
NSABP B31 [19] $n = 2043$	AC + TH + H vs AC + T	34% vs 17%	4.1% vs 0.8%	19%
NCCTG N9831 [22] $n = 2766$	AC + TH + H vs AC + T + H vs AC + T	5.8–10.4% vs 4.0–7.8% vs 4.0–5.1%	3.3% vs 2.8% vs 0.3%	n/a
BCIRG 006 [18] $n = 3222$	AC + T vs AC + TH + H vs TCaH(2)	11% vs 19% vs 9%	0.7% vs 2.0% vs 0.4%	n/a
HERA [20] $n = 5102$	Adj chemo (3) → H vs Adj chemo alone	7.1% vs 2.2%	0.6% vs 0.06%	4.3%
FinHer [23] $n = 232$	V or T + H vs V or T (4) → FEC × 3	3.5% vs 8.6%	0% vs 3.4%	n/a

Note that 6.7% did not receive H after A due to unacceptable drops in LVEF; included a non-anthracycline arm. In addition, 96% of chemotherapy was A containing. No prior anthracycline before H exposure; H exposure limited to 9 weeks

A anthracycline, *C* cyclophosphamide, *T* taxane, *H* trastuzumab, *Ca* carboplatin, *V* vinorelbine, *F* 5-flourouracil, *E* epirubicin, *n/a* information not available

and the modulation of mitochondrial integrity via the Bcl-X family proteins that leads to ATP depletion and to contractile dysfunction [26]. There is also emerging evidence for a role of NRG/ErbB signaling in regulation of sympathetic tone, which may also play a role in the observed effects on cardiac function [65].

Lapatinib is an oral receptor tyrosine kinase inhibitor of HER2 and EGFR and is estimated to have a risk of cardiotoxicity of 1.6%. In clinical study, asymptomatic cardiac events were reported in 53 patients (1.4%), and symptomatic events occurred in 7 (0.2%). In patients treated with prior anthracyclines, trastuzumab, or neither, the incidence of cardiac events was 2.2%, 1.7%, and 1.5%, respectively. The mean time to onset of cardiac events was 13 weeks [27].

Bevacizumab is a humanized monoclonal antibody directed against vascular endothelial growth factor (VEGF) and is not longer an approved regimen for breast cancer. Cardiac toxicity associated with bevacizumab appears to be relatively low. In the major phase III trials in metastatic breast cancer, reported rates of CTCAE grade 3/4 congestive heart failure were 0.8–2.2% in a mostly anthracycline-pretreated population [28]. To date, clinical trial data do not suggest significant increases in cardiac toxicity during treatment with bevacizumab, even in the setting of concurrent treatment with other cardiotoxic agents.

At present, the most frequently used modality for detecting LVD is the periodic measurement of LVEF by either echocardiography or multigated acquisition scanning. However, LVEF measurement is a relatively insensitive tool for detecting cardiotoxicity at an early stage because there is little change in resting LVEF until a critical amount of myocardial damage has taken place, and it may only be apparent after compensatory mechanisms are exhausted. In addition, measurement of LVEF presents a number of challenges related to image quality, assumption of left ventricular geometry, load dependency, and expertise. Multiple-gated acquisition (MUGA) scan can reduce interobserver variability; however disadvantages include exposure to radioactivity as well as limitations in information that can be obtained about cardiac structure and diastolic function. Magnetic resonance imaging (MRI) is considered the gold standard for the evaluation of LV volumes, mass, and function. However, lack of availability and high cost limit its routine use. Novel ultrasound imaging techniques, such as contrast echocardiography and real-time 3D echocardiography, are under investigation.

The treatment of LVD induced by anticancer drugs includes standard therapy for heart failure with ACE inhibitors (ACE-I) and beta blockers (BB), which may be highly effective [29, 30]. Randomized prospective clinical trials are evaluating the use of prophylactic ACE inhibitors and beta blockers in the prevention of chemotherapy-induced LVD [31]. The OVERCOME trial showed that the combined treatment with enalapril and carvedilol may prevent heart failure in patients treated for hematologic malignancies [31]. The MANTICORE study is evaluating the efficacy of perindopril and bisoprolol in the prevention of trastuzumab-mediated left ventricular remodeling in HER2-positive breast cancer [32]. Dexrazoxane, an iron-chelating agent and topoisomerase II inhibitor, significantly reduces anthracycline-related cardiotoxicity in adults with different solid tumors including breast cancer and in children with acute lymphoblastic leukemia and Ewing's sarcoma [33]. Dexrazoxane is not routinely used in clinical practice, and it is recommended as a cardioprotectant only for patients with metastatic breast cancer who have already received more than 300 mg/m^2 of doxorubicin.

Ischemia

Although rare, acute coronary syndromes including myocardial infarction have been associated with administration of cytotoxic, hormonal, and targeted agents for cancer treatment. Antimetabolites and inhibitors of microtubule polymerization are most frequently responsible for ischemic heart disease. The antimetabolite 5-Fluorouracil (FU) is associated with cardiac ischemia, including angina pectoris and acute myocardial infarction [34]. Ischemia can take place in patients without underlying coronary artery disease (CAD) (incidence, 1.1%), but the incidence is higher in patients with known CAD (4.5%) [35]. Cardiac events typically occur early (within 2–5 days of starting therapy) and with return of risk to baseline after cessation of the 5-FU and implementation of preventative medical therapy. High doses (>800 mg/m^2) and continuous infusions of 5-FU have been associated with higher rates of cardiotoxicity (7.6%) as compared with bolus injections (2%) [36, 37]. Other commonly cited risk factors include history of cardiovascular disease, prior mediastinal radiation, and the concurrent use of additional chemotherapy [38]. The incidence and risk factors of cardiotoxicity of capecitabine, an oral 5-FU analog, are poorly defined. From the four retrospective reviews published, the incidence of cardiotoxicity ranges from 3 to 9% [39–42]. Coronary artery thrombosis, arteritis, or vasospasm secondary to drug exposure have been proposed as the most likely underlying mechanisms of acute coronary syndromes associated with 5-FU and capecitabine. Other alternative mechanisms could be involved, including direct toxicity on myocardium, interaction with coagulation system, and autoimmune responses [43].

Paclitaxel administration has been associated with cases of myocardial ischemia and infarction. In a large study of approximately 1000 patients, the incidence of cardiac toxicity was 14% [44]. The etiology of myocardial ischemia associated with paclitaxel is thought to be multifactorial, with other drugs and underlying heart disease as possible contributing factors [45]. In addition, the Cremophor EL vehicle in which paclitaxel is formulated may play a role in its cardiac toxicity, which has been attributed to its induction of histamine release [45].

Endocrine agents, such as tamoxifen [46], and aromatase inhibitors [47], which are widely used in the treatment of hormone receptor-positive breast cancer, are associated with rare cardiac ischemia risk. Cardiac events, including myocardial infarction and cardiac failure, have been reported at very low frequency in the major adjuvant trials comparing use of AIs to a control arm of 5 years of tamoxifen [48]. Differential changes in lipid profile have been proposed as an etiology for these observations; however, a strong signal linking AIs and relevant changes in lipid levels is lacking.

The management of cardiac ischemia and coronary heart disease is similar to the management of patients with coronary artery disease without cancer, with an emphasis after intervention on platelet inhibition [49].

Venous Thromboembolism

Venous thromboembolism represents one of the most important causes of morbidity and mortality in cancer patients. According to population-based case-control studies, the 2-year cumulative incidence of VTE is between 0.8 and 8%. The increased risk of recurrent VTE in cancer patients is greatest in the first few months after malignancy is diagnosed and can persist for many years after an initial episode of symptomatic VTE [50–54]. Because the natural history of cancer is dynamic, the risk for VTE may increase and subside over time as a result of hospitalization, chemotherapy, metastasis, remission, and many other factors. Potential factors that may contribute to chemotherapy-induced thrombogenesis include the release of procoagulants and cytokines by chemotherapy-induced tumor cell damage, and direct endothelial damage, as well as hepatotoxicity from chemotherapeutic agents leading to decreased production of normally produced anticoagulants [55].

Breast anticancer agents correlated with an increased risk of VTE include antiangiogenic agents, cisplatin, and tamoxifen. The anti-vascular endothelial growth factor agent bevacizumab has been associated with an increased risk of VTE in one meta-analysis [56], in contrast with three other analyses that showed no increased risk of VTE in patients treated with bevacizumab [57–59]. Hurwitz showed that the risk of grade 3–5 bleeding in patients treated with anticoagulant after a VTE was low and was not increased by bevacizumab treatment [59]. These results are concordant with other reports indicating that patients with cancer can be safely treated with anticoagulation therapy while on chemotherapy [60] and that the risk of serious bleeding is not increased by bevacizumab [57, 61].

Based on the results of several studies, routine VTE prophylaxis for advanced cancer patients receiving chemotherapy is not recommended but may be considered and discussed with high-risk cancer patients [62], while prophylaxis with low-molecular-weight heparin or fondaparinux in hospitalized cancer patients confined to bed with an acute medical complication is recommended.

QT Prolongation

Prolongation of the QT interval can lead to life-threatening cardiac arrhythmias, including torsades de pointes (TdP) [63]. Although prolongation of the QT interval is not the best predictor of proarrhythmic risk, it represents the principal clinical surrogate marker by which to evaluate the arrhythmic risk of a drug, and it has led to withdrawal of several anticancer drugs from the market. QT prolongation has been reported as infrequent in association with many anticancer therapies used in the course of treatment for breast cancer. Tamoxifen has the most well-established effect at on QT interval, where the mechanism appears to involve a direct effect on the expression and activity of channels involved in cardiac repolarization [64]. While TdP is uncommon during the treatment of breast cancer, patients with a history of QT interval prolongation, patients who are taking antiarrhythmics, or patients with relevant cardiovascular disease, bradycardia, thyroid dysfunction, or electrolyte disturbances should be screened and monitored. Periodic monitoring with on-treatment ECGs and electrolytes should be considered.

Conclusion

The therapeutic options for patients with breast cancer now include increasingly complex combinations of medications, radiation therapy, and surgical intervention. Many highly effective agents in contemporary oncology, including anthracyclines, trastuzumab, and anti-VEGF, are associated with potential adverse cardiac effects and are likely to have significant effects on patient outcomes. The development of cardiovascular disease during the course of breast cancer treatment can adversely impact the management of the underlying malignancy. Therefore, understanding cardiac toxicity is crucial to optimize outcome. Given the growth of novel biologic therapies, efforts are needed to promote strategies for risk detection and management and to avoid dangerous toxicities that may impede development as well as patient access to new agents. Progress in understanding of treatment-related cardiac toxicity requires the development of clear definitions of cardiac toxicity and standardized measurements that predict long-term outcomes. Studies are also needed to more accurately predict which patients are at highest risk of developing treatment-related cardiotoxicity; these studies might include genomic testing that identifies those at highest risk. Thus, more research is needed to assess and manage patients with heart disease and breast cancer. To that end it is necessary to forge a dynamic partnership between oncologists and cardiologists with the development of a new generation of "cardio-oncology" investigators with the aim of obtaining optimal patient outcomes.

References

1. Ewer MS, Vooletich MT, Durand JB, et al. Reversibility of trastuzumab-related cardiotoxicity: new insights based on clinical course and response to medical treatment. J Clin Oncol. 2005;23:7820–6.
2. Sawyer DB, Peng X, Chen B, et al. Mechanisms of anthracycline cardiac injury: can we identify strategies for cardioprotection? Prog Cardiovasc Dis. 2010;53:105–13.
3. Crone SA, Zhao YY, Fan L, Gu Y, Minamisawa S, Liu Y, et al. ErbB2 is essential in the prevention of dilated cardiomyopathy. Nat Med. 2002;8(5):459–65.

4. Meyer D, Birchmeier C. Multiple essential functions of neuregulin in development. Nature. 1995;378:386–90.

5. Seidman A, Hudis C, Pierri MK, et al. Cardiac dysfunction in the trastuzumab clinical trials experience. J Clin Oncol. 2002;20:1215–21.

6. Singal PK, Deally CM, Weinberg LE. Subcellular effects of adriamycin in the heart: a concise review. J Mol Cell Cardiol. 1987;19(8):817–28.

7. Kwok JC, Richardson DR. Anthracyclines induce accumulation of iron in ferritin in myocardial and neoplastic cells: inhibition of the ferritin iron mobilization pathway. Mol Pharmacol. 2003;63(4):849–61.

8. Jones RL, Swanton C, Ewer MS. Anthracycline cardiotoxicity. Expert Opin Drug Saf. 2006;5:791–809.

9. Raschi E, Vasina V, Ursino MG, et al. Anticancer drugs and cardiotoxicity: insights and perspectives in the era of targeted therapy. Pharmacol Ther. 2010;125:196–218.

10. Cardinale D, Sandri MT, Martinoni A, et al. Left ventricular dysfunction predicted by early troponin I release after high-dose chemotherapy. J Am Coll Cardiol. 2000;36:517–22.

11. Cardinale D, Sandri MT, Martinoni A, et al. Myocardial injury revealed by plasma troponin I in breast cancer treatment with high-dose chemotherapy. Ann Oncol. 2002;13:710–5.

12. Deng S, Wojnowski L. Genotyping the risk of anthracycline-induced cardiotoxicity. Cardiovasc Toxicol. 2007;7:129–34.

13. Batist G, Ramakrishnan G, Rao CS, et al. Reduced cardiotoxicity and preserved antitumor efficacy of liposome-encapsulated doxorubicin and cyclophosphamide compared with conventional doxorubicin and cyclophosphamide in a randomized, multicenter trial of metastatic breast cancer. J Clin Oncol. 2001;19:1444–54.

14. Harris L, Batist G, Belt R, et al. Liposome-encapsulated doxorubicin compared with conventional doxorubicin in a randomized multicenter trial as first-line therapy of metastatic breast carcinoma. Cancer. 2002;94:25–36.

15. Goldberg MA, Antin JH, Guinan EC, et al. Cyclophosphamide cardiotoxicity: an analysis of dosing as a risk factor. Blood. 1986;68:1114–8.

16. Gottdiener JS, Appelbaum JR, Ferrans VJ, Deisseroth A, Ziegler J. Cardiotoxicity associated with high-dose cyclophosphamide therapy. Arch Intern Med. 1981;141:758–63.

17. Martin M, Pienkowski T, Mackey J, et al. Adjuvant docetaxel for node-positive breast cancer. N Engl J Med. 2005;352:2302–13.

18. Slamon D, Eiermann W, Robert N, et al. Adjuvant trastuzumab in HER2-positive breast cancer. N Engl J Med. 2011;365(14):1273–83.

19. Romond EH, Perez EA, Bryant J, et al. Trastuzumab plus adjuvant chemotherapy for operable HER2-positive breast cancer. N Engl J Med. 2005;353:1673–84.

20. Piccart-Gebhart MJ, Procter M, Leyland-Jones B, et al. Trastuzumab after adjuvant chemotherapy in HER2-positive breast cancer. N Engl J Med. 2005;353:1659–72.

21. Slamon DJ, Leyland-Jones B, Shak S, et al. Use of chemotherapy plus a monoclonal antibody against HER2 for metastatic breast cancer that overexpresses HER2. N Engl J Med. 2001;344:783–92.

22. Tan-Chiu E, Yothers G, Romond E, et al. Assessment of cardiac dysfunction in a randomized trial comparing doxorubicin and cyclophosphamide followed by paclitaxel, with or without trastuzumab as adjuvant therapy in node-positive, human epidermal growth factor receptor 2-overexpressing breast cancer: NSABP B-31. J Clin Oncol. 2005;23:7811–9.

23. Joensuu H, Kellokumpu-Lehtinen PL, Bono P, et al. FinHer Study Investigators Adjuvant docetaxel or vinorelbine with or without trastuzumab for breast cancer. N Engl J Med. 2006;354(8):809–20.

24. Chien KR. Herceptin and the heart: a molecular modifier of cardiac failure. N Engl J Med. 2006;354:789–90.

25. Sliwkowski MX, Lofgren JA, Lewis GD, et al. Nonclinical studies addressing the mechanism of action of trastuzumab (Herceptin). Semin Oncol. 1999;26:60–70.

26. Shell SA, Lyass L, Trusk PB, et al. Activation of AMPK is necessary for killing cancer cells and sparing cardiac cells. Cell Cycle. 2008;7:1769–75.
27. Perez EA, Koehler M, Byrne J, et al. Cardiac safety of lapatinib: pooled analysis of 3689 patients enrolled in clinical trials. Mayo Clin Proc. 2008;83:679–86.
28. Miller K, Wang M, Gralow J, et al. Paclitaxel plus bevacizumab versus paclitaxel alone for metastatic breast cancer. N Engl J Med. 2007;357:2666–76.
29. Cardinale D, Colombo A, Sandri MT, et al. Prevention of high-dose chemotherapy-induced cardiotoxicity in high-risk patients by angiotensin-converting enzyme inhibition. Circulation. 2006;114:2474–81.
30. Cardinale D, Colombo A, Lamantia G, et al. Anthracycline-induced cardiomyopathy. Clinical relevance and response to pharmacologic therapy. J Am Coll Cardiol. 2010;55:213–20.
31. Bosch X, Esteve J, Sitges M, et al. Prevention of chemotherapy-induced left ventricular dysfunction with enalapril and carvedilol: rationale and design of the OVERCOME trial. J Card Fail. 2011;17:6438.
32. Pituskin E, Haykowsky M, Mackey JR, et al. Rationale and design of the Multidisciplinary Approach to Novel Therapies In Cardiology Oncology REsearch Trial (MANTICORE 101 Breast): a randomized, placebo-controlled trial to determine if conventional heart failure pharmacotherapy can prevent trastuzumab-mediated left ventricular remodelling among patients with HER+ early breast cancer using cardiac MRI. BMC Cancer. 2011;11:318.
33. Huh WW, Jaffe N, Durand JB, et al. Comparison of doxorubicin cardiotoxicity in pediatric sarcoma patients when given with dexrazoxane versus continuous infusion. Pediatr Hematol Oncol. 2010;27:546–57.
34. Gradishar WJ, Vokes EE. 5-Fluorouracil cardiotoxicity: a critical review. Ann Oncol. 1990;1:409–14.
35. Labianca R, Beretta G, Clerici M, et al. Cardiac toxicity of 5-fluorouracil: a study on 1083 patients. Tumori. 1982;68:505–10.
36. Meyer CC, Calis KA, Burke LB, Walawander CA, Grasela TH. Symptomatic cardiotoxicity associated with 5-fluorouracil. Pharmacotherapy. 1997;17:729–36.
37. de Forni M, Malet-Martino MC, Jaillais P, et al. Cardiotoxicity of high-dose continuous infusion fluorouracil: a prospective clinical study. J Clin Oncol. 1992;10:1795–801.
38. Jensen SA, Sorensen JB. Risk factors and prevention of cardiotoxicity induced by 5-fluorouracil or capecitabine. Cancer Chemother Pharmacol. 2006;58:487–93.
39. Van Cutsem E, Hoff PM, Blum JL, Abt M, Osterwalder B. Incidence of cardiotoxicity with the oral fluoropyrimidine capecitabine is typical of that reported with 5-fluorouracil. Ann Oncol. 2002;13:484–5.
40. Ng M, Cunningham D, Norman AR. The frequency and pattern of cardiotoxicity observed with capecitabine used in conjunction with oxaliplatin in patients treated for advanced colorectal cancer (CRC). Eur J Cancer. 2005;41:1542–6.
41. Saif MW, Tomita M, Ledbetter L, Diasio RB. Capecitabine-related cardiotoxicity: recognition and management. J Support Oncol. 2008;6:41–8.
42. Walko CM, Lindley C. Capecitabine: a review. Clin Ther. 2005;27:23–44.
43. Frickhofen N, Beck FJ, Jung B, Fuhr HG, Andrasch H, Sigmund M. Capecitabine can induce acute coronary syndrome similar to 5-fluorouracil. Ann Oncol. 2002;13:797–801.
44. Trimble EL, Adams JD, Vena D, et al. Paclitaxel for platinum-refractory ovarian cancer: results from the first 1000 patients registered to National Cancer Institute Treatment Referral Center 9103. J Clin Oncol. 1993;11:2405–10.
45. Rowinsky EK, McGuire WP, Guarnieri T, Fisherman JS, Christian MC, Donehower RC. Cardiac disturbances during the administration of Taxol. J Clin Oncol. 1991;9:1704–12.
46. Braithwaite RS, Chlebowski RT, Lau J, et al. Meta-analysis of vascular and neoplastic events associated with tamoxifen. J Gen Intern Med. 2003;18:937–47.
47. Nabholtz JM, Gligorov J. Cardiovascular safety profiles of aromatase inhibitors: a comparative review. Drug Saf. 2006;29:785–801.

48. Cuppone F, Bria E, Verma S, et al. Do adjuvant aromatase inhibitors increase the cardiovas-
    cular risk in postmenopausal women with early breast cancer? Meta-analysis of randomized
    trials. Cancer. 2008;112:260–7.
49. Chen CL, Parameswaran R. Managing the risks of cardiac therapy in cancer patients. Semin
    Oncol. 2013;40(2):210–7.
50. Winter PC. The pathogenesis of venous thromboembolism in cancer: emerging links with
    tumour biology. Hematol Oncol. 2006;24:126–33.
51. Petralia GA, Lemoine NR, Kakkar AK. Mechanisms of disease: the impact of antithrombotic
    therapy in cancer patients. Nat Clin Pract Oncol. 2005;2:356–63.
52. Lip GY, Chin BS, Blann AD. Cancer and the prothrombotic state. Lancet Oncol.
    2002;3:27–34.
53. Yusuf SW, Razeghi P, Yeh ET. The diagnosis and management of cardiovascular disease in
    cancer patients. Curr Probl Cardiol. 2008;33:163–96.
54. Khorana AA. Risk assessment for cancer-associated thrombosis: what is the best approach?
    Thromb Res. 2012;129:S10–5.
55. Czaykowski PM, Moore MJ, Tannock IF. High risk of vascular events in patients with
    urothelial transitional cell carcinoma treated with cisplatin-based chemotherapy. J Urol.
    1998;160:2021–4.
56. Nalluri SR, Chu D, Keresztes R, et al. Risk of venous thromboembolism with the angiogenesis
    inhibitor bevacizumab in cancer patients: a meta-analysis. JAMA. 2008;300:2277–85.
57. Scappaticci FA, Skillings JR, Holden SN, et al. Arterial thromboembolic events in patients
    with metastatic carcinoma treated with chemotherapy and bevacizumab. J Natl Cancer Inst.
    2007;99:1232–9.
58. Calvo V, Ramirez N, Saura C, et al. Risk of venous and arterial thromboembolic events in
    patients with metastatic breast cancer treated with bevacizumab: a meta-analysis. J Clin Oncol
    2010;28:124s Suppl:abstr 1043.
59. Hurwitz HI, Saltz LB, Van Cutsem E, et al. Venous thromboembolic events with chemother-
    apy plus bevacizumab: a pooled analysis of patients in randomized phase II and III studies. J
    Clin Oncol. 2011;29(13):175764.
60. Khorana AA, Connolly GC. Assessing risk of venous thromboembolism in patients with
    cancer. J Clin Oncol. 2009;27:483947.
61. Leighl N, Bennouna J, Kuo H. Safety of bevacizumab treatment in non-small cell lung cancer
    (NSCLC) subjects receiving full-dose anticoagulation (FDAC) treated on protocol BO17704.
    Eur J Cancer. 2007;391 Suppl 5:abstr 6610.
62. Agnelli G, Gussoni G, Bianchini C, et al. Nadroparin for the prevention of thromboembolic
    events in ambulatory patients with metastatic or locally advanced solid cancer receiving
    chemotherapy: a randomised, placebo-controlled, double-blind study. Lancet Oncol.
    2009;10:9439.
63. Suter TM, Ewer MS. Cancer drugs and the heart: importance and management. Eur Heart
    J. 2013;34(15):1102–11.
64. Slovacek L, Ansorgova V, Macingova Z, Haman L, Petera J. Tamoxifen-induced QT interval
    prolongation. J Clin Pharm Ther. 2008;33(4):453–5.
65. Hedhli N, Kalinowski A, S Russel K. Cardiovascular effects of neuregulin-1/ErbB signaling:
    role in vascular signaling and angiogenesis. Curr Pharm Des 2014; 20(39): 4899–905

Chapter 11
Cardiac Toxic Chemotherapy and Cancer Survivorship

Dava Szalda, Monica Ahluwalia, and Joseph R. Carver

Introduction

With remarkable progress in cancer diagnosis and therapy, there are growing numbers of cancer survivors with almost 15 million current survivors in the United States whose number is estimated to grow to 19 million by 2024 [1, 2]. This population is composed of adult survivors of pediatric cancer and adult survivors of adult cancer. Because of the recognition that cardiovascular morbidity and mortality play an important role in outcomes of cancer survivors, especially those exposed to potentially cardiac toxic cancer therapy, understanding the unique cardiac needs of cancer survivors and existing evidence for care is essential to comprehensive cardio-oncology and general survivorship care. Cancer survivors are a heterogeneous group of patients in that they may have had pre-existing cardiac conditions or risk factors and varied treatment exposures that impact the risk of chemotherapeutic regimens and radiation exposure. Treatment information, along with current age, family history, and other modifiable risk factors (i.e., smoking or

Electronic supplementary material: The online version of this chapter (doi:10.1007/978-3-319-43096-6_11) contains supplementary material, which is available to authorized users.

D. Szalda
Abramson Cancer Center, Cancer Survivorship Program, Pediatric Oncology,
The Children's Hospital of Philadelphia, Philadelphia, PA, USA
e-mail: dava.szalda@uphs.upenn.edu

M. Ahluwalia
Department of Internal Medicine, Perelman School of Medicine,
University of Pennsylvania, Philadelphia, PA, USA
e-mail: monica.ahluwalia@nyumc.org

J.R. Carver (✉)
Abramson Cancer Center, University of Pennsylvania, Philadelphia, PA, USA
e-mail: joseph.carver2@uphs.upenn.edu

obesity), continue to be important considerations for patients. This heterogeneity, coupled with the potentially long asymptomatic latency period from treatment completion to symptomatic recognition, has meant that universally accepted guidelines for surveillance and prevention have been slow to develop.

Adult survivors of pediatric cancer are addressed as a distinct group, and their care will also be covered in this chapter. Though childhood cancer is thankfully rare and childhood cancer survivors make up a small percentage of the overall number of cancer survivors, childhood cancer survivors are growing rapidly in number. Over 80 % of children diagnosed with cancer today will be cured [3]. For these survivors, treatment regimens, particularly treatment intensity, is distinct from treatment of adult cancers, and these survivors ideally have decades of survivorship in which they are increasingly vulnerable to cardiovascular disease. Indeed, the Childhood Cancer Survivor Study, the largest and most complete cohort study of childhood cancer survivors, has found that childhood cancer survivors suffer from chronic conditions at alarming rates, with cardiovascular disease being a major cause of morbidity and mortality [4, 5], and more often than not, these late-occurring cardiac problems become apparent at times when survivors are no longer followed by their oncologists. A recent scientific statement from the American Heart Association by Lipshultz et al. provides an exhaustive review of all current data regarding the long-term cardiovascular toxicity of cancer therapy in children, adolescents, and young adults. This review includes detailed descriptions of pathophysiology, natural history, monitoring, and management [6].

Cancer treatments (chemotherapy and therapeutic radiation) can result in diverse late-appearing (i.e. following treatment completion) cardiovascular issues affecting the vascular system as well as all of the cardiac structures. Manifestations are often initially asymptomatic and potentially can affect all structures of the heart, with a disease-free latency period that may last decades before the emergence of overt, symptomatic disease and an incidence that increases in most instances with increased cumulative dosing and duration of survival. Cardiomyopathy secondary to chemotherapeutic agents including anthracyclines and HER2-targeted therapies has been the most well described and studied [7, 8]. Radiation exposure may lead to premature atherosclerosis and valvular, pericardial, and conduction system disease [9, 10]. In addition, other vascular structures exposed to therapeutic radiation can develop premature atherosclerosis, e.g. carotid disease after mantle radiation and renal artery disease after retroperitoneal radiation exposure [11]. Asymptomatic disease manifested by echocardiographic abnormalities and/or subtle clinical examination signs are more common than symptomatic disease and, depending on the definitions applied, can be found in up to 50 % of all survivors of anthracycline or radiation-based therapy [12, 13]. Although there is an acceptance of the potential risks and need for surveillance, there is still currently a lack of agreement about the details of standards for follow-up and testing.

In 2005, the American Society of Clinical Oncology (ASCO) convened an expert panel to develop guidelines for the ongoing cardiac surveillance and care of adult and pediatric survivors of cancer. Because of a lack of direct, high-quality evidence on the benefits of screening and treatment, the document, published in

2007, became an evidence review that summarized the then-current literature regarding late-cardiopulmonary effects among cancer survivors [14]. A more recent update from Memorial Sloan Kettering Cancer Center was published in 2013 [15]. Since then, many professional organizations have attempted to stratify risk in cancer survivors and provide recommendations for follow-up care based on best available evidence and expert consensus. These include, but are limited to, the Heart Failure Association of the European Society of Cardiology, the European Society of Medical Oncology, the Children's Oncology Group (COG), and the National Comprehensive Cancer Network (NCCN). At the time of writing of this chapter, a preliminary article from the International Cardio-Oncology Society is in press, and a combined workgroup from ASCO and the ACC/AHA to develop guidelines has been convened.

What has been the problem? Since the original ASCO endeavor, we still lack solid randomized clinical trial evidence that demonstrates an improvement in outcomes related to screening and cardioprotection, a persistent belief that cancer treatment-associated cardiac disease is different from non-cancer-related cardiac disease, a medical-legal fear that guidelines will increase liability for care providers and financial concerns about over-testing. In addition, there is still a lack of consensus about definitions, type of cardiac imaging, and biomarker testing strategy.

Cardiac toxicity from anthracycline chemotherapy in adult survivors of adult cancer is manifested mainly by a dilated cardiomyopathy and characterized by a reduction in systolic function as measured by a reduction in left ventricular ejection fraction (LVEF) or fractional shortening (FS). This may be preceded by isolated diastolic dysfunction, a decrease in global longitudinal strain (GLS), or right ventricular dysfunction. Cardiac toxicity from anthracycline-based chemotherapy in survivors of pediatric cancer develops as a restrictive process with diastolic dysfunction and early preservation of systolic cardiac function.

Cardiac toxicity from platinum-based chemotherapy includes a high prevalence of hypertension and metabolic syndrome and premature vascular disease consistently demonstrated compared to matched untreated cohorts [16].

Cardiac toxicity from radiation includes restrictive cardiomyopathy and valvular, pericardial, coronary, and conduction system disease.

Chemotherapy and radiation damage the heart through many potential mechanisms, including oxidative stress, mitochondrial dysfunction, myofilament degradation, endothelial cell damage and dysfunction, and progenitor cell depletion/dysfunction. Because of an innate cardiac "functional reserve," damage can occur without the manifestation of overt symptoms. After treatment completion, there is a variable period of asymptomatic risk, i.e., latency period, that may persist for decades. This duration of asymptomatic latency and progression of disease is likely related to genetic factors because everyone does not develop cardiotoxicity, even with the progressive hemodynamic burden of stress related to comorbidity and environmental factors. There has been exciting new research characterizing genetic abnormalities that are associated with an increased risk for anthracycline-related

Table 11.1 Stages of heart failure

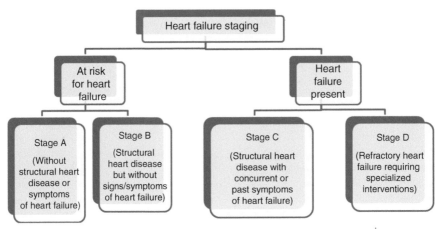

cardiac toxicity [17–19]. The alteration in cardiac reserve is a target for investigation to predict and diagnose asymptomatic cardiac toxicity.

It is logical to extend the American College of Cardiology (ACC)/American Heart Association (AHA) definition and guidelines for care delineating four stages of heart failure [20] to the cancer survivor population. This is especially useful since the natural history of cancer treatment-related cardiac toxicity moves along a pathway from asymptomatic abnormalities of left ventricular function, ACC/AHA stages (A/B), to symptomatic disease, ACC/AHA stages (C/D). This construct is detailed in Table 11.1, and the working postulate is that early intervention at stages A/B can prevent progression to C/D [21, 22]. This construct also takes advantage of evidence-based recommendations for the care of heart failure patients with already accepted risk-benefit analyses and published strength of recommendations. This classification also has been incorporated into the management of pediatric heart failure [23].

Risk Assessment: An Overview

For left ventricular systolic dysfunction, we propose an approach that incorporates the ACC/AHA staging when evaluating and managing the care of cancer survivors. It is accepted that the risk of anthracycline-induced cardiac toxicity increases with cumulative dosing. The higher the dose of anthracycline the higher the risk of cardiac toxicity. There is disagreement about the cutoff in dosing to define high risk and for purposes of our classification, we have chosen a doxorubicin dose >240 mg/m^2 or its equivalent. A detailed discussion about acute treatment phase cardioprotective strategies (beta blockers/ACE inhibitors/ARBs, continuous infusion, anthracycline formulation choice, use of dexrazoxane, etc.) is beyond the scope of this chapter.

From a population standpoint, the direct relationship between cumulative dose exposure and cardiac risk has predictive value and helps to define a high-risk population; however, for the individual survivor, there is wide variation in risk, i.e., toxicity may occur at low doses so that there is no "safe" dose [24–26] or may not occur at high doses. The amount of excess risk, derived from a meta-analysis of eight trials, demonstrated that anthracyclines increased the risk of clinical cardiac toxicity 5.43-fold, subclinical cardiac toxicity by 6.25-fold, any cardiac toxicity by 2.27-fold, and the risk of cardiac death by 4.94-fold compared with non-anthracycline regimens [27]. "High risk" has been associated with several factors: (1) sex, such that women are at higher risk compared to men; (2) age, such that risk is higher at extremes of age (children and elderly); and (3) preexisting risk factors for or diagnosis of cardiovascular disease. Associated mediastinal radiation also increases the risk associated with chemotherapy [28].

For all forms of radiation-induced cardiac toxicity, it is generally accepted that the approximate risk is 1 % at 5 years and doubles every 5 years. Clinically significant radiation changes more commonly occur 10 or more years posttreatment completion and are unusual but possible before that time. At 20 years posttreatment completion, the risk for clinically significant cardiomyopathy, CAD, valvular disease, pericardial disease, and carotid artery stenosis is 8 %, 10 %, 7 %, 1 %–3 %, and 6 %, respectively.

In assessing and defining risk, radiation treatment that involves the chest (mediastinal, mantle, left side for breast cancer, craniospinal, or total body radiation) should be considered as an additional risk factor for premature or accelerated atherosclerotic vascular disease and may be considered as an additional potent risk factor comparable to diabetes, cigarette smoking, and hypertension, to guide risk stratification and set treatment targets for those risk factors that can be modified, e.g., aggressive lipid management to "secondary" prevention targets.

Screening Strategies

With knowledge of the impact of cardiac toxicity on long-term survivors of cancer, early detection of asymptomatic cardiac toxicity has become a primary goal. Current standards for screening patients and for cardiac monitoring rely primarily on the measurement of left ventricular ejection fraction (LVEF) by echocardiography or multigated acquisition scanning.

To date, there are no evidence-based guidelines for cardiac toxicity monitoring after treatment completion. There are "guidelines" based on consensus with weak evidence for both adults and pediatric survivors that are listed and referenced in Table 11.2. Screening guideline development has been slowed by the focus on a single test and the assumption that cardiac toxicity risk is binary. A combination of tests, e.g., imaging and biomarker(s) coupled with a comprehensive history and

Table 11.2 Existing survivorship guidelines[a]

• American Society of Clinical Oncology
– J Clin Oncol 2007; 25:3991–4008
• European Society of Medical Oncology
– Ann Oncol 2010;21:277–282
• Heart Failure Association of the European Society of Cardiology
– Eur J Heart Fail 2011;13:1–10
• American Society of Echocardiography/European Association of Cardiovascular Imaging
– J AM Soc Echocardiography 2014;27:91–939
• NCCN Clinical Practice Guidelines in Oncology: Survivorship
– Anthracycline-induced cardiac toxicity (2015)
• Harmonization of Surveillance Guidelines
– Lancet Oncology 2015;16: e123–e136
• American Society of Clinical Oncology Working Group
– (in progress)
• International Cardio-Oncology Society Working Group
– (in progress)

[a]Modified from Sara Armenian, MD

physical examination rather than a single test, may be the most effective population-based strategy that achieves an appropriate balance between lack of screening and over-screening. In the continuum of cardiac toxicity, every long-term survivor is at risk for the future development of cardiac disease. The main goals of screening are to identify the presence of structural heart disease and the patient's place in the continuum. This theoretically allows early intervention to prevent progression by identifying the presence of asymptomatic cardiovascular disease before symptomatic progression and resultant cardiovascular morbidity. Many of the outstanding questions regarding type, frequency, and intensity of screening survivors are being considered by an ASCO-charged working group to compliment the current existing "guidelines" listed in Table 11.2.

The Role of Biomarkers

The measurement of cardiac biomarkers (troponin I and T, B-type natriuretic peptide [BNP], and N-terminal pro-BNP [NTproBNP]) to predict late cardiac toxicity has been explored [29]. Biomarkers are attractive as a screening tool because of the ease of measurement, low cost compared to imaging, and ability to use in a serial or longitudinal manner. It is also conceivable that they have potential predictive value allowing early diagnosis and then early initiation of preventive strategies or altered monitoring schedules prior to the development of overt heart failure. Troponin in its various forms has been studied during the treatment phase as a predictor of early and late cardiac toxicity with inconsistent results that have prevented universal adoption of its use in existing "guidelines" [30].

Natriuretic peptides such as BNP and NTproBNP are secreted from the myocardium in response to increased hemodynamic stress and have been widely used in the management of heart failure. Elevated levels of these peptides have been found in asymptomatic patients treated with anthracyclines and the elevation precedes the development of overt heart failure. However, natriuretic peptides have not shown to be consistently effective for population-based screening, with little incremental value over standard clinical variables. Their major strength, however, may be in their negative predictive value, as it is atypical to have clinically significant structural heart disease with LV dysfunction and a normal BNP or NTproBNP level [7, 30]. Current consensus opinion concludes that the strength of the evidence is not strong enough to make this a standard recommendation in screening and follow-up of cancer survivors. Other biomarkers currently being investigated during the acute cancer treatment phase as predictors of late toxicity include topoisomerase 2B, myeloperoxidase, growth-differentiation factor 15, soluble fms-like tyrosine kinase receptor-1, and galectin-3 [31].

The Role of Echocardiography

The single most useful diagnostic test in the evaluation of cardiac function before, during, and after cancer treatment has been the two-dimensional echocardiogram coupled with Doppler flow studies to quantitate systolic and diastolic function, cardiac chamber dimensions, wall thickness/mass, valvular disease, and the pericardium. In addition to systolic function, the echocardiogram provides a comprehensive assessment of diastolic function that also is critical, as early abnormalities that precede decreases in systolic function have long-term consequences in the anthracycline-treated population. Furthermore, echocardiograms provide insight into the degree of cardiac remodeling from hypertension, wall motion abnormalities from CAD, and valvular/pericardial disease that may result from radiation exposure.

Cardiac toxicity via echocardiography has been defined as an LVEF decline of ≥ 5 to $<53\%$ with heart failure symptoms or an asymptomatic decrease of LVEF ≥ 10 to $<53\%$ [32].

All current echocardiographic-derived measurements of left ventricular function (LVEF and FS) are load dependent and comorbidity dependent (fluid overload, sepsis, ischemic heart disease, or other drug therapy) and limited by multiple technical considerations. As a measure of global LV function, they are currently unable to consistently detect subtle, early changes in regional myocardial wall motion.

A normal LVEF or FS does not exclude cardiac dysfunction. There is a critical need to develop more robust and sensitive measures of LV dysfunction to improve our current methods of monitoring patients. Currently, there is an expanding interest in the measurement of tissue Doppler-derived strain. Each adult survivor of pediatric or adult cancer who was treated with at-risk therapy, e.g., anthracyclines or chest radiation, has ACC/AHA stage A heart failure and, as such, has defined goals of therapy that can be used to target modifiable cardiovascular risk factors. The goal of screening is to recognize and then prevent progression to the more advanced stages B, C, and D. Within this population, a high- and low-risk group can be identified to help guide frequency of assessment and surveillance.

Newer methods to assess cardiac function have been extensively reported and include cardiac MRI, three-dimensional echocardiography, and various tissue Doppler-derived measurements of regional myocardial strain. Strain imaging in the adult cancer survivor population demonstrates abnormalities that occur and persist in survivors despite preserved LVEF. To date, no modality has emerged as the "winner." A recent extensive review of the current state of imaging in cancer patients endorsed by the American Society of Echocardiography and the European Association of Cardiovascular Imaging has been published [32].

Screening for CAD

Tests available to screen for CAD include the electrocardiogram (ECG), exercise treadmill test, exercise myocardial perfusion imaging, exercise (stress) echocardiography, electron-beam computed tomography (CT) scanning for coronary calcium, coronary CT angiography, cardiac magnetic resonance imaging, and carotid intima-media thickness measurement. The sensitivity, specificity, and predictive accuracy of these tests for the noncancer population have been reviewed in detail [33].

The US Preventive Services Task Force guidelines for CAD detection in asymptomatic patients in the noncancer population do not recommend routine ECG, exercise treadmill test, exercise myocardial perfusion imaging, exercise (stress) echocardiography, and other nontraditional testings (scanning for coronary calcium, coronary CT angiography, magnetic resonance imaging, measurement of carotid intima-media thickness) for either the presence of severe coronary artery stenosis or the prediction of coronary heart disease (CHD) events in adults at low risk for CHD events. For higher-risk patients, they found inadequate evidence that testing (beyond that obtained by a detailed cardiac history and assessment of conventional CHD risk factors) would result in interventions that lead to improved CHD-related health outcomes [34, 35].

However, these recommendations did not specifically address the survivor population at risk for radiation-induced premature CAD, which differs from atherosclerotic CAD in pathophysiology, onset (beginning at 8–10 years posttreatment completion), and lesion location (ostial or proximal left main, left anterior descending, or right coronary artery). Therefore, application of their recommendations to the survivor population may not be generalizable, but may be used to help in decision making and should guide the needed future research in this area. We are

Table 11.3 High risk characteristics[a]

• Patient Factors	• Treatment Factors
– Age (<15 years and >65 years)	– Acute cardiac toxicity during treatment, includes asymptomatic decrease in LVEF
– Female gender	– Cumulative anthracycline dose >240 mg/m^2 doxorubicin or its equivalent
– Any cardiac symptoms or abnormal physical exam	– Chest radiation >30 Gy
– Associated cardiac co-morbidity (hypertension, CAD, LV dysfunction)	– Combination chest radiation with any anthracycline
– Obesity	– Pre-modern (before 1975) radiation treatment
	– Length of follow-up 10 years or more post treatment end

CAD coronary artery disease, *LV* left ventricular, *LVEF* left ventricular ejection fraction
[a]Any 1 factor implies "high risk" Stage A

sensitized to the increased risk of CAD in the post-radiation-treated cancer survivor and have a low threshold to pursue screening (stress testing, coronary CT angiography) for any symptoms that may even remotely suggest coronary ischemia.

Is There a High-Risk Population?

It can be assumed that every survivor exposed to anthracyclines and/or chest radiation is at stage A and "at risk." Subsequent sub-characterization as low- or high-risk should be matched and drive the frequency and intensity of screening. Patient and treatment high-risk variables are listed in Table 11.3. The presence of any one variable defines a high-risk patient who should be considered at stage A.

Guidelines/Recommendations: The Landscape

Long-term survivors of cancer have a myriad of health issues that are increased in prevalence compared to age-matched siblings or controls; among these, cardiac toxicity is the most prevalent noncancer condition. This recognition that there are long-term health concerns after chemotherapy prompted the Institute of Medicine to publish two reports providing general recommendations for ongoing care and research for survivors of childhood and adult cancers [36, 37]. Specific recommendations about the nature and frequency of cardiac testing were not addressed.

The Children's Oncology Group also has published revised guidelines [38] for long-term care for pediatric cancer survivors. The guidelines are expert panel, consensus-derived, based on a recognized risk, with monitoring frequency matched to risk. After baseline screening, specific testing is recommended from yearly to every 5 years based on age at treatment, dose of anthracycline, and associated exposure to radiotherapy. In addition, the panel recognized that the risk of CAD associated with radiotherapy is manifested between 5 and 10 or more years after treatment completion, and they recommend testing strategies. For survivors of adult cancer, the landscape is less clear. Current existing guidelines include the ASCO, European Society of Medical Oncology, Heart Failure Society of the European Society of Cardiology, American Society of Echocardiography/European Association of Cardiovascular Imaging, and the National Cooperative Cancer Network (NCCN) and are referenced in Table 11.2. All include a baseline CV assessment at the start of potentially cardiac toxic therapy, assessment of the treatment of associated comorbidity prior to, during, and after treatment. They suffer from varied definitions of cardiac toxicity, the role of cardioprotective strategies during and after cancer treatment, and the frequency and modality of posttreatment completion follow-up. All recommend monitoring of cardiovascular risk factors and reinforce the value of a healthy lifestyle. The "concordances" of the "harmonization" group for pediatric survivors described above could easily be extended to the adult survivors of adult cancer [39].

Surveillance Suggestions

This section describes a general approach to the screening and care of adult cancer survivors and does not represent an absolute standard of care but provides a clinically relevant approach to guide the care of these patients based on existing data defining cardiac risk and the value of therapeutic intervention. These recommendations can be used as a roadmap allowing for individual practitioner discretion and are subject to change as knowledge and technological advances are made. The goal is the early detection of preclinical lesions/disease that are actionable, in other words, discovery when interventions should have the greatest beneficial impact. Although there are no universal guidelines, we reinforce the concept that the echocardiogram is the modality of choice for the long-term monitoring of cardiac structure and function in cancer survivors exposed to potentially cardiac toxic treatments.

For all patients, the approach can be simplified into five questions that guide subsequent testing:

1. What are the details of previous cancer treatment?
2. What is the patient's cardiovascular risk independent of treatment?
3. What is the patient's current functional status?
4. Is there any current or prior clinical evidence of structural heart disease or CAD?
5. How does the knowledge from 1 to 4 predict risk and dictate potential cardioprotective strategies based on existing knowledge and associated comorbidity?

Assess Prior Cancer Therapy

A detailed treatment summary should be obtained that includes the cancer diagnosis, age at diagnosis, all treatments, previous cardiac testing, and treatment-related cardiac complications. Particular attention should be made to cumulative dose of anthracycline, use of trastuzumab, and field, dose, and site of radiation. One user-friendly and detailed online treatment summary form is offered by Oncolink™ and is available at: http://livestrongcareplan.org/pdf/CancerTherapyTreatmentSummary.pdf.

Assess Risk Status Independent of Treatment

Patients should be specifically asked about traditional cardiac risk factors and comorbidity (which magnify and increase the risk for cardiac toxicity), current medications, and lifestyle/behavior. History should include detailed conversation about diet, physical activity, and tobacco use. Current BMI and blood pressure should be obtained with routine physical exam. A fasting lipid measurement should be obtained with routine blood work. A thorough family history helps to define the potential for atherosclerotic disease and inherited cardiomyopathy.

A complete physical examination should include determination of blood pressure in both arms in the supine, sitting, and standing positions because there is an increase in autonomic dysfunction after chemotherapy and radiotherapy. Body mass index and waist circumference should be recorded. Examination of the jugular pulse provides information about filling pressures, and examination of the ocular fundus provides information about the overall arterial vasculature and the presence of other cardiac risk factors. Fluid status assessment, cardiac palpation, and auscultation should be included. Any abnormality should result in a referral for cardiology consultation.

Fasting lipid levels should be measured at baseline, given the high incidence of obesity, metabolic syndrome, and potential atherosclerosis in cancer survivors [40]. Prior exposure to therapeutic radiation or platinum-based chemotherapy each individually helps define "high risk," and treatment should be targeted to the highest tolerable statin dose or the achievement of an LDL <70. In addition to counseling about healthy lifestyle and risk factor modification, treatment guidelines aligned with stage A should be applied: treatment of diabetes and hypertension, encouraging smoking cessation, encouraging regular exercise, discouraging excessive alcohol intake and recreational drug use, and controlling the metabolic syndrome. Patient education about symptom recognition and requirement for immediate follow-up for any subtle change in performance or new symptom development should be provided.

Assess Current Functional Status at Initial and Follow-Up Examinations

At each encounter, a thorough history should be obtained, with special focus on dyspnea, cough, chest pain, palpitations, edema, orthopnea, orthostatic symptoms, and syncope. Attention should be paid to symptoms and minor, subtle longitudinal changes in exercise and performance status.

For patients previously exposed to therapeutic radiation, there is an increased risk of premature cerebro-arterial vascular disease manifested as transient ischemic attacks and stroke; patients should be specifically asked about transient neurologic symptoms, such as weakness, speech problems, or visual changes [41].

Assess Cardiac Structure

We propose that all at-risk survivors should have a baseline ECG, two-dimensional transthoracic echocardiogram, and NTproBNP level measured at initial examination. Coupled with a thorough history and physical examination, screening for the major structural manifestations of cardiac toxicity is accomplished. It is recommended that echocardiographic-derived LV systolic function be quantified and not "eyeballed" and that contrast be used when the endocardial borders are not well defined. We propose the use of NTproBNP for its negative predictive value. With no abnormal results on these three tests, the patient is at stage A.

Each stage A patient can be subclassified as low or high risk, according to Table 11.3. For the low-risk stage A patient, in the absence of new symptoms or a change in performance status, reevaluation can be scheduled approximately every 2 years. At each visit, in addition to a detailed history and thorough physical examination, measurement of a NTproBNP level may be helpful as a follow-up screening tool, given its negative predictive value. This blood test is easier to perform, has less dependence on technician skill, does not require insurance pre-authorization, and is less expensive than any imaging modality. No regular cardiac imaging is recommended in the absence of a change in performance status, development of new cardiac symptoms, or new abnormal examination findings, and normal NTproBNP. We currently have been using a Vscan (GE™) handheld cardiac ultrasound to confirm the absence of global left ventricular dysfunction during follow-up visits. This adds 1–2 min to the office visit, does not require precertification by insurance or appointment scheduling with the echocardiographic lab, and has no economic impact to the patient. When normal, we have also avoided measurement of NTproBNP and serial echocardiograms.

For any low-risk stage A survivor who has borderline normal findings on ECG (minor ST-T wave changes, nonspecific intraventricular conduction delay, or arrhythmias) or who has borderline normal echocardiogram findings (LVEF at lower limit of normal for the laboratory or mild diastolic dysfunction), we treat cardiovascular comorbidity and then reevaluate with a follow-up ECG and echo-cardiogram at 1 year. If the results have normalized, the patient remains stage A and can be managed according to the aforementioned outline. If these borderline abnormalities persist, the patient has progressed to stage B and is managed accordingly.

High-risk stage A and stage B patients should be followed yearly, and we encourage a baseline evaluation by a cardiologist knowledgeable in the late effects of cancer treatment for these patients. At follow-up, any change in performance, symptoms, examination findings, or elevation of the NTproBNP level should result in further evaluation with a formal transthoracic echocardiogram. In the absence of any change in status or biomarker level, echocardiograms can be repeated at 5-year intervals or at the discretion of the treating practitioner.

The patients who have received chest radiation less than 30 Gy without chemotherapy are managed as low-risk stage A patients with the addition of treating lipids to secondary prevention targets (low-density lipoprotein less than 70 mg/dl, high-density lipoprotein more than 45 mg/dl). These patients can be evaluated every 2 years. Special emphasis regarding symptoms related to CAD and carotid disease, as well as diligence in looking for subtle changes in exercise activity and endurance, should be part of their routine evaluation. Those who received 30 Gy or more of therapeutic radiation should be considered high-risk stage A and reevaluated yearly. In the absence of any change in status or evidence of vascular disease on physical examination, there is no current recommendation for stress testing or coronary artery calcium scoring. Any subtle change in overall status or any hint of exertion-related symptoms, regardless of radiation dose, should trigger stress testing.

Because there is a documented increased risk of atherosclerotic risk factors, vascular disease, and arterial events in patients treated with platinum-based chemotherapy, aggressive management of cardiac risk factors is recommended along with regular reinforcement of weight control, smoking cessation, lipid control, and temperance with alcohol.

Special Caveats

With the development of hypertension, preferred treatment should be with angiotensin-converting enzyme inhibitors/angiotensin receptor blockers and β-blockers to take advantage of their potential beneficial effects on cardiac remodeling.

For cancer survivors who have been exposed to potentially cardiac toxic chemotherapy or chest radiation, cardiac decompensation is a concern during pregnancy. The hemodynamic stress is due to an increase in blood volume approaching 50 % that begins soon after gestation and peaks at 26–30 weeks. However, limited analysis shows that risk is low [42]. Because cardiac dysfunction may first become apparent during pregnancy, we encourage management input from a cardiologist before, during, and after pregnancy. Increases in cardiac output and heart rate begin early, and evaluation in the first trimester is helpful in predicting the subsequent course. Because the increase in maternal blood volume peaks at 26–30 weeks of pregnancy, we routinely reassess these patients early in the third trimester and communicate directly with their obstetrician for labor, delivery, and postpartum management.

Any low-risk stage A survivor who has a cancer recurrence and/or further malignancy requiring additional chemotherapy or radiotherapy should subsequently be considered and managed as high-risk stage A, with consideration for a cardiology consultation to help guide treatment decisions prior to, during, and after treatment.

Survivors of allogeneic stem cell transplantation are at risk for the late development of accelerated atherosclerosis and the metabolic syndrome [43], and they should be followed up according to the high-risk stage A pathway.

Carotid artery stenosis also is a recognized radiation treatment complication with an increased late incidence of transient ischemia and stroke [44, 45]. Carotid bruits may be audible on physical examination. A baseline carotid duplex study can be obtained 5 years after treatment completion.

All patients should also be given a treatment summary and survivorship care plan that outlines their future cardiac follow-up in addition to the remainder of their survivorship care. Ideally this care plan is updated at appropriate intervals should a change in status occur. This care plan should include information on healthy lifestyle and signs/symptoms that should be brought to a practitioner's attention.

We have reviewed some of the common cardiac conditions and cardiac risk in cancer survivors and provided a practical framework for addressing these issues clinically. The following clinical vignettes explore common patient presentations and the "big" issues that may occur in the longitudinal outpatient care of adult cancer survivors. This information will be helpful to cardiologists, cardio-oncologists, oncologists, as well as primary care specialists in nursing and medicine who care for this population. Each case will address presentation, evaluation, treatment, and anticipatory guidance for survivors and incorporate known clinical guidelines when available.

Cases

Case 1 A 28-year-old male diagnosed with nodular sclerosing Hodgkin lymphoma (NSHL) at age 10 years presents to your office. He received six cycles of ABVD chemotherapy without CV side effects and remains in complete remission. His last "EF" was 33 % at treatment completion. He remains asymptomatic and is physically active. He jogs more than 2 miles a week. His performance status is 0. On physical examination, his vital signs include a blood pressure of 110/74 mmHg and heart rate 66 beats per minute. His body mass index is 21.3 kg/m^2. His cardiovascular exam is unremarkable. Electrocardiogram revealed normal sinus rhythm and normal axis.

Hodgkin lymphoma accounts for 10 % of all lymphomas and 0.6 % of all cancers diagnosed annually worldwide. Prognosis and treatment are largely dependent on staging of the lymphoma. Treatment protocols consist of a combination of chemotherapy and/or radiation therapy. As more patients are being cured of lymphoma with advancements in treatment options, 5-year survival has improved. As a result, treatment-related toxicities primarily contribute to late-term morbidities and mortality including secondary malignancies, cardiac toxicity, or radiation-induced hypothyroidism.

What Are His Cardiovascular Risks?

Cardiovascular toxicity is the most common nonmalignant cause of mortality in survivors of cancer treatment with a hazard ratio (HR) of 10.9 (95 % CI 4.5–26.0) for the development of heart failure compared to siblings [5]. ABVD is a standard chemotherapy regimen for Hodgkin's lymphoma and consists of doxorubicin, bleomycin, vinblastine, and dacarbazine. Bleomyocin can cause pulmonary toxicity that can be a noncardiac cause of dyspnea. Anthracycline-based chemotherapy can cause left ventricular dysfunction (cardiomyopathy). Based on his anthracycline dose, most would place him in a high-risk category (see Table 11.3). Luckily this patient did not receive radiation therapy, but this is an important point to confirm with Hodgkin's lymphoma survivors as treatment regimens vary based on stage of disease/response to initial treatment and protocol/treatment era.

What Instructions Would You Provide?

The patient should receive information and counseling on treatment side effects. Surveillance should primarily focus on preventative health, i.e., primary prevention. Thus, patients should be counseled on routine health habits: diet, achieving/maintaining an "ideal" weight, exercise, and avoidance of tobacco. He may continue to perform activity as tolerated but should be monitored closely for long-term toxicities of chemotherapy as described above. We generally promote regular aerobic "cardio" exercise and discourage isometric exercise (beyond simple muscle toning) because of the effects of isometric exercise on raising systolic blood pressure and increasing myocardial stress.

What Tests Would You Send?

There is limited information on routine testing with cardiac biomarkers and cardiac imaging for screening purposes to detect cardiac injury. Initial assessment should include a complete blood count, basic metabolic panel, and lipid screen. Baseline electrocardiogram and echocardiogram are recommended. Currently, measurement of NTproBNP and troponin is optional and left to the discretion and bias of the medical professional.

Follow-Up

The patient should receive routine follow-up with a primary care physician and preferably someone who is familiar with survivorship care. Screening frequency has not been well established in low-risk patients who remain asymptomatic. Therefore, further testing is not advised in this patient population other than annual visits, but the patient having ongoing communication with a practitioner who is familiar with cancer survivors will allow for additional testing as clinically indicated. There are expert and consensus guidelines for cardiac follow-up in subgroups of patients who develop stage B/C/D disease, and these patients should be referred to a cardiologist for disease-specific management.

For all cancer survivors, *life-long* annual check for blood pressure, glucose, and fasting lipid panel with an emphasis on cardiovascular disease prevention should be performed.

What if He Was a Woman and Asked You About Getting Pregnant?

In the absence of any current CV issues—and assuming she has the ability to get pregnant—we generally reevaluate patients with knowledge of gestation and then late in second trimester, at the time of peak increase in blood volume, which is consistent with the Children's Oncology Group Long-Term Follow-Up guidelines. We stress communication and joint management with a high-risk obstetrician about fluid management at delivery and postpartum to avoid over-hydration.

Case 2 Same patient as Case 1 who had additional mantle radiation in addition to anthracycline-based chemotherapy.

With the Exposure to Therapeutic Radiation: How Would You Modify the Answers to the Above Questions?

Mantle radiation increases the risk not only for myocardial disease but late conduction, valvular, pericardial, and vascular disease related to the exposed field. For mantle radiation, the vascular risk is CAD with a relative risk of myocardial infarction or sudden death reported at 6.7 % in a cohort of Hodgkin's survivors at a mean of 11 years post-radiation completion [46].

For all possible cardiac toxicity, Mulrooney et al. reported an increased risk of heart failure with a HR of 5.9 (95 % CI 3.4–9.6), myocardial infarction HR of 5.0 (95 % CI 2.3–10.4), pericardial disease HR of 6.3 (95 % CI 3.3–11.9), and valvular disease HR of 4.8 (95 % CI 3.0–7.6). The risk of cardiac toxicity is increased with higher doses of radiation administered. Additionally, Mulrooney also demonstrated that radiation therapy administered with anthracycline-based chemotherapy results in a higher incidence of congestive heart failure and valvular disease [47].

There is an agreement that the risk of CAD is increased post therapeutic radiation exposure and that the risk, like that of anthracycline chemotherapy for cardiomyopathy, is related to cumulative dosing and increased with associated traditional cardiac risk factors. All published studies suffer because they are predominantly retrospective, small, from a single center, mix a variety of radiation treatment techniques, and describe/compare a spectrum of screening techniques. To date, we still believe that testing for silent ischemia should be based on risk factors and clinical presentation—with individual decision making based on these clinical findings.

The most appropriate modality for CAD screening is still uncertain [48, 49].

Although NCCN recommends a stress test/echocardiogram 10 years after radiation treatment completion, we still rely on clinical judgment for decision making. In addition, testing may be performed earlier with screening intervals depending on baseline screening results, presence of symptoms, cardiovascular risk factors, and their modification coupled with the amount and historical period of mediastinal radiation. Although there are several limitations to cardiac computed tomography angiography (CTA) including radiation dose, contrast administration, and less reliability to evaluate smaller vessels, small studies suggest that CTA with calcium scoring as an alternative to stress testing for the evaluation for coronary artery disease in patients previously treated with chest radiation [49].

For this patient, he should have testing for any symptom that sounds like CAD according to the "best test" (expertise and availability) at his local institution—either nuclear stress, coronary CTA, stress echo, or stress MRI.

If the radiotherapy field includes the head and neck, the carotid arteries and thyroid are at risk for late toxicity, and this has cardiovascular implications. In this population, we recommend obtaining a baseline carotid duplex study early in follow-up encounters. Thyroid function should be checked annually as thyroid dysfunction may occur 1–10 years from initial treatment, and thyroid cancer surveillance should be considered by physical exam or formal ultrasound depending on practitioner discretion.

For this patient, asymptomatic carotid disease might also be a consideration based on prior treatment and the current presence of carotid bruits.

We would also recommend aggressive lipid management to secondary prevention targets. For females at risk, who are in their childbearing years and capable of becoming pregnant, we like to wait until after family completion to initiate statin therapy.

After radiation therapy, the presence of one isolated cardiac toxicity is unusual, i.e., isolated conduction disease, pericardial disease, myocardial disease, coronary disease, or valvular disease generally do not occur alone but usually in some combination; thus, the presence of aortic valve disease and conduction disease (LBBB) is not surprising and is a common occurrence.

We continue to offer him yearly follow-up.

Case 3 The same male with NSHL returns for follow-up 10 years after initial evaluation. He is totally without functional impairment and has no exertional symptoms.

Exam now shows bilateral carotid bruit, paradoxical splitting of the second heart sound and a 2/6 SEM along the LSB followed by a 1/4 decrescendo diastolic murmur.

ECG shows sinus rhythm and new left bundle branch block (LBBB).

The presumed diagnosis is aortic stenosis and insufficiency and possible associated carotid disease.

He needs a transthoracic echocardiogram to quantitate the degree of aortic valve disease and to reassess his left ventricular function as well as a carotid duplex study.

Studies were completed: There was non-obstructive atherosclerotic disease bilaterally in the carotid arteries and mild-moderate aortic stenosis with aortic valve area of 1.5 cm² (mean/peak gradient 10/28 mmHg).

Management includes risk factor reduction with at least yearly follow-up. He should be educated about "red flag" symptoms suggesting progression of aortic valve and conduction disease.

Case 4 A 35-year-old female was diagnosed with non-Hodgkin's mediastinal lymphoma at age 30 years and treated with R-CHOP and mantle radiation. At her baseline, and most recent past evaluation by you, she was asymptomatic with no cardiac abnormality.

She now returns at her "5-year anniversary" at age 35 years. She tells you that she has reduced jogging distance and duration because of subtle fatigue and maybe some associated shortness of breath.

Vital signs and examination are virtually unchanged and unremarkable.

What is the cause of her symptoms? The differential includes late effects from anthracycline chemotherapy (cardiomyopathy) versus CAD and ischemia related to XRT or chronotropic incompetence with failure to achieve an increased cardiac output with exercise due to her prior treatment. In any event, she now has stage C disease.

Studies should include a repeat ECG, CAD investigation, PFTs, and an echocardiogram to look at valvular disease, pericardium, and LV function. Treatment depends on the results of these investigations and ranges from medical management of left ventricular dysfunction to treatment of ischemia with either medical therapy or revascularization.

ECG showed sinus rhythm with diffuse nonspecific T wave flattening. Voltage was normal. PFTs were normal. A stress echocardiogram showed a reduction in LVEF from prior 60 % to current 40 % at rest with normal increment of LVEF with exercise and no wall motion abnormality.

The testing suggests LV systolic dysfunction as a working diagnosis. Treatment includes standard pharmacologic measures for heart failure with continued aggressive risk factor management and frequent follow-up.

Case 5 A 28-year-old male was diagnosed with CLL. He was treated with multi-agent chemotherapy (including doxorubicin 240 mg/m², cyclophosphamide,

ARA-C, and etoposide) followed by 10/10 sibling-matched allogeneic stem cell transplant.

He has all of the risks described in Case 1 with additional risk conferred by stem cell transplant. Excluding graft-versus-host disease (GVHD), in general, those patients post allotransplant show an increased incidence of metabolic syndrome, diabetes, and hypertension. We tend to be more aggressive in screening and management of these risks.

He returns after 2 years.

He has no symptoms but on exam his blood pressure is 160/96 and his BMI is 30.

He has hypertension. It is recognized that there is a marked increase in cardiovascular risk when modifiable cardiac risk factors are also present. Armstrong reported that the coexistence of exposure and hypertension increased the relative risk of heart failure among survivors with anthracycline exposure with hypertension which was 88.5 (95 % CI 45.2–161.8) and is more than a simple effect [50].

Armenian et al. showed the additive and somewhat proportional effect of traditional cardiac risk factors in patients with prior hematopoietic stem cell transplant: from 4.7 % with no factors to 7.0 % and 11.2 % with one factor and >1 factor, respectively [51].

We would start therapy with either an ACE inhibitor/ARB or beta blocker to control blood pressure and to take advantage of any potential cardioprotective effect of these drugs. We would redouble our efforts to aggressively manage his lipids and provide more frequent follow-up.

Case 6 A 55-year-old female presents for cardiovascular risk evaluation. She was diagnosed with left hormone receptor-positive breast cancer at 48 years of age. She was treated with a lumpectomy and 5000 cGy radiation and 5 years of tamoxifen. She is now on an aromatase inhibitor. She has no functional limitation, vital signs are normal, and her cardiac examination is unremarkable.

Breast cancer is the most common cancer in women worldwide, with more than one million new diagnoses each year. The overall 5-year survival rate is approximately 90 %. Radiation for early-stage breast cancer can reduce the rates of local recurrence and of death from breast cancer and has led to a large proportion of survivors who have received radiation as a part of their treatment.

Today, there are an estimated 2.8 million survivors of breast cancer who have an increased risk of cardiovascular disease and that has become the leading cause of death in this group of survivors [52, 53]. As such, prevention and management of cardiac risk has become an important focal point.

What Are Her Cardiovascular Risks?

For the majority of women who survive breast cancer, late cardiac toxicity resulting from their cancer therapies may have a greater impact on their overall survival than recurrent breast cancer.

Treatment-Related Factors: Medical Therapy

She did not receive anthracycline-based chemotherapy. As a hormone receptor-positive breast cancer patient, she received adjuvant tamoxifen and/or an aromatase inhibitor. Tamoxifen is a nonsteroidal triphenylethylene derivative that binds to the estrogen receptor. It has both estrogenic and antiestrogenic actions, depending on the target tissue. It is strongly antiestrogenic on mammary epithelium hence its use in both the prevention and treatment of breast cancer. Clinical trials assessing the effects of tamoxifen on breast cancer recurrence have not demonstrated an increased cardiovascular risk and, in fact, some reduction in cardiovascular risk due to favorable lipid-lowering effects, i.e., lower LDL and raised HDL [54].

Aromatase inhibitors (AIs) are also commonly used as adjuvant therapy in postmenopausal women with hormone receptor-positive early breast cancer. AIs stop the production of estrogen, and long-term safety data show that AIs may have a more favorable overall safety profile compared with tamoxifen (less hot flushes, endometrial cancer, and fewer cardiovascular events including thromboembolism). AIs lack any lipid-lowering effect [55], and when women are transitioned from tamoxifen to an AI, a lipid panel should be measured after therapy initiation.

Overall, cardiovascular risk appears low with either of these types of hormonal therapy.

Radiation Therapy

As previously noted, radiation-related heart disease may affect any cardiac structure resulting in coronary artery disease, myocardial dysfunction, pericarditis, conduction disease, and valvular heart disease. Although there has been controversy, it is now generally accepted that left-sided radiation has significant risk compared to right-sided radiation, and the risk is increased with increasing dosing. With information about the radiation field (i.e., left vs. right breast, breast only, or breast plus internal mammary chain), it may be possible to estimate dose of radiation to the heart to assist in risk stratification. Dose-volume histograms for the whole heart or specific cardiac structures can be useful in understanding the risk of ischemic heart disease and cardiac events—the latter may be obtained for more recent radiation exposure but do not exist for treatment dating back to at least the last decade.

Rates of major coronary events, like other radiation-related effects of cancer therapy, increase linearly with the mean dose to the heart. There is no apparent threshold at which this begins, i.e., there should be considered no safe dose of radiation and even low-dose radiation can lead to increased risk. Moreover, this increased dose-dependent risk occurs independent of tumor type but may be magnified with comorbid CV risk factors.

Patient-Level Factors

Evaluation of pre-existing medical conditions, as in the general population, are essential to estimate overall late CV risk and may drive screening decisions; more comorbidity equals more risk and a lower threshold for testing.

What Tests Would You Order?

In this women coming for initial assessment, a baseline ECG and echocardiogram may be obtained as well as a baseline NTproBNP level. Because risk factor reduction is a primary concern, measurement of fasting lipids is essential.

What Instructions Do You Give?

Women should be counseled as to their excess risk of cardiovascular disease due to radiation. She is 55 years old, has no other cardiovascular risk factors, and was exposed to 5000 cGy XRT to her left chest. Depending on the radiation techniques used to shield her heart, there is a small absolute risk of late cardiac toxicity that is no more than 1–2 % over the next 20+ years.

We would reinforce a healthy lifestyle and be aggressive in managing her lipids.

Follow-Up

Risk factor management may be managed by a primary care doctor or specialized survivorship clinic for routine survivorship care. Periodic cardiology collaboration may be valuable.

Case 7 A 55-year-old female presents for cardiovascular risk evaluation. She was diagnosed with left hormone receptor-positive, HER2/neu-positive breast cancer at 45 years of age. She was treated with lumpectomy followed by chemotherapy that included doxorubicin [240 mg/m2] and cyclophosphamide (AC) × 4, trastuzumab/ Taxol (TH) × 4, a year of trastuzumab, 5 years of tamoxifen and is now on an aromatase inhibitor. She had serial echocardiograms prior to and after anthracycline treatment and every 3 months during trastuzumab treatment. There was no change in LV systolic function—LVEF remained constant through the end of treatment. She remains in complete remission 9 years post treatment completion.

How Is She Different from Case 6?

She was exposed to potentially cardiac toxic chemotherapy. To date, the incidence of late-appearing cardiomyopathy from trastuzumab alone is close to zero. Therefore, her late cardiac toxicity risk is from anthracycline exposure and the risk is cardiomyopathy. The classic relationship for the risk of developing cardiac toxicity was described by Von Hoff who showed an association with the total cumulative dose of anthracycline. We have subsequently learned that the real-world risk, although generally proportional to the total accumulated dose, actually can occur in a less linear fashion and may be more time dependent. It is increasingly recognized that asymptomatic abnormalities in noninvasive studies can be found in greater frequency and at a lower cumulative anthracycline dose than previously reported. Although less studied than doxorubicin, the incidence of cardiac toxicity with daunorubicin, idarubicin, mitoxantrone, and epirubicin (a semisynthetic derivative) is similar with equivalent dosing regimens.

What Instructions Would You Give Her?

Adopt a healthy lifestyle—no smoking, maintain weight, exercise, and treat modifiable risk factors. She should avoid extreme stressors, e.g., running a marathon, especially if not adequately trained.

We would provide education about recognition and reporting of subtle symptoms that would suggest LV dysfunction including any change in functional capacity or new symptoms of breathlessness, palpitation, or chest pain.

In view of her risk, she should be evaluated yearly by a health-care professional knowledgeable about the late cardiac toxicity associated with anthracycline exposure.

Case 8 Same woman as in Case 7 except that during active treatment, she had asymptomatic drop in LVEF to 42 % with 6-month post treatment completion LVEF returned to pretreatment baseline EF of 58 %.

What Are Her Cardiovascular Risks?

With demonstrable LV systolic dysfunction during treatment, she has a life-long risk for LV dysfunction, even if the EF normalizes after treatment.

If she received heart failure medication, this should be continued indefinitely as there is a documented risk of relapse after stopping these medications.

What Testing Should She Have at This Time?

Since she is going to continue a heart failure regimen, there is little need for serial testing of LV function or in measuring or trending serial biomarkers.

If her EF is ≤35 %, there should be consideration for prophylactic ICD.

What Instructions Would You Give Her?

In addition to what is listed in Case 7, prompt recognition of any change in status should be emphasized.

She should not stop or let any intervening doctor stop heart failure medication.

What Is Her Follow-Up Plan?

In the absence of a change in status, yearly follow-up is recommended.

Case 9   Same woman as in Case 8. Now age 58 years on cardiac medications (ACE inhibitor and beta blocker) with new diagnosis of AML with hemoglobin of 6.9 g. Only complaint is fatigue. No exertional chest pain or shortness of breath. No fluid retention or subjective awareness of dysrhythmia.

What Are Her Cardiovascular Risks?

The drop in hemoglobin is a relative stress test, and the absence or presence of cardiac decompensation may help predict the future risk of treatment-related cardiac toxicity. Because of her prior exposure to 240 mg/m^2 of doxorubicin and her prior history of anthracycline-induced cardiac dysfunction, induction therapy should not include an anthracycline. It is well established that a rechallenge with anthracyclines in a patient with anthracycline-induced cardiac toxicity has a high risk.

During induction, consolidation, and transplant (if that is the course), there are frequent and sometimes dramatic fluctuations in fluid status, renal and hepatic function, and blood pressure. Associated sepsis may impact continuous dosing of her heart failure medications. Any decision to hold any of these drugs during these "crises" should be routinely reassessed as clinical status improves with re-institution of baseline medications to avoid long-term interruption of these therapies.

Because fluid resuscitation is common along with hydration for chemotherapy, over-hydration is a common occurrence, and this can be easily assessed and avoided with serial monitoring of weight.

What Are the Gaps in Survivorship Care in 2017?

There are three major gaps that impact the care of cancer survivors exposed to potentially cardiac toxic cancer treatment. In a broad sense, they are related to knowledge and personnel and process:

1. The lack of validation of markers, biomarkers and/or imaging, that reliably predict late cardiac toxicity and the development of cardioprotective strategies in this high-risk population.
2. Currently there is a lack of care providers knowledgeable about the late cardiac effects of cancer treatment to deal effectively with this exponentially growing population.
3. Lack of universal adoption of treatment summaries to help guide future risk assessment; this assumes some degree of patient education about these risks at treatment completion.

Directions for Future Research

With current understanding of the complexity of care for long-term cancer survivors, a model of comprehensive, multi-specialty care teams and cardio-oncology has emerged [56]. Future research should be focused on defining a care delivery model that is consistent with the projected healthcare work force and scalable to the rapidly increasing survivor population. In the future, we will need to make more use of telemedicine and allied health personnel.

For long-term survivors of cancer, the factors affecting the rate of progression from stage A to symptomatic, structural cardiovascular disease are still incompletely defined. Global risk models specific to community-based populations predicting the risk of heart failure have been validated [57]. There is a need for refinement to develop a comparable and easily useable tool specific for late chemotherapy cardiac toxicity.

With wide individual variation in the development of late cardiac toxicity, a genetic predisposition seems like a likely factor; although there has been preliminary identification of target genes and mutations, this important link is just in its infancy and lags behind the volume of research related to biomarkers and imaging. The establishment of an international group to organize the banking of blood samples coupled with long-term clinical follow-up to accelerate the process and knowledge is critical.

Future screening recommendations require an accurate quantification of the risk of sudden death as the first manifestation of radiation-induced CAD in the survivor population and whether revascularization intervention in asymptomatic patients has true benefit. Existing bias has emerged from small series of patients, generally treated with premodern radiotherapy techniques and before the contemporary treatment of coronary risk factors. Understanding the risk also would help to define the role of nontraditional testing in this population.

Finally, the predictive value of biomarkers, such as the monitoring of troponins/BNP during high-dose chemotherapy, and the benefit of early intervention have not been consistent. A large-scale study to define the true benefit of single or multiple biomarkers and early intervention also is needed.

Many of the current knowledge gaps and questions posed could be resolved by adequately addressing both early and late cardiac toxicity routinely in cancer clinical trials [58].

We suggest that clinicians maintain a heightened awareness of the prevalence and need for surveillance and early treatment for all long-term cancer survivors who were exposed to potentially cardiac toxic therapy. We reiterate that no evidence-based guidelines currently exist but recognize that there is a real risk for late cardiac toxicity. We provide these recommendations for long-term follow-up and care until there is ample research and data to create evidence-based guidelines.

References

1. Parry C, Kent EE, Mariotto AB, et al. Cancer survivors: a booming population. Cancer Epidemiol Biomarkers Prev. 2011;20:1996–2005.
2. American Cancer Society. Cancer treatment and survivorship facts & figures 2014–2015. Atlanta: American Cancer Society; 2014.
3. Smith MA, Altekruse SF, Adamson PC, et al. Declining childhood and adolescent cancer mortality. Cancer. 2014;120:2497–506.
4. Oeffinger KC, Mertens AC, Sklar CA, et al. Chronic health conditions in adult survivors of childhood cancer. N Eng J Med. 2006;355:1572–82.
5. Armstrong GT, Kawashima T, Leisenring W, et al. Aging and risk of severe life threatening, and fatal events in the Childhood Cancer Survivor Study. J Clin Oncol. 2014;32:1218–27.
6. Lipshultz SE, Adams J, Colan SD, et al. Long-term cardiovascular toxicity in children, adolescents, and young adults who receive cancer therapy: pathophysiology, course, monitoring, management, prevention and research directions. A scientific statement from the American Heart Association. Circulation. 2013;128:1927–95.
7. Eschenhagen T, Force T, Ewer MS, et al. Cardiovascular side effects of cancer therapies: a position statement from the Heart Failure Association of the European Society of Cardiology. Eur J Heart Fail. 2011;1:1–10.
8. Bovelli D, Plataniokis G, Roila F. Cardiotoxicity of chemotherapeutic agents and radiotherapy-related heart disease. ESMO clinical practice guidelines. Ann Oncol. 2010;21 Suppl 5:277–82.
9. Galper SL, Yu JB, Mauch PM, et al. Clinically significant cardiac disease in patients with Hodgkin lymphoma treated with mediastinal irradiation. Blood. 2011;111:412–8.

10. Hull MC, Morris CG, Pepine CJ, et al. Valvular dysfunction and carotid, subclavian, and coronary artery disease in survivors of Hodgkin lymphoma treated with radiation therapy. JAMA. 2003;290:2831–7.
11. Ng AK. Review of the cardiac long-term effects of therapy for Hodgkin lymphoma. Br J Haematol. 2011;154:23–31.
12. Lipshultz SE, Lipsitz SR, Sallan SE, et al. Chronic progressive cardiac dysfunction years after doxorubicin therapy for childhood acute lymphoblastic leukemia. J Clin Oncol. 2005;23:2629–36.
13. Sorensen K, Levitt GA, Bull C, et al. Late anthracycline cardiotoxicity after childhood cancer: a prospective longitudinal study. Cancer. 2003;97:1991–8.
14. Carver JR, Shapiro CL, Ng A, et al. ASCO Cancer Survivorship Expert Panel. American Society of Clinical Oncology clinical evidence review on the emerging care of adult cancer survivors: cardiac and pulmonary late effects. J Clin Oncol. 2007;25:3991–4009.
15. Steingart RM, Yadav N, Manrique C, et al. Cancer survivorship: Cardiotoxic therapy in the adult cancer patient; Cardiac outcomes with recommendations for patient management. Semin Oncol. 2013;40:690–708.
16. Moore RA, Adel N, Riedel E, et al. High incidence of thromboembolic events in patients treated with cisplatin-based chemotherapy: a large retrospective analysis. J Clin Oncol. 2011;29:3466–73.
17. Armenian SH, Ding Y, Mills G, et al. Genetic susceptibility to anthracycline-related congestive heart failure in survivors of haematopoietic cell transplantation. Br J Haematol. 2013;163:205–13.
18. Lipshultz SE, Lipsitz SR, Kutok JL, et al. Impact of hemochromatosis gene mutations on cardiac status in doxorubicin-treated survivors of childhood high-risk leukemia. Cancer. 2013;119:3555–62.
19. Aminkeng F, Bhavsar AP, Visscher H, et al. A coding variant in RARG confers susceptibility to anthracycline-induced cardiotoxicity in childhood cancer. Nat Genetics. 2015;47:1079–84.
20. Jessup M, Abraham WT, Casey DE, et al. 2009 focused update: ACC/AHA guidelines for the diagnosis and management of heart failure in adults: a report of the American College of Cardiology Foundation/American Heart Association Task Force on Practice Guidelines. J Am Col Cardiol. 2009;53:1343–82.
21. Wang TJ, Evans JC, Benjamin EJ, et al. Natural history of asymptomatic left ventricular systolic dysfunction in the community. Circulation. 2003;108:977–82.
22. The SOLVD Investigators. Effect of enalapril on mortality and the development of heart failure in asymptomatic patients with reduced left ventricular ejection fractions. N Eng J Med. 1992;327:685–91.
23. Rosenthal D, Chrisant MR, Edens E, et al. International Society for Heart and Lung Transplantation: practice guidelines for management of heart failure in children. J Heart Lung Transplan. 2004;23:1313–33.
24. Amigioni M, Giannattosio C, Frashini D, et al. Low anthracyclines doses-induced cardiotoxicity in acute lymphoblastic leukemia long-term female survivors. Ped Blood Cancer. 2010;55:1343–7.
25. Vandecruys E, Mondelaers V, De Wolf D, et al. Late cardiotoxicity after low dose of anthracycline therapy for acute lymphoblastic leukemia in childhood. J Cancer Surviv. 2012;6:95–101.
26. Smith LA, Cpornelius VR, Plummer CS, et al. Cardiotoxicity of anthracycline agents for the treatment of cancer: systemic review and meta-analysis of randomized cancer trials. BMC Cancer. 2010;10:337.
27. Lipshultz SE, Adams MJ. Cardiotoxicity after childhood cancer: beginning with an end in mind. J Clin Oncol. 2010;28:1276–80.
28. Cardinale D, Sandri MT. Role of biomarkers in chemotherapy-induced cardiotoxicity. Prog Cardiovasc Dis. 2010;53:121–9.

29. Ky B, Carver JR. Biomarker approach to the detection and cardioprotective strategies during anthracycline chemotherapy. Heart Fail Clin. 2011;7:323–31.
30. Thygesen K, Mair J, Mueller C, et al. Recommendations for the use of natriuretic proteins in acute cardiac care; a position statement from the Study Group on biomarkers in Cardiology of the ESC Working Group on Acute Cardiac Care. Eur Heart J. 2012;33:2001–16.
31. Putt M, Hahn VS, Januzzi JL, et al. Longitudinal changes in multiple biomarkers are associated with cardiotoxicity in breast cancer patients treated with doxorubicin, taxanes and trastuzumab. Clin Chem. 2015;61:1164–72.
32. Plano JC, Galderisi M, Barac A, et al. Expert consensus for multimodality imaging evaluation of adult patients during and after cancer therapy: a report from the American Society of Echocardiography and the European Association of Cardiovascular Imaging. J Am Soc Echocardiogr. 2014;27:911–39.
33. Greenland P, Alpert JS, Beller GA, et al. The 2010 Joint American College of Cardiology Foundation/American Heart Association guidelines for the assessment of cardiovascular risk in asymptomatic adults. J Am Coll Cardiol. 2010;56:50–103.
34. U.S. Preventive Services Task Force. Screening for coronary artery disease: recommendation statement. Ann Int Med. 2004;140:569–72.
35. U.S. Preventive Services Task Force. Using non-traditional risk factors in coronary heart disease risk assessment: recommendation statement. Ann Int Med. 2009;151:474–82.
36. Hewitt M, Weiner SL, Simone JV. Childhood cancer survivorship: Improving care and quality of life. Washington, DC: National Academics Press; 2003.
37. Hewitt M, Greenfield S, Stovall E, editors. From cancer patient to cancer survivor: Lost in transition. Washington, DC: National Academics Press; 2006.
38. Children's Oncology Group. Long-term follow-up guidelines for survivors of childhood and adolescent and young adult cancer. Vesion 4.0, 2014. www.survivorshipguidelines.org.
39. Armenian SH, Hudson MM, Mulder RL, et al. Recommendations for cardiomyopathy surveillance for survivors of childhood cancer: a report from the International Late Effects of Childhood Cancer Guideline Harmonization Group. Lancet Oncol. 2015;16:e123–36.
40. deHaas EC, Oosting SF, Lefrandt JD, et al. The metabolic syndrome in cancer survivors. Lancet Oncol. 2010;11:193–203.
41. Bowers DC, Liu Y, Leisenting W, et al. Late-occurring stroke among long-term survivors of chronic leukemia and brain tumors: a report from the Childhood Cancer Survivor Study. J Clin Oncol. 2006;24:5277–80.
42. Edgar AB, Wallace HB. Pregnancy in women who had childhood cancer. Eur J Cancer. 2007;43:1890–4.
43. Baker KS, Armenian S, Bhatia S. Long-term consequences of hematopoietic stem-cell transplantation: current state of the science. Bio Blood Marrow Transplant. 2010;1(Suppl):S90–6.
44. Dorresteijn LD, Marres HA, Bartelink H, et al. Radiotherapy of the neck as a risk factor for stroke. Ned Tijdschr Geneeskd. 2005;149:1249–53.
45. Plummer C, Henderson RD, O'Sullivan SJ. Ischemic stroke and transient ischemic attack after head and neck radiotherapy: a review. Stroke. 2011;42:2410–8.
46. Seddon B, Cook A, Gothard L, et al. Detection of defects in myocardial perfusion imaging in patients with early breast cancer treated with radiotherapy. Radiother Oncol. 2002;64:53–63.
47. Mulrooney DA, Yeazel MW, Kawashima T, et al. Cardiac outcomes in a cohort of adult survivors of childhood and adolescent cancer: retrospective analysis of the Childhood Cancer Survivor Study cohort. BMJ. 2009;339:b4606.
48. Heidenreich PA, Schnittger I, Strauss HW, et al. Screening for coronary artery disease after mediastinal irradiation for Hodgkin's disease. J Clin Oncol. 2007;25:43–9.
49. Kupeli S, Hazirolan T, Varnan A, et al. Evaluation of coronary artery disease by computed tomography in patients treated for childhood Hodgkin's lymphoma. J Clin Oncol. 2010;28:1025–30.
50. Armstrong GT, Oeffinger KC, Chen C, et al. Modifiable risk factors and major cardiac events among adult survivors of childhood cancer. J Clin Oncol. 2013;31:3673–80.

51. Armenian SH, Sun CL, Vase T, et al. Cardiovascular risk factors in hematopoietic stem cell transplantation survivors: role in development of subsequent cardiovascular disease. Blood. 2012;120:4505–12.
52. Patnaik JL, Byers T, DiGuiseppi C, et al. The influence of comorbidities on overall survival among older women diagnosed with breast cancer. J Natl Cancer Inst. 2011;103:1101–11.
53. Hooning MJ, Botma A, Aleman BM, et al. Long-term risk of cardiovascular disease in 10-year survivors of breast cancer. J Natl Cancer Inst. 2007;99:365–75.
54. Bruning PF, Bonfrer JM, Hart AA, et al. Tamoxifen, serum lipoproteins and cardiovascular risk. Br J Cancer. 1988;58:487–99.
55. Pritchard KI, Abramson BL. Cardiovascular health and aromatase inhibitors. Drugs. 2006;66:1727–40.
56. Albini A, Pennesi G, Donatelli I, et al. Cardiotoxicity of anticancer drugs: the need for cardio-oncology and cardio-oncological prevention. J Natl Cancer Inst. 2010;102:14–25.
57. Kalogereropoulis A, Psaty BM, Vasan RS, et al. Validation of the Health ABC Heart Failure model for incident heart failure risk prediction: the Cardiovascular Health Study. Circ Heart Fail. 2010;3:495–502.
58. Verma S, Ewer MS. Is cardiotoxicity being adequately assessed in current trials of cytotoxic and targeted agents in breast cancer? Ann Oncol. 2011;22:1011–8.

Chapter 12
Geriatric Cardio-oncology

Anne Blaes and Chetan Shenoy

Introduction

The incidence of cancer increases with age. As cancer therapies improve and the population as a whole increases, there are rising numbers of elderly patients with cancer. More than half of patients newly diagnosed with cancer are age 65 years or older [1]. In January 2012, it was estimated that more than eight million cancer survivors were older than 65 years, comprising 59 % of the prevalent population of cancer survivors. Estimations predict that by 2050, there will be over 19 million cancer survivors over the age of 85 years [2]. To complicate matters, elderly patients have been underrepresented in cancer clinical trials [3]. Patients older than 65 years historically represented only 38 % of enrolled patients on clinical trials [4]. Concern for toxicity, particularly cardiac-related toxicity and treatment-related mortality, has led to lower-intensity regimens in older patients. These factors ultimately have led to relatively few scientific data on how current cancer therapies impact the aging population.

Electronic supplementary material: The online version of this chapter (doi:10.1007/978-3-319-43096-6_12) contains supplementary material, which is available to authorized users.

A. Blaes (✉)
Division of Hematology, Oncology and Transplantation, Department of Medicine,
University of Minnesota, Minneapolis, MN, USA
e-mail: blaes004@umn.edu

C. Shenoy
Division of Cardiology, Department of Medicine, University of Minnesota,
Minneapolis, MN, USA
e-mail: cshenoy@umn.edu

Impact of Aging

Aging cancer patients are particularly vulnerable to cardiotoxicity from cancer treatment because of their baseline risk resulting from their age [5–7]. In general, older patients have a number of factors, including concomitant medical conditions (comorbidities) and physiologic and functional changes that can affect prognosis, treatment, and outcomes of cancer [6–8]. Approximately 80 % of older adults have one comorbid condition, and 50 % have at least two comorbid conditions. This number increases to over 70 % in patients over 80 years of age [9].

For many of these patients, one of their comorbid illnesses is underlying cardiac disease; in men, approximately 20 % between 60 and 79 years of age and 32 % over 80 years of age have coronary artery disease. In women, approximately 10 % between 60 and 79 years of age and 19 % over 80 years of age have coronary artery disease [10]. When cardiovascular disease is defined as coronary artery disease, heart failure, stroke, or hypertension, the prevalence for men is 69 % between 60 and 79 years of age and 85 % over 80 years of age. Similarly, in women, approximately 68 % of women between 60 and 79 years of age and 86 % over 80 years of age have cardiovascular disease [10].

Not surprisingly, cardiovascular risk factors are frequently present in cancer patients: in a hospital-based registry of >19,000 cancer patients, 38 % of patients had hypertension and 11 % had diabetes mellitus [11]. Data from the SEER-Medicare database show that patients with non-Hodgkin lymphoma aged 65 years or older have a high prevalence of cardiovascular risk factors—diabetes in 32 %, hypercholesterolemia in 54 %, and hypertension in 73 % [12]. In a study of 205 patients with non-Hodgkin lymphoma aged 80 years or older, 87 % had at least one comorbidity, and 50 % had cardiovascular disease [13].

The presence of comorbidities can lead to polypharmacy and potential drug interactions with chemotherapy [6, 7, 14, 15]. The presence of comorbidities may also lead to alterations in cancer outcome [8]. Additionally, kidney and liver function decline with age [6]. Ultimately, these factors may lead to modifications in treatment. These factors may also lead to excess cardiac toxicity depending on the clearance of the used drug [16]. Chemotherapy medications can also result in direct cardiac injury [5, 6, 17]. The sequential impact of these factors, illustrated in Fig. 12.1 and previously described by Shenoy et al., can be conceptualized as a "snowball effect," whereby the "snowball" formed of older age and age-related factors is "set into motion" by a cancer diagnosis and then "momentum" is gained as the cancer drugs result in direct injury on tissues or functional status is changed by the cancer [6]. Ultimately, this leads to symptoms and cardiovascular manifestations.

In order to help care for the aging population with cancer, a multidimensional, interdisciplinary diagnostic process focusing on looking at an older person's medical, psychosocial, and functional capacity has been recommended [7]. This coordinated care has been recommended through comprehensive geriatric assessments (CGAs) [18, 19]. A number of recent publications have examined various CGAs.

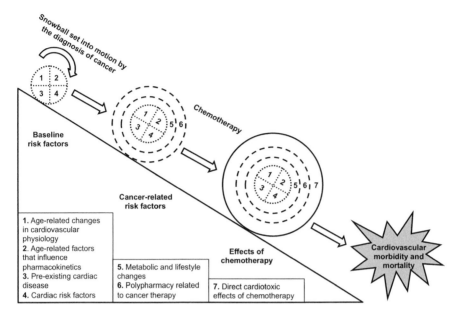

Fig. 12.1 The "snowball effect" leading to cardiovascular complications of breast cancer therapy in older patients. Reproduced with permission from Shenoy et al. [6]

The common themes of the various tools are to provide a comprehensive assessment of the patient looking at functional status, cognitive abilities, emotional conditions, comorbid conditions including cardiovascular disease and heart failure, nutritional status, polypharmacy, as well as the existing social and environmental situation of the patient (Table 12.1).

While there are a number of tools available, the International Society of Geriatric Oncology has provided consensus guidelines that the following domains be evaluated in a geriatric assessment: functional status, comorbidity, cognition, mental health status, fatigue, social status, nutrition, and presence of geriatric syndromes defined as dementia, delirium, failure to thrive, incontinence, osteoporosis, neglect/abuse, falls, constipation, polypharmacy, pressure ulcers, and sarcopenia [19]. Classic oncology tools like the Eastern Cooperative Oncology Group (ECOG) or Karnofsky performance status have been shown to reflect poorly the functional impairment in the geriatric population [20]. Incorporating a geriatric assessment tool into the care of the geriatric cardio-oncology patient is important. The use of CGAs has been shown to improve overall survival, quality of life, and physical function, and to decrease hospitalizations and nursing home placement in the geriatric population [21–24]. CGAs also have the potential to predict several relevant treatment-related complications (post-op complications, toxicity related to systemic treatment) [25]. There are several ongoing clinical trials in oncology looking at the utility of CGAs in improving functional status, quality of life, and outcomes in elderly patients with a variety of cancers (NCT02025062,

Table 12.1 Factors influencing cancer care in the elderly

Functional status
Cognitive abilities
Emotional conditions
Comorbid conditions
Nutritional status
Polypharmacy
Alterations in pharmacokinetics
Social environment
Fatigue
Presence of a geriatric syndrome[a]

[a]Geriatric syndromes are dementia, delirium, failure to thrive, incontinence, osteoporosis, neglect/abuse, falls, constipation, pressure ulcers, and sarcopenia

NCT02000011, NCT01188330, NCT02072733, NCT01829958, NCT02315469). The results of these studies are much anticipated.

In addition to the increasing prevalence of coronary heart disease with age [10], the geriatric cancer population is also more susceptible to cardiac injury from cancer treatment [6]. Many cancer agents have known cardiac toxicities [26]. These can include left ventricular dysfunction (decrease in cardiac contractile function) and heart failure, myocardial ischemia and infarction, hypertension, and arrhythmias such as QT prolongation [6, 26–32]. Less common injuries including myocarditis, pericarditis, and atrial fibrillation also occur. Multiple recent reviews have described in detail the pathophysiology, diagnosis, and management of this cardiotoxicity [26, 27, 29–32]. Data is limited, however, regarding how age impacts these adverse effects of cancer therapy.

One factor contributing to our limited understanding of the effects of age on cardiovascular effects of cancer treatment is the limited experience with geriatric populations in clinical trials [3, 4]. Despite a high incidence of cancer in the elderly, older patients make up only 20 % of those in phase 2 clinical trials and approximately 38 % of overall clinical trials for cancer [33]. While clinical trials remain the main approach for evaluating the cardiac safety and efficacy of cancer treatment, few elderly are actually enrolled in these trials. Until elderly-specific data are available, we are left extrapolating data from studies of all ages to the geriatric population.

Disease Specifics

One of the most commonly used classes of chemotherapeutic drugs known to cause cardiac injury and most specifically heart failure are the anthracyclines (e.g., doxorubicin, epirubicin, and idarubicin) [34, 35]. Anthracyclines are used as part of curative intent therapy most commonly in breast cancer, lymphoma, sarcoma, and leukemia [27, 36]. Doxorubicin cardiac injury, causing type 1 cardiomyopathy, is serious and can be associated with impaired survival. The risk of cardiomyopathy from doxorubicin is proportional to cumulative dose also, in addition to age. The incidence of congestive heart failure is estimated to be 2 % at 200 mg/m^2, 5 % at 400 mg/m^2, 16 % at 500 mg/m^2, and 26 % at 550 mg/m^2 [37–39]. However, those over 65 years old had a twofold increased risk of doxorubicin-related congestive heart failure as compared to those younger than 65 years when adjusting for a history of cardiac disease, ejection fraction, performance status, and gender [39, 40]. The risk of congestive heart failure also appeared to be threefold higher in the elderly receiving 400 mg/m^2 or higher [39, 40].

Breast Cancer

Approximately 50–60 % of patients newly diagnosed with breast cancer are women aged >65 years [41]. In examining 31,748 elderly women with early-stage breast cancer using the Surveillance, Epidemiology, and End Results (SEER)-Medicare database, women who received any chemotherapy were 2.5 times more likely to develop cardiomyopathy than if they received no chemotherapy [42]. When looking specifically at anthracycline chemotherapy, the incidence of cardiotoxicity was 1.55 % for patients not receiving chemotherapy and 4.09 % for patients receiving anthracyclines (odds ratio, 3.51; 95 % confidence interval [CI], 2.63–4.69) in the first year after breast cancer diagnosis. After 5 years of follow-up, the cumulative incidence had increased to 4.97 % in patients not receiving chemotherapy and 10.23 % in patients receiving an anthracycline-containing regimen. In a follow-up study by Pinder et al. of 43,448 women ages 66–80 years with a diagnosis of breast cancer, 38 % of the group who had anthracycline exposure developed congestive heart failure by year 10 compared to 33 % in the non-anthracycline group and 29 % in the no-chemotherapy group [43]. Risk factors for the development of congestive heart failure in this patient population included advancing age, black race, use of trastuzumab, stage of cancer, and a personal history of hypertension, diabetes mellitus, coronary artery disease, peripheral vascular disease, and chronic obstructive pulmonary disease. Similarly, in an evaluation of the SEER-Medicare database looking at elderly women ages of 67 and 94 years (mean 76 years) between 2000 and 2007, the incidence of heart failure or cardiomyopathy 3 years after a breast cancer diagnosis was 20.2 % in those who received anthracyclines without trastuzumab [44].

In approximately a quarter of women with breast cancer, their tumors overexpress the human epidermal growth factor-2 (HER2) oncogene. In this case, trastuzumab is recommended. Trastuzumab is a monoclonal antibody that targets the human epidermal growth factor (HER2 or ErbB2). It is used in both the adjuvant and metastatic settings [45, 46]. Trastuzumab has been associated with type 2 cardiomyopathy, in which contractility loss occurs as opposed to cardiac myocyte death as is seen with the anthracyclines [47]. In the initial trials of trastuzumab in the metastatic setting, the incidence of cardiac dysfunction when trastuzumab was given alone, with paclitaxel, or with an anthracycline was 3–7 %, 13 %, and 27 %, respectively [46]. Subsequent trials in the adjuvant setting suggest the rates of grade 3 or 4 heart failure are 0–3.9 % in trastuzumab-treated patients as compared to 0–1.3 % in those not receiving trastuzumab [45]. In the PHARE trial, the rates were higher in those who received trastuzumab over 12 months versus 6 months (5.7 % vs. 1.9 %, $p < 0.0001$), demonstrating an association in terms of cardiotoxicity with more trastuzumab exposure [48].

In real-world evaluations of cardiac dysfunction and trastuzumab in the elderly population, the rates of cardiac dysfunction appear much higher than expected [44, 49–51]. Some of this may be explained by the fact that women in the clinical trials were typically younger and healthier. In one evaluation of the SEER-Medicare database looking at elderly women ages 67–94 years (mean 76 years) between 2000 and 2007, the incidence of heart failure or cardiomyopathy 3 years after a breast cancer diagnosis was 18.1 % in those with no chemotherapy, 30 % in those who received trastuzumab alone, and 41.9 % in those who received trastuzumab and anthracyclines [44]. In a subsequent retrospective population-based study of 12,500 women diagnosed with locoregional breast cancer treated in eight integrated health systems that looked at women with a mean age of 60 years and a median follow-up of 4.4 (2.6–6.9) years, the 5-year cumulative risk of heart failure for women who received anthracyclines and trastuzumab was 7.5 % in those less than 55 years, 11.4 % women ages 55–64 years, 35.6 % women ages 65–74 years, and 40.7 % in those over the age of 75 years [49]. In this analysis, the risk was not felt to be attributable to anthracyclines alone. While these analyses have limitations and may have some misclassification, it certainly appears that the elderly population is at a higher risk for cardiotoxicity both with anthracyclines and trastuzumab; this risk may also continue to increase even 10 years after the completion of therapy.

There are now several new agents used to treat HER2-positive breast cancers including lapatinib, pertuzumab, and trastuzumab emtansine. Lapatinib, an orally active tyrosine kinase inhibitor that affects both HER2 and the epidermal growth factor receptor, appears to have a safer cardiac profile than trastuzumab, even in those who have received prior anthracyclines [52]. Though age was not specifically evaluated as a risk factor, treatment-related cardiac events have occurred <1 % of the time [52, 53]. Cardiac toxicity also does not appear to be higher when lapatinib is given in conjunction with trastuzumab compared with when trastuzumab is given alone [54–58]. Trastuzumab emtansine (TDM-1), an antibody drug conjugate composed of trastuzumab and a derivative of the antimitotic agent maytansine, and pertuzumab, a monoclonal antibody that binds to a different epitope of the HER2 extracellular domain than does trastuzumab, both approved by the Federal Drug Administration in 2012 and 2013, also do not appear to increase the rates of cardiac dysfunction. While neither long-term data nor geriatric-specific data are available, the early studies of TDM-1 and pertuzumab do not appear to increase the risk of cardiac dysfunction with rates of cardiomyopathy being 0–1.6 % [59–61]. In one study, combinations of pertuzumab in conjunction with anthracyclines appear safe from a cardiac perspective [62]. There is, however, limited follow-up available at this time. Finally, there are newer clinical trials published looking at the use of trastuzumab with less combination chemotherapy. Tolaney et al. demonstrated excellent clinical outcomes in using 12 weekly doses of paclitaxel with trastuzumab followed by every-3-week trastuzumab to complete 12 months [63]. This regimen appears safe and effective and, given there is less systemic combination chemotherapy, has the potential for less cardiac toxicity. Long-term cardiac follow-up is warranted.

In addition to the cardiac concerns from doxorubicin and trastuzumab-based therapies in breast cancer patients, approximately three-fourths of breast cancer cases are hormone-responsive tumors, in which endocrine therapy using tamoxifen or aromatase inhibitors will be prescribed. Aromatase inhibitors have been shown to reduce both disease recurrence and breast cancer-related mortality in women with ER-positive, early disease [64]. The major clinical trials that have examined the efficacy and safety of the aromatase inhibitors include the Arimidex, Tamoxifen, Alone, or in Combination (ATAC) study [64], the Breast International Group (BIG 1–98) [65], and the Intergroup Exemestane Study (IES) [66]. In these studies, the use of aromatase inhibitors was associated with higher rates of hypertension, hypercholesterolemia, angina pectoris, and ischemic cardiovascular disease [66–68]. After 33 months of follow-up of the ATAC trial, there were 2.3 % ischemic cardiovascular disease events, 0.8 % myocardial infarction, and 1.7 % angina rates associated with the aromatase inhibitor anastrazole compared to 1.9 %, 0.8 %, and 1.0 % rates, respectively, with tamoxifen [69]. In the BIG 1–98 trial, cardiac event rates were 4.1 % at 25.8 months and 5.5 % at 51 months with letrozole compared to 3.8 and 5.0 % with tamoxifen [70]. In the exemestane study, the incidence of ischemic cardiovascular disease was higher for exemestane (9.9 %) compared with tamoxifen (8.6 %) [66]. Two recent meta-analyses have suggested a small increase in cardiovascular events in patients taking AIs as compared to those on tamoxifen [68, 71]. In women with a history of cardiovascular disease, the use of anastrazole was associated with a 17 % incidence of cardiac events; this ultimately resulted in a black-box warning of anastrazole for those with a history of cardiovascular disease. These studies were not specifically in elderly women; however, the median age in the ATAC trial at the time of the 10-year analysis was 72 years and was similar in the other trials in which postmenopausal women were enrolled. Given women are now taking adjuvant endocrine therapy for not only 5 years but up to 10 years and are using aromatase inhibitors in the chemoprevention setting [72], there is concern about the long-term effects of aromatase inhibitors on the vascular system. It is important for clinicians to monitor lipids and other cardiovascular risk factors while on adjuvant endocrine therapy.

Non-Hodgkin Lymphoma

Risk factors for the development of non-Hodgkin lymphoma (NHL) have been identified and are not specific for age. However, age, specifically over 60 years, was the most important factor independently associated with outcome. An advanced age resulted in lower response rates and a decrease in survival [73].

From a therapy perspective, the standard approach to diffuse large B-cell lymphoma, one of the most common subtypes of NHL, is a combination of chemotherapy using anthracyclines. In a large analysis of the elderly using the SEER database, 9438 patients with DLBCL were evaluated [74]. Despite doxorubicin being a backbone of chemotherapy for those with diffuse large B-cell lymphoma, only 42 % received doxorubicin. Any doxorubicin use was associated with a 29 % increase in risk of CHF; CHF risk was associated with an increased number of doxorubicin claims, increasing age, prior heart disease, comorbidities, diabetes, and hypertension [74]. This was also confirmed in another study looking at early-stage diffuse large B-cell lymphoma, regardless of whether individuals received radiation therapy [75].

While alternative non-anthracycline-containing regimens have been studied in prospective studies, these combinations of therapy resulted in lower complete response rates and shorter survival compared with anthracycline-containing regimens [76, 77]. The substitution of liposomal doxorubicin has also been studied in the elderly. In these small studies, it appears to be an acceptable alternative, even in those with known cardiac disease in which ejection fractions remained stable [78]. However, the follow-up of these patients was limited. In those patients with an absolute contraindication to anthracycline in which their ejection fraction is below 30 %, there are non-anthracycline-containing regimens that could be considered, such as CEPP (B) [79]. Consideration of the use of an angiotensin-converting enzyme inhibitor or beta-blocker concomitantly with chemotherapy could be considered as will be discussed below.

Sarcomas

Ewing sarcoma typically occurs in young adults, while other types of sarcoma such as leiomyosarcomas tend to occur in older adults, in which anthracyclines and platinums are the backbone of therapy. Little literature exists on the cardiac impact of these treatment regimens on elderly patients with sarcomas. A number of sarcoma regimens substitute liposomal doxorubicin for standard doxorubicin, thus theoretically reducing the cardiac damage seen from this class of drugs. Monitoring left ventricular ejection fraction is still recommended when any anthracycline is recommended. Similarly, while the platinum chemotherapy drugs are known to cause endothelial dysfunction in childhood cancer survivors, it is unclear whether this complication applies to the elderly.

Tyrosine kinase inhibitors have been studied in the treatment of some subtypes of sarcoma, including leiomyosarcomas [80]. Tyrosine kinase inhibitors have been associated with a small increase in congestive heart risk. The overall incidence of all-grade and high-grade CHF associated with tyrosine kinase inhibitors was 3.2 % (95 % CI 1.8 %, 5.8 %) and 1.4 % (95 % CI 0.9 %, 2.3 %), respectively, in a recent meta-analysis of over 10,000 patients [81]. Age did not appear to be associated with increased risk, nor did tumor subtype.

Finally, sarcomas and lymphomas can manifest as cardiac tumors.

Ovarian Cancer

Ovarian cancer is the leading mortality of gynecologic cancers. More than half of these cases occur in women over the age of 65 years, with the primary treatment consisting of debulking surgery and postoperative chemotherapy with platinum and paclitaxel chemotherapies. Despite the disease occurring primarily in elderly women, in an analysis of all Southwestern Oncology Group trials of 16,396 patients in 164 trials in the 1990s, only 30 % of those individuals in the trials were over the age of 65 years [3]. Similarly, in another analysis of elderly women with ovarian cancer using the SEER registries, 9 % of the women in clinical trials using new therapies were over the age of 75 years. Elderly women are underrepresented in clinical trials [82]. Elderly women also appear to have poorer outcomes than their younger counterparts with only half receiving standard platinum chemotherapy, regardless of comorbidity [83].

From a cardiac perspective, the primary risk for elderly women with ovarian cancer consists of their surgical risk and then their chemotherapy exposure. The platinum and paclitaxel regimens are not known to be particularly cardiotoxic at any age. There are studies suggesting the platinum chemotherapies can cause endothelial dysfunction and can result in increased clotting risks [84, 85]; however, these features are not unique to the elderly population. In recurrent ovarian cancer, chemotherapy consisting of bevacizumab, liposomal doxorubicin, gemcitabine, and topotecan can be utilized. It appears the risk of hypertension and arterial thrombosis may be increased in the elderly [86]. For liposomal doxorubicin, it appears that doses up to 550 mg/m^2 are safe from a cardiac perspective [87]. When administered at modified doses of 45 mg/m^2 every 4 weeks, no cardiac toxicity has been observed [88]. In these studies, however, no description of the impact on the elderly was outlined [88]. In similar analyses, frequent determinations of LVEF, as routinely done for other anthracyclines, did not appear to have any clinical value in patient follow-up. In these studies though, the median age was 53 years; it is thus difficult to conclude what monitoring is necessary in the elderly receiving prolonged liposomal doxorubicin [89, 90].

Other Cancers

Lung cancer, bladder cancer, and colon cancer are all common cancers for which the prevalence increases as the population ages. Traditionally cardiotoxic medications such as anthracyclines and trastuzumab are not typically used in these cancers.

Platinum therapies, known to increase clotting risk and endothelial dysfunction, may be used. In many of these diseases, further work with selective tyrosine kinase inhibitors as well as vascular endothelial-growth factor inhibitors continue are being studied. Many of these medications, particularly bevacizumab and regorafenib, are known to cause hypertension. Additionally, multiple new agents have been approved recently for melanoma including BRAF inhibitors vemurafenib and dabrafenib. Both of these medications are known to cause QT prolongation [91]. Hypertension and QT prolongation are side effects not unique to the aging population. However, as individuals age, it is also more likely that they may have hypertension or be on concurrent medications that may result in arrhythmias. As a result, monitoring for side effects remains vital in the care of these patients. Further ongoing work is being done evaluating the association between many of these targeted therapies and incident heart failure.

Unique Situations

Hematopoietic stem cell transplantation (HSCT) is a potential cure for various hematologic malignancies, which carries a risk of treatment-related complications and mortality. To lower these risks, reduced intensity conditioning regimens have now been adapted, allowing older patients up to the age of 70 years to become eligible for stem cell transplantation.

Currently available data suggest that cardiac complications from HSCT are infrequent, occurring <1 % of the time [92]. However, the median age of patients in this study was 22 years [92], and it is likely that older patients will have a higher incidence of cardiac complications. The geriatric patient often presents with comorbidities indicating that a complete geriatric assessment may be beneficial. There are little data available on the role of CGAs in the hematopoietic stem cell transplantation population. Through the HSCT-specific comorbidity index, a cardiac comorbidity (defined as the presence of coronary artery disease, congestive heart failure, myocardial infarction, or an ejection fraction <50 %) is considered as a low-risk comorbidity. Further, recent data suggests that those with an ejection fraction <50 % can still be eligible for HSCT, and patients with borderline left ventricular systolic dysfunction can safely undergo HSCT without alterations in overall survival or treatment-related complications [93].

Prevention of Chemotherapy-Related Cardiac Complications

Risk factors for chemotherapy-related cardiac complications should be assessed in all patients diagnosed with cancer who are being considered for cancer therapy whether it be the administration of biologics, chemotherapy, or radiation therapy.

Given that advancing age has consistently been associated with cardiac complications from chemotherapy using anthracyclines or trastuzumab-based treatments, it is highly recommended that all elderly patients scheduled for anthracyclines or trastuzumab-based therapies should receive a multidisciplinary consultation for risk stratification, risk modification, and primary prevention of cardiotoxicity [5, 6]. These patients should ideally consult with a multidisciplinary team consisting of oncologists, cardiologists, primary care physicians, geriatricians, pharmacists, and nurses [94]. Consideration for a consultation should also occur in geriatric cancer patients with a cardiovascular history who are being prescribed tyrosine kinase inhibitors, chest radiation, left-sided breast radiation, or combination systemic chemotherapy. Depending on the individual risk for cardiotoxicity, the multidisciplinary team should discuss the choices of cardiotoxic standard-of-care therapies or less cardiotoxic—but potentially less effective—alternatives [95]. A lower-intensity chemotherapy regimen, however, should not be prescribed based simply on a patient's risk factors or concern for potential cardiac complication as this has been shown to alter clinical cancer outcomes. Cardiologists should address the extent of baseline cardiac evaluation, the frequency of surveillance to detect cardiotoxicity, and possible use of cardioprotective therapy such as beta-blockers and angiotensin-converting enzyme inhibitors for the primary prevention of cardiotoxicity [6].

Current prevention strategies are based primarily on pretreatment evaluation of cardiac left ventricular ejection fraction. However, this approach has been shown in multiple studies to have a low clinical impact, primarily due to the low prevalence of asymptomatic left ventricular systolic dysfunction [96–108]. Alternative strategies that show promise in risk stratification include strain imaging by echocardiography and the assessment of cardiac fibrosis by cardiac magnetic resonance imaging. However, data are sorely lacking regarding the role of these newer imaging techniques in the risk stratification and prevention of cardiotoxicity in the older adult.

Polypharmacy is a significant issue in caring for the geriatric population [6, 7]. Drug interactions should be avoided; careful review of a patient's medications, prescription and over the counter, is imperative in ensuring additional toxicities will not occur [109, 110]. Consultation with pharmacists at the time of oncology evaluation has been shown to reduce medication errors as well as minimize drug interactions and subsequent toxicity [111–113].

In deciding on potentially cardiotoxic drugs, alternative classes of drugs may be available that are equally efficacious and less cardiotoxic [114]. When possible, these agents should be considered in the geriatric population. Analogs of doxorubicin such as epirubicin [115–119], idarubicin [120, 121], and liposomal doxorubicin [122, 123] have been shown to have less cardiac complications than doxorubicin. The overall cumulative lifetime dose of doxorubicin or its analogs should also be considered; consideration should be given to not exceed 450 mg/m^2 lifetime cumulative dose of doxorubicin in those over the age of 65 years [99, 124]. Calculators are available to calculate cumulative doxorubicin equivalent dosing when using doxorubicin analogs. Alternative schedules for doxorubicin administration may also be helpful in reducing cardiac toxicity. A continuous schedule of doxorubicin has been shown to be less cardiac toxic than a bolus schedule in adults [125–129], while a shorter schedule rather than a longer schedule for trastuzumab has been demonstrated to be less cardiotoxic [48].

In addition to changes in doxorubicin dosing and administration, the use of cardioprotective agents has also been studied in combination with chemotherapy. The best-studied cardioprotective agent is dexrazoxane. This iron chelator has been evaluated and found to protect the hearts of older women with metastatic breast cancer receiving >300 mg/m^2 of doxorubicin or >540 mg/m^2 of epirubicin for cardiac protection [130]. The medication has not, however, been more widely used due to concerns about its roles in clinical efficacy and secondary malignancies. Other cardiac protective agents such as angiotensin-converting enzyme inhibitors, beta-blockers such as carvedilol, and lipid-lowering agents have been evaluated to help prevent cardiac dysfunction [131–138]. There are also several ongoing clinical trials looking at the impact of these medications on preventing cardiac toxicity, particularly in breast cancer (NCT01009918, NCT02177175, NCT01724450). While none of these studies were performed in a geriatric population, the current studies are not excluding the elderly, and the published studies appear to be effective in minimizing risks of cardiac dysfunction when given in conjunction with chemotherapy in patients of all ages.

Patients should be counseled about lifestyle changes such as smoking cessation, physical exercise, and weight loss that can also potentially prevent cardiovascular complications.

Surveillance

Surveillance during and after potentially cardiotoxic therapy is critical because early detection and treatment of cardiac dysfunction can prevent further cardiotoxicity and improve cardiac outcomes [139]. The earlier the onset of treatment, the better will be the results. An asymptomatic decrease in left ventricular ejection fraction is universally accepted as an indication for treatment with angiotensin-converting enzyme inhibitors and beta-blockers. While data are not available specifically for the elderly, it is likely that these treatments are equally effective in them.

While age is considered an important risk factor for cardiotoxicity, surveillance recommendations are generally not tailored to the elderly. The International Society of Geriatric Oncology recommends regular monitoring of the left ventricular ejection fraction by echocardiography or multiple-gated acquisition scan after every two to three cycles of anthracyclines in patients age 70 years or older [40]. They also recommend consideration of liposomal formulations, prolonged infusions, or use of dexrazoxane if there is a decrease of more than 10 % in left ventricular ejection fraction, even if it remains within the normal range.

This recommendation applies especially to patients with hypertension, diabetes, or coronary artery disease [40].

Cardiac monitoring with echocardiography or radionuclide ventriculography (multiple-gated acquisition [MUGA] scans) is the standard of care among patients receiving trastuzumab-based chemotherapy. The National Comprehensive Cancer Network (NCCN) guidelines recommend cardiac monitoring at baseline and at 3, 6, and 9 months after initiating trastuzumab therapy. In a recent study from the SEER-Medicare and the Texas Cancer Registry-Medicare-linked databases, the patterns of cardiac monitoring of 2203 patients aged 66 or older with breast cancer who were treated with adjuvant trastuzumab-based chemotherapy were studied [140]. The investigators found that 64 % of the patients had inadequate monitoring, defined as the absence of a baseline (within 4 months before first trastuzumab dose) cardiac evaluation (with echocardiogram or MUGA scan) and subsequent follow-up cardiac evaluation at least every 4 months while receiving trastuzumab therapy [140]. Because trastuzumab-related cardiotoxicity is reversible, efforts to improve the adequacy of cardiac monitoring are needed, particularly in the elderly.

Consideration should be given to cumulative radiation exposure and the risk of secondary cancers with the use of MUGA scans for surveillance. Guidelines such as those from the International Society of Geriatric Oncology and the United Kingdom National Cancer Research Institute for cardiac monitoring after trastuzumab therapy recommend the use of the same imaging modality throughout the course of treatment [40, 141]. A breast cancer patient receiving adjuvant trastuzumab therapy is recommended to undergo cardiac monitoring before starting treatment, every 3 months during and upon completion of treatment, and every 6 months for at least 2 years following completion of therapy [142]. More frequent monitoring is recommended if trastuzumab is withheld for a significant drop in left ventricular ejection fraction [142]. With 12 months of adjuvant trastuzumab therapy as the standard of care, this translates into a minimum of nine studies. With an average typical effective ionizing radiation dose of 8 mSv per multiple-gated acquisition scan [143, 144], the use of multiple-gated acquisition scans would result in a cumulative effective dose of 72 mSv. Based on published estimates of the radiation-related cancer risk from technetium-99 m myocardial perfusion studies [145], a 50-year-old female who undergoes nine multiple-gated acquisition scans would be estimated to have a lifetime risk of 0.64 % for a radiation-related secondary cancer. While the risk in the elderly is lower than this estimate due to the lower overall life expectancy, it is not an insignificant risk considering the excellent survival rates for patients diagnosed with breast cancer today—a 5-year relative survival rate of 89 % and a 10-year relative survival rate of 82 % [146]. To avoid this risk, echocardiography and cardiac magnetic resonance imaging should be considered as the imaging modalities for surveillance.

Serum cardiac biomarkers, such as N-terminal prohormone brain natriuretic peptide and troponin, are being studied for the early detection of cardiotoxicity, but further investigation is needed before they can be recommended for clinical use [147].

Future Directions

There is a need for systematic research and evidence-based guidelines on the risk prediction models, early biomarkers of toxicity, monitoring, surveillance, and treatment of older patients with cancer receiving potentially cardiotoxic therapy. There are several ongoing studies looking at the impact of comprehensive geriatric assessments on cancer care. The results of these studies will be extremely valuable in determining how to best risk-stratify and treat elderly patients with cancer while preserving their quality of life and functional outcomes. Increasing recruitment of older patients to cancer trials by eliminating an upper age limit to clinical trial eligibility and mandating adequate representation of the elderly is also important in determining how new therapies will impact our aging population.

Funding institutions should encourage research that is designed specifically to study cardiac complications of cancer therapy in the elderly. Establishing the utility of the currently available techniques and biomarkers for the prediction, detection, and prognostication of cardiotoxicity in the elderly should be a high priority. New noninvasive and cost-effective diagnostic tools should be developed for the risk stratification and early identification of preclinical cardiotoxicity in the elderly.

References

1. Parry C, Kent EE, Mariotto AB, Alfano CM, Rowland JH. Cancer survivors: a booming population. Cancer Epidemiol Biomarkers Prev. 2011;20(10):1996–2005.
2. Rowland JH, Bellizzi KM. Cancer survivorship issues: life after treatment and implications for an aging population. J Clin Oncol. 2014;32(24):2662–8.
3. Hutchins LF, Unger JM, Crowley JJ, Coltman Jr CA, Albain KS. Underrepresentation of patients 65 years of age or older in cancer-treatment trials. N Engl J Med. 1999;341 (27):2061–7.
4. Unger JM, Coltman Jr CA, Crowley JJ, et al. Impact of the year 2000 Medicare policy change on older patient enrollment to cancer clinical trials. J Clin Oncol. 2006;24(1):141–4.
5. Accordino MK, Neugut AI, Hershman DL. Cardiac effects of anticancer therapy in the elderly. J Clin Oncol. 2014;32(24):2654–61.
6. Shenoy C, Klem I, Crowley AL, et al. Cardiovascular complications of breast cancer therapy in older adults. Oncologist. 2011;16(8):1138–43.
7. Lichtman SM, Hurria A, Jacobsen PB. Geriatric oncology: an overview. J Clin Oncol. 2014;32(24):2521–2.
8. Hewitt M, Rowland JH, Yancik R. Cancer survivors in the United States: age, health, and disability. J Gerontol A Biol Sci Med Sci. 2003;58(1):82–91.
9. Centers for Disease Control and Prevention. The State of Aging and Health in America. 2013. http://www.cdc.gov/aging/pdf/state-aging-health-in-america-2013.pdf. Accessed 15 Mar 2015.
10. Mozaffarian D, Benjamin EJ, Go AS, et al. Heart disease and stroke statistics-2015 update: a report from the American heart association. Circulation. 2015;131(4):e29–322.
11. Piccirillo JF, Tierney RM, Costas I, Grove L, Spitznagel Jr EL. Prognostic importance of comorbidity in a hospital-based cancer registry. JAMA. 2004;291(20):2441–7.

12. Carver JR, Schuster SJ, Glick JH. Doxorubicin cardiotoxicity in the elderly: old drugs and new opportunities. J Clin Oncol. 2008;26(19):3122–4.

13. Thieblemont C, Grossoeuvre A, Houot R, et al. Non-Hodgkin's lymphoma in very elderly patients over 80 years. A descriptive analysis of clinical presentation and outcome. Ann Oncol. 2008;19(4):774–9.

14. Satariano WA, Ragland DR. The effect of comorbidity on 3-year survival of women with primary breast cancer. Ann Intern Med. 1994;120(2):104–10.

15. Yancik R, Wesley MN, Ries LA, Havlik RJ, Edwards BK, Yates JW. Effect of age and comorbidity in postmenopausal breast cancer patients aged 55 years and older. JAMA. 2001;285(7):885–92.

16. Terret C, Zulian GB, Naiem A, Albrand G. Multidisciplinary approach to the geriatric oncology patient. J Clin Oncol. 2007;25(14):1876–81.

17. Yeh ET. Cardiotoxicity induced by chemotherapy and antibody therapy. Annu Rev Med. 2006;57:485–98.

18. Puts MT, Hardt J, Monette J, Girre V, Springall E, Alibhai SM. Use of geriatric assessment for older adults in the oncology setting: a systematic review. J Natl Cancer Inst. 2012;104 (15):1133–63.

19. Wildiers H, Heeren P, Puts M, et al. International Society of Geriatric Oncology consensus on geriatric assessment in older patients with cancer. J Clin Oncol. 2014;32(24):2595–603.

20. Repetto L, Fratino L, Audisio RA, et al. Comprehensive geriatric assessment adds information to Eastern Cooperative Oncology Group performance status in elderly cancer patients: an Italian Group for Geriatric Oncology Study. J Clin Oncol. 2002;20(2):494–502.

21. Cohen HJ, Feussner JR, Weinberger M, et al. A controlled trial of inpatient and outpatient geriatric evaluation and management. N Engl J Med. 2002;346(12):905–12.

22. Ellis G, Whitehead MA, O'Neill D, Langhorne P, Robinson D. Comprehensive geriatric assessment for older adults admitted to hospital. Cochrane Database Syst Rev. 2011;7, CD006211.

23. Ellis G, Whitehead MA, Robinson D, O'Neill D, Langhorne P. Comprehensive geriatric assessment for older adults admitted to hospital: meta-analysis of randomised controlled trials. BMJ. 2011;343:d6553.

24. Stuck AE, Siu AL, Wieland GD, Adams J, Rubenstein LZ. Comprehensive geriatric assessment: a meta-analysis of controlled trials. Lancet. 1993;342(8878):1032–6.

25. Falandry C, Weber B, Savoye AM, et al. Development of a geriatric vulnerability score in elderly patients with advanced ovarian cancer treated with first-line carboplatin: a GINECO prospective trial. Ann Oncol. 2013;24(11):2808–13.

26. Yeh ET, Bickford CL. Cardiovascular complications of cancer therapy: incidence, pathogenesis, diagnosis, and management. J Am Coll Cardiol. 2009;53(24):2231–47.

27. Jones RL, Ewer MS. Cardiac and cardiovascular toxicity of nonanthracycline anticancer drugs. Expert Rev Anticancer Ther. 2006;6(9):1249–69.

28. Altena R, de Haas EC, Nuver J, et al. Evaluation of sub-acute changes in cardiac function after cisplatin-based combination chemotherapy for testicular cancer. Br J Cancer. 2009;100 (12):1861–6.

29. Monsuez JJ, Charniot JC, Vignat N, Artigou JY. Cardiac side-effects of cancer chemotherapy. Int J Cardiol. 2010;144(1):3–15.

30. Albini A, Pennesi G, Donatelli F, Cammarota R, De Flora S, Noonan DM. Cardiotoxicity of anticancer drugs: the need for cardio-oncology and cardio-oncological prevention. J Natl Cancer Inst. 2010;102(1):14–25.

31. Altena R, Perik PJ, van Veldhuisen DJ, de Vries EG, Gietema JA. Cardiovascular toxicity caused by cancer treatment: strategies for early detection. Lancet Oncol. 2009;10(4):391–9.

32. Curigliano G, Mayer EL, Burstein HJ, Winer EP, Goldhirsch A. Cardiac toxicity from systemic cancer therapy: a comprehensive review. Prog Cardiovasc Dis. 2010;53(2):94–104.

33. Aapro MS, Kohne CH, Cohen HJ, Extermann M. Never too old? Age should not be a barrier to enrollment in cancer clinical trials. Oncologist. 2005;10(3):198–204.

34. Bird BR, Swain SM. Cardiac toxicity in breast cancer survivors: review of potential cardiac problems. Clin Cancer Res. 2008;14(1):14–24.
35. Singal PK, Iliskovic N. Doxorubicin-induced cardiomyopathy. N Engl J Med. 1998;339 (13):900–5.
36. Fisher RI, Gaynor ER, Dahlberg S, et al. Comparison of a standard regimen (CHOP) with three intensive chemotherapy regimens for advanced non-Hodgkin's lymphoma. N Engl J Med. 1993;328(14):1002–6.
37. Lefrak EA, Pitha J, Rosenheim S, Gottlieb JA. A clinicopathologic analysis of adriamycin cardiotoxicity. Cancer. 1973;32(2):302–14.
38. Von Hoff DD, Layard MW, Basa P, et al. Risk factors for doxorubicin-induced congestive heart failure. Ann Intern Med. 1979;91(5):710–7.
39. Swain SM, Whaley FS, Ewer MS. Congestive heart failure in patients treated with doxorubicin: a retrospective analysis of three trials. Cancer. 2003;97(11):2869–79.
40. Aapro M, Bernard-Marty C, Brain EG, et al. Anthracycline cardiotoxicity in the elderly cancer patient: a SIOG expert position paper. Ann Oncol. 2011;22(2):257–67.
41. Yancik R, Ries LA. Aging and cancer in America. Demographic and epidemiologic perspectives. Hematol Oncol Clin North Am. 2000;14(1):17–23.
42. Doyle JJ, Neugut AI, Jacobson JS, Grann VR, Hershman DL. Chemotherapy and cardiotoxicity in older breast cancer patients: a population-based study. J Clin Oncol. 2005;23(34):8597–605.
43. Pinder MC, Duan Z, Goodwin JS, Hortobagyi GN, Giordano SH. Congestive heart failure in older women treated with adjuvant anthracycline chemotherapy for breast cancer. J Clin Oncol. 2007;25(25):3808–15.
44. Chen J, Long JB, Hurria A, Owusu C, Steingart RM, Gross CP. Incidence of heart failure or cardiomyopathy after adjuvant trastuzumab therapy for breast cancer. J Am Coll Cardiol. 2012;60(24):2504–12.
45. Slamon D, Eiermann W, Robert N, et al. Adjuvant trastuzumab in HER2-positive breast cancer. N Engl J Med. 2011;365(14):1273–83.
46. Slamon DJ, Leyland-Jones B, Shak S, et al. Use of chemotherapy plus a monoclonal antibody against HER2 for metastatic breast cancer that overexpresses HER2. N Engl J Med. 2001;344 (11):783–92.
47. Ewer MS, Lippman SM. Type II chemotherapy-related cardiac dysfunction: time to recognize a new entity. J Clin Oncol. 2005;23(13):2900–2.
48. Pivot X, Romieu G, Bonnefoi H, et al. Abstract S5-3: PHARE Trial results of subset analysis comparing 6 to 12 months of trastuzumab in adjuvant early breast cancer. Cancer Res. 2012;72(24 Suppl):S5-3-S5-3.
49. Bowles EJ, Wellman R, Feigelson HS, et al. Risk of heart failure in breast cancer patients after anthracycline and trastuzumab treatment: a retrospective cohort study. J Natl Cancer Inst. 2012;104(17):1293–305.
50. Chavez-MacGregor M, Zhang N, Buchholz TA, et al. Trastuzumab-related cardiotoxicity among older patients with breast cancer. J Clin Oncol. 2013;31(33):4222–8.
51. Brower V. Cardiotoxicity debated for anthracyclines and trastuzumab in breast cancer. J Natl Cancer Inst. 2013;105(12):835–6.
52. Geyer CE, Forster J, Lindquist D, et al. Lapatinib plus capecitabine for HER2-positive advanced breast cancer. N Engl J Med. 2006;355(26):2733–43.
53. Perez EA, Koehler M, Byrne J, Preston AJ, Rappold E, Ewer MS. Cardiac safety of lapatinib: pooled analysis of 3689 patients enrolled in clinical trials. Mayo Clin Proc. 2008;83 (6):679–86.
54. Blackwell KL, Burstein HJ, Storniolo AM, et al. Randomized study of lapatinib alone or in combination with trastuzumab in women with ErbB2-positive, trastuzumab-refractory metastatic breast cancer. J Clin Oncol. 2010;28(7):1124–30.
55. Valachis A, Nearchou A, Polyzos NP, Lind P. Cardiac toxicity in breast cancer patients treated with dual HER2 blockade. Int J Cancer. 2013;133(9):2245–52.

56. Moreno-Aspitia A, Dueck AC, Ghanem-Canete I, et al. RC0639: phase II study of paclitaxel, trastuzumab, and lapatinib as adjuvant therapy for early stage HER2-positive breast cancer. Breast Cancer Res Treat. 2013;138(2):427–35.
57. Morris PG, Iyengar NM, Patil S, et al. Long-term cardiac safety and outcomes of dose-dense doxorubicin and cyclophosphamide followed by paclitaxel and trastuzumab with and without lapatinib in patients with early breast cancer. Cancer. 2013;119(22):3943–51.
58. Robidoux A, Tang G, Rastogi P, et al. Lapatinib as a component of neoadjuvant therapy for HER2-positive operable breast cancer (NSABP protocol B-41): an open-label, randomised phase III trial. Lancet Oncol. 2013;14(12):1183–92.
59. Krop IE, LoRusso P, Miller KD, et al. A phase II study of trastuzumab emtansine in patients with human epidermal growth factor receptor 2-positive metastatic breast cancer who were previously treated with trastuzumab, lapatinib, an anthracycline, a taxane, and capecitabine. J Clin Oncol. 2012;30(26):3234–41.
60. Verma S, Miles D, Gianni L, et al. Trastuzumab emtansine for HER2-positive advanced breast cancer. N Engl J Med. 2012;367(19):1783–91.
61. Hurvitz SA, Dirix L, Kocsis J, et al. Phase II randomized study of trastuzumab emtansine versus trastuzumab plus docetaxel in patients with human epidermal growth factor receptor 2-positive metastatic breast cancer. J Clin Oncol. 2013;31(9):1157–63.
62. Schneeweiss A, Chia S, Hickish T, et al. Pertuzumab plus trastuzumab in combination with standard neoadjuvant anthracycline-containing and anthracycline-free chemotherapy regimens in patients with HER2-positive early breast cancer: a randomized phase II cardiac safety study (TRYPHAENA). Ann Oncol. 2013;24(9):2278–84.
63. Tolaney SM, Barry WT, Dang CT, et al. Adjuvant paclitaxel and trastuzumab for node-negative, HER2-positive breast cancer. N Engl J Med. 2015;372(2):134–41.
64. Baum M, Budzar AU, Cuzick J, et al. Anastrozole alone or in combination with tamoxifen versus tamoxifen alone for adjuvant treatment of postmenopausal women with early breast cancer: first results of the ATAC randomised trial. Lancet. 2002;359(9324):2131–9.
65. Colleoni M, Giobbie-Hurder A, Regan MM, et al. Analyses adjusting for selective crossover show improved overall survival with adjuvant letrozole compared with tamoxifen in the BIG 1–98 study. J Clin Oncol. 2011;29(9):1117–24.
66. Coombes RC, Hall E, Gibson LJ, et al. A randomized trial of exemestane after two to three years of tamoxifen therapy in postmenopausal women with primary breast cancer. N Engl J Med. 2004;350(11):1081–92.
67. Mouridsen H, Keshaviah A, Coates AS, et al. Cardiovascular adverse events during adjuvant endocrine therapy for early breast cancer using letrozole or tamoxifen: safety analysis of BIG 1–98 trial. J Clin Oncol. 2007;25(36):5715–22.
68. Cuppone F, Bria E, Verma S, et al. Do adjuvant aromatase inhibitors increase the cardiovascular risk in postmenopausal women with early breast cancer? Meta-analysis of randomized trials. Cancer. 2008;112(2):260–7.
69. Howell A, Cuzick J, Baum M, et al. Results of the ATAC (Arimidex, Tamoxifen, Alone or in Combination) trial after completion of 5 years' adjuvant treatment for breast cancer. Lancet. 2005;365(9453):60–2.
70. Coates AS, Keshaviah A, Thurlimann B, et al. Five years of letrozole compared with tamoxifen as initial adjuvant therapy for postmenopausal women with endocrine-responsive early breast cancer: update of study BIG 1–98. J Clin Oncol. 2007;25(5):486–92.
71. Younus M, Kissner M, Reich L, Wallis N. Putting the cardiovascular safety of aromatase inhibitors in patients with early breast cancer into perspective: a systematic review of the literature. Drug Saf. 2011;34(12):1125–49.
72. Cuzick J, Sestak I, Forbes JF, et al. Anastrozole for prevention of breast cancer in high-risk postmenopausal women (IBIS-II): an international, double-blind, randomised placebo-controlled trial. Lancet. 2014;383(9922):1041–8.
73. Vose JM, Armitage JO, Weisenburger DD, et al. The importance of age in survival of patients treated with chemotherapy for aggressive non-Hodgkin's lymphoma. J Clin Oncol. 1988;6 (12):1838–44.

74. Hershman DL, McBride RB, Eisenberger A, Tsai WY, Grann VR, Jacobson JS. Doxorubicin, cardiac risk factors, and cardiac toxicity in elderly patients with diffuse B-cell non-Hodgkin's lymphoma. J Clin Oncol. 2008;26(19):3159–65.
75. Pugh TJ, Ballonoff A, Rusthoven KE, et al. Cardiac mortality in patients with stage I and II diffuse large B-cell lymphoma treated with and without radiation: a surveillance, epidemiology, and end-results analysis. Int J Radiat Oncol Biol Phys. 2010;76(3):845–9.
76. Liang R, Todd D, Chan TK, Chiu E, Lie A, Ho F. COPP chemotherapy for elderly patients with intermediate and high grade non-Hodgkin's lymphoma. Hematol Oncol. 1993;11 (1):43–50.
77. Sonneveld P, de Ridder M, van der Lelie H, et al. Comparison of doxorubicin and mitoxantrone in the treatment of elderly patients with advanced diffuse non-Hodgkin's lymphoma using CHOP versus CNOP chemotherapy. J Clin Oncol. 1995;13(10):2530–9.
78. Zaja F, Tomadini V, Zaccaria A, et al. CHOP-rituximab with pegylated liposomal doxorubicin for the treatment of elderly patients with diffuse large B-cell lymphoma. Leuk Lymphoma. 2006;47(10):2174–80.
79. Chao NJ, Rosenberg SA, Horning SJ. CEPP(B): an effective and well-tolerated regimen in poor-risk, aggressive non-Hodgkin's lymphoma. Blood. 1990;76(7):1293–8.
80. Hensley ML, Sill MW, Scribner Jr DR, et al. Sunitinib malate in the treatment of recurrent or persistent uterine leiomyosarcoma: a Gynecologic Oncology Group phase II study. Gynecol Oncol. 2009;115(3):460–5.
81. Qi WX, Shen Z, Tang LN, Yao Y. Congestive heart failure risk in cancer patients treated with vascular endothelial growth factor tyrosine kinase inhibitors: a systematic review and meta-analysis of 36 clinical trials. Br J Clin Pharmacol. 2014;78(4):748–62.
82. Talarico L, Chen G, Pazdur R. Enrollment of elderly patients in clinical trials for cancer drug registration: a 7-year experience by the US Food and Drug Administration. J Clin Oncol. 2004;22(22):4626–31.
83. Wright J, Doan T, McBride R, Jacobson J, Hershman D. Variability in chemotherapy delivery for elderly women with advanced stage ovarian cancer and its impact on survival. Br J Cancer. 2008;98(7):1197–203.
84. Carver JR, Ng A, Meadows AT, Vaughn DJ. Cardiovascular late effects and the ongoing care of adult cancer survivors. Dis Manag. 2008;11(1):1–6.
85. Travis LB, Beard C, Allan JM, et al. Testicular cancer survivorship: research strategies and recommendations. J Natl Cancer Inst. 2010;102(15):1114–30.
86. Scappaticci FA, Skillings JR, Holden SN, et al. Arterial thromboembolic events in patients with metastatic carcinoma treated with chemotherapy and bevacizumab. J Natl Cancer Inst. 2007;99(16):1232–9.
87. Yildirim Y, Gultekin E, Avci ME, Inal MM, Yunus S, Tinar S. Cardiac safety profile of pegylated liposomal doxorubicin reaching or exceeding lifetime cumulative doses of 550 mg/m^2 in patients with recurrent ovarian and peritoneal cancer. Int J Gynecol Cancer. 2008;18 (2):223–7.
88. Steppan I, Reimer D, Sevelda U, Ulmer H, Marth C, Zeimet AG. Treatment of recurrent platinum-resistant ovarian cancer with pegylated liposomal doxorubicin--an evaluation of the therapeutic index with special emphasis on cardiac toxicity. Chemotherapy. 2009;55 (6):391–8.
89. Uyar D, Kulp B, Peterson G, Zanotti K, Markman M, Belinson J. Cardiac safety profile of prolonged (>or = 6 cycles) pegylated liposomal doxorubicin administration in patients with gynecologic malignancies. Gynecol Oncol. 2004;94(1):147–51.
90. Grenader T, Goldberg A, Gabizon A. Monitoring long-term treatment with pegylated liposomal doxorubicin: how important is intensive cardiac follow-up? Anti-Cancer Drugs. 2010;21(9):868–71.
91. Bronte E, Bronte G, Novo G, Bronte F, Bavetta MG, Lo Re G, et al. What links BRAF to the heart function? New insights from the cardiotoxicity of BRAF inhibitors in cancer treatment. Oncotarget. 2015;6(34):35589–601.

92. Murdych T, Weisdorf DJ. Serious cardiac complications during bone marrow transplantation at the University of Minnesota, 1977–1997. Bone Marrow Transplant. 2001;28(3):283–7.

93. Hurley P, Konety S, Cao Q, Weisdorf D, Blaes A. Hematopoietic stem cell transplantation in patients with systolic dysfunction: can it be done? Biol Blood Marrow Transplant. 2015;21(2):300–4.

94. Cohen HJ. A model for the shared care of elderly patients with cancer. J Am Geriatr Soc. 2009;57 Suppl 2:S300–2.

95. Lenihan DJ, Cardinale D, Cipolla CM. The compelling need for a cardiology and oncology partnership and the birth of the International CardiOncology Society. Prog Cardiovasc Dis. 2010;53(2):88–93.

96. Avelar T, Pauliks LB, Freiberg AS. Clinical impact of the baseline echocardiogram in children with high-risk acute lymphoblastic leukemia. Pediatr Blood Cancer. 2011;57(2):227–30.

97. Bryant A, Sheppard D, Sabloff M, et al. A single-institution analysis of the utility of pre-induction ejection fraction measurement in patients newly diagnosed with acute myeloid leukemia. Leuk Lymphoma. 2015;56(1):135–40.

98. Conrad AL, Gundrum JD, McHugh VL, Go RS. Utility of routine left ventricular ejection fraction measurement before anthracycline-based chemotherapy in patients with diffuse large B-cell lymphoma. J Oncol Pract. 2012;8(6):336–40.

99. Jensen BV, Skovsgaard T, Nielsen SL. Functional monitoring of anthracycline cardiotoxicity: a prospective, blinded, long-term observational study of outcome in 120 patients. Ann Oncol. 2002;13(5):699–709.

100. Jeyakumar A, DiPenta J, Snow S, et al. Routine cardiac evaluation in patients with early-stage breast cancer before adjuvant chemotherapy. Clin Breast Cancer. 2012;12(1):4–9.

101. Karanth NV, Roy A, Joseph M, de Pasquale C, Karapetis C, Koczwara B. Utility of prechemotherapy echocardiographical assessment of cardiac abnormalities. Support Care Cancer. 2011;19(12):2021–6.

102. Mina A, Rafei H, Khalil M, Hassoun Y, Nasser Z, Tfayli A. Role of baseline echocardiography prior to initiation of anthracycline-based chemotherapy in breast cancer patients. BMC Cancer. 2015;15(1):10.

103. Porea TJ, Dreyer ZE, Bricker JT, Mahoney Jr DH. Evaluation of left ventricular function in asymptomatic children about to undergo anthracycline-based chemotherapy for acute leukemia: an outcome study. J Pediatr Hematol Oncol. 2001;23(7):420–3.

104. Sabel MS, Levine EG, Hurd T, et al. Is MUGA scan necessary in patients with low-risk breast cancer before doxorubicin-based adjuvant therapy? Multiple gated acquisition. Am J Clin Oncol. 2001;24(4):425–8.

105. Shureiqi I, Cantor SB, Lippman SM, Brenner DE, Chernew ME, Fendrick AM. Clinical and economic impact of multiple gated acquisition scan monitoring during anthracycline therapy. Br J Cancer. 2002;86(2):226–32.

106. Steuter J, Bociek R, Loberiza F, et al. Utility of prechemotherapy evaluation of left ventricular function for patients with lymphoma. Clin Lymphoma Myeloma Leuk. 2015;15(1):29–34.

107. Toggweiler S, Odermatt Y, Brauchlin A, et al. The clinical value of echocardiography and acoustic cardiography to monitor patients undergoing anthracycline chemotherapy. Clin Cardiol. 2013;36(4):201–6.

108. Watts RG, George M, Johnson Jr WH. Pretreatment and routine echocardiogram monitoring during chemotherapy for anthracycline-induced cardiotoxicity rarely identifies significant cardiac dysfunction or alters treatment decisions: a 5-year review at a single pediatric oncology center. Cancer. 2012;118(7):1919–24.

109. Engdal S, Klepp O, Nilsen OG. Identification and exploration of herb-drug combinations used by cancer patients. Integr Cancer Ther. 2009;8(1):29–36.

110. McCune JS, Hatfield AJ, Blackburn AA, Leith PO, Livingston RB, Ellis GK. Potential of chemotherapy-herb interactions in adult cancer patients. Support Care Cancer. 2004;12(6):454–62.

111. Vantard N, Ranchon F, Schwiertz V, et al. EPICC study: evaluation of pharmaceutical intervention in cancer care. J Clin Pharm Ther. 2015;40(2):196–203.

112. Lopez-Martin C, Garrido Siles M, Alcaide-Garcia J, Faus FV. Role of clinical pharmacists to prevent drug interactions in cancer outpatients: a single-centre experience. Int J Clin Pharm. 2014;36(6):1251–9.

113. Yeoh TT, Si P, Chew L. The impact of medication therapy management in older oncology patients. Support Care Cancer. 2013;21(5):1287–93.

114. Jones S, Holmes FA, O'Shaughnessy J, et al. Docetaxel with cyclophosphamide is associated with an overall survival benefit compared with doxorubicin and cyclophosphamide: 7-year follow-up of US oncology research trial 9735. J Clin Oncol. 2009;27(8):1177–83.

115. Brambilla C, Rossi A, Bonfante V, et al. Phase II study of doxorubicin versus epirubicin in advanced breast cancer. Cancer Treat Rep. 1986;70(2):261–6.

116. A prospective randomized phase III trial comparing combination chemotherapy with cyclophosphamide, fluorouracil, and either doxorubicin or epirubicin. French Epirubicin Study Group. J Clin Oncol. 1988;6(4):679–88.

117. Gasparini G, Dal Fior S, Panizzoni GA, Favretto S, Pozza F. Weekly epirubicin versus doxorubicin as second line therapy in advanced breast cancer. A randomized clinical trial. Am J Clin Oncol. 1991;14(1):38–44.

118. Italian Multicentre Breast Study with Epirubicin, Ambrosini G, Balli M, Garusi G, Demicheli R, Jirillo A. Phase III randomized study of fluorouracil, epirubicin, and cyclophosphamide v fluorouracil, doxorubicin, and cyclophosphamide in advanced breast cancer: an Italian multicentre trial. J Clin Oncol. 1988;6(6):976–82.

119. Jain KK, Casper ES, Geller NL, et al. A prospective randomized comparison of epirubicin and doxorubicin in patients with advanced breast cancer. J Clin Oncol. 1985;3(6):818–26.

120. Lopez M, Contegiacomo A, Vici P, et al. A prospective randomized trial of doxorubicin versus idarubicin in the treatment of advanced breast cancer. Cancer. 1989;64(12):2431–6.

121. Villani F, Galimberti M, Comazzi R, Crippa F. Evaluation of cardiac toxicity of idarubicin (4-demethoxydaunorubicin). Eur J Cancer Clin Oncol. 1989;25(1):13–8.

122. Safra T. Cardiac safety of liposomal anthracyclines. Oncologist. 2003;8 Suppl 2:17–24.

123. van Dalen EC, Michiels EM, Caron HN, Kremer LC. Different anthracycline derivates for reducing cardiotoxicity in cancer patients. Cochrane Database Syst Rev. 2010;3, CD005006.

124. Barrett-Lee PJ, Dixon JM, Farrell C, et al. Expert opinion on the use of anthracyclines in patients with advanced breast cancer at cardiac risk. Ann Oncol. 2009;20(5):816–27.

125. Legha SS, Benjamin RS, Mackay B, et al. Reduction of doxorubicin cardiotoxicity by prolonged continuous intravenous infusion. Ann Intern Med. 1982;96(2):133–9.

126. Weiss AJ, Metter GE, Fletcher WS, Wilson WL, Grage TB, Ramirez G. Studies on adriamycin using a weekly regimen demonstrating its clinical effectiveness and lack of cardiac toxicity. Cancer Treat Rep. 1976;60(7):813–22.

127. Chlebowski RT, Paroly WS, Pugh RP, et al. Adriamycin given as a weekly schedule without a loading course: clinically effective with reduced incidence of cardiotoxicity. Cancer Treat Rep. 1980;64(1):47–51.

128. Hortobagyi GN, Frye D, Buzdar AU, et al. Decreased cardiac toxicity of doxorubicin administered by continuous intravenous infusion in combination chemotherapy for metastatic breast carcinoma. Cancer. 1989;63(1):37–45.

129. Shapira J, Gotfried M, Lishner M, Ravid M. Reduced cardiotoxicity of doxorubicin by a 6-hour infusion regimen. A prospective randomized evaluation. Cancer. 1990;65(4):870–3.

130. Hensley ML, Hagerty KL, Kewalramani T, et al. American Society of Clinical Oncology 2008 clinical practice guideline update: use of chemotherapy and radiation therapy protectants. J Clin Oncol. 2009;27(1):127–45.

131. Cardinale D, Bacchiani G, Beggiato M, Colombo A, Cipolla CM. Strategies to prevent and treat cardiovascular risk in cancer patients. Semin Oncol. 2013;40(2):186–98.

132. Blaes AH, Gaillard P, Peterson BA, Yee D, Virnig B. Angiotensin converting enzyme inhibitors may be protective against cardiac complications following anthracycline chemotherapy. Breast Cancer Res Treat. 2010;122(2):585–90.

133. Cardinale D, Colombo A, Sandri MT, et al. Prevention of high-dose chemotherapy-induced cardiotoxicity in high-risk patients by angiotensin-converting enzyme inhibition. Circulation. 2006;114(23):2474–81.
134. Kalay N, Basar E, Ozdogru I, et al. Protective effects of carvedilol against anthracycline-induced cardiomyopathy. J Am Coll Cardiol. 2006;48(11):2258–62.
135. Seicean S, Seicean A, Plana JC, Budd GT, Marwick TH. Effect of statin therapy on the risk for incident heart failure in patients with breast cancer receiving anthracycline chemotherapy: an observational clinical cohort study. J Am Coll Cardiol. 2012;60(23):2384–90.
136. Bosch X, Rovira M, Sitges M, et al. Enalapril and carvedilol for preventing chemotherapy-induced left ventricular systolic dysfunction in patients with malignant hemopathies: the OVERCOME trial (preventiOn of left Ventricular dysfunction with Enalapril and caRvedilol in patients submitted to intensive ChemOtherapy for the treatment of Malignant hEmopathies). J Am Coll Cardiol. 2013;61(23):2355–62.
137. Oliva S, Cioffi G, Frattini S, et al. Administration of angiotensin-converting enzyme inhibitors and beta-blockers during adjuvant trastuzumab chemotherapy for nonmetastatic breast cancer: marker of risk or cardioprotection in the real world? Oncologist. 2012;17(7):917–24.
138. Seicean S, Seicean A, Alan N, Plana JC, Budd GT, Marwick TH. Cardioprotective effect of beta-adrenoceptor blockade in patients with breast cancer undergoing chemotherapy: follow-up study of heart failure. Circ Heart Fail. 2013;6(3):420–6.
139. Cardinale D, Colombo A, Lamantia G, et al. Anthracycline-induced cardiomyopathy: clinical relevance and response to pharmacologic therapy. J Am Coll Cardiol. 2010;55(3):213–20.
140. Chavez-MacGregor M, Niu J, Zhang N, et al. Cardiac monitoring during adjuvant trastuzumab-based chemotherapy among older patients with breast cancer. J Clin Oncol. 2015;33(19):2176–83.
141. Jones AL, Barlow M, Barrett-Lee PJ, et al. Management of cardiac health in trastuzumab-treated patients with breast cancer: updated United Kingdom National Cancer Research Institute recommendations for monitoring. Br J Cancer. 2009;100(5):684–92.
142. Herceptin (Trastuzumab) Prescribing Information. http://www.gene.com/download/pdf/herceptin_prescribing.pdf. Date checked 10 Mar 2015.
143. Einstein AJ, Berman DS, Min JK, et al. Patient-centered imaging: shared decision making for cardiac imaging procedures with exposure to ionizing radiation. J Am Coll Cardiol. 2014;63 (15):1480–9.
144. Chen J, Einstein AJ, Fazel R, et al. Cumulative exposure to ionizing radiation from diagnostic and therapeutic cardiac imaging procedures: a population-based analysis. J Am Coll Cardiol. 2010;56(9):702–11.
145. Berrington de Gonzalez A, Kim KP, Smith-Bindman R, McAreavey D. Myocardial perfusion scans: projected population cancer risks from current levels of use in the United States. Circulation. 2010;122(23):2403–10.
146. DeSantis CE, Lin CC, Mariotto AB, et al. Cancer treatment and survivorship statistics, 2014. CA Cancer J Clin. 2014;64(4):252–71.
147. Colombo A, Cipolla C, Beggiato M, Cardinale D. Cardiac toxicity of anticancer agents. Curr Cardiol Rep. 2013;15(5):362.

Chapter 13
Future Clinical and Professional Directions in Cardio-oncology

Ana Barac and Erica L. Mayer

Introduction

The emergence and growth of the field of cardio-oncology has been driven and strongly influenced by unprecedented advances in the fields of oncology and cardiology. The twenty-first century is witnessing a revolution in targeted cancer therapeutics, leading to significant increases in survivorship of many cancers, and an increasingly changing paradigm moving cancer from an "acute disease" to a chronic condition in which host characteristics and overall health determine cancer therapy options and choices. As described in many of the chapters in this book, existing and emerging cancer therapies may be highly effective against malignancy; however they may also put patients at risk of both short- and long-term cardiovascular complications. Increasingly, providing care to cancer patients requires close collaboration between oncology and cardiology colleagues, both in guiding cardiovascular preventive and therapeutic strategies in cancer patients prior to and during active cancer treatment and monitoring and treating cardiovascular complications in the cancer survivor population. Since the earliest observations of cardiac toxicity in patients receiving anthracyclines, the field has expanded tremendously, incorporating careful analyses of potential toxicities of novel agents,

Electronic supplementary material: The online version of this chapter (doi:10.1007/978-3-319-43096-6_13) contains supplementary material, which is available to authorized users.

A. Barac (✉)
MedStar Heart and Vascular Institute, Medstar Washington Hospital Center, Washington, DC, USA
e-mail: ana.barac@medstar.net

E.L. Mayer
Dana-Farber Cancer Institute, Harvard Medical School, Boston, MA, USA
e-mail: erica_mayer@dfci.harvard.edu

evaluating the use of imaging and biomarkers for risk stratification, considering modern cardioprotective strategies, and evaluating the epidemiology of cardiac toxicity in real-world populations. At the same time, modern general cardiovascular preventive and treatment strategies have resulted in increased life expectancy, and the development of cardiovascular technologies has opened new frontiers of early diagnosis and interventions. It is the growth of these highly subspecialized areas of cardiology and oncology that will continue to critically shape the field of cardio-oncology.

Despite the important advances in this area, many limitations and challenges exist both in the care of patients and in the clinical and academic support of the field. It is hoped that greater recognition of the importance of multidisciplinary cardio-oncology care will further the development of this emerging field, ultimately leading to improved outcomes for patients undergoing cancer treatment and for cancer survivors.

Clinical Collaboration

In response to patient needs, an increasing number of cardio-oncology clinics have been created in the United States. In many, if not most instances, these programs reflect home-grown collaborative efforts between oncology and cardiovascular health providers aiming to improve detection and treatment of cardiovascular complications of cancer therapies, reduce risk, and optimize overall patient outcomes. These programs have tended to be associated with highly specialized, tertiary care, oncology institutions such as NCI Comprehensive Cancer Centers, with a paucity of programs in the community oncology practices, where the majority of cancer patients receive care. Active collaboration is also occurring in research, reflected in the exponential increase in the number of publications in the field of cardio-oncology that importantly move the field forward [1].

Recent investigations have highlighted gaps in cardiovascular service for cancer patients. Examinations have been published from both US and ex-US academic centers describing the clinical management of breast cancer patients with documented declines in ventricular function after exposure to anthracyclines and/or the anti-HER2 monoclonal antibody trastuzumab. These analyses have demonstrated only a fraction of the affected patient population are receiving guideline-recommended heart failure medication and only half are being referred for cardiology consultation [2, 3].

Therefore, significant opportunity clearly exists to improve collaboration between the medical specialties and optimize care of this patient population. Barriers to utilization of cardiovascular services by oncologists have not been well described, may be diverse, and deserve further study. Critical broadening of interdisciplinary exchange is needed to advance the future of cardio-oncology with inclusion of diverse stakeholders, health-care providers, scientists and

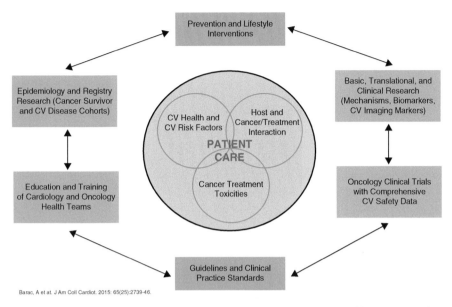

Barac, A et al. J Am Coll Cardiol. 2015; 65(25):2739-46.

Fig. 13.1 Overview of the spectrum of cardio-oncology: bench to bedside to community.
Partnerships across and within the disciplines of cardiology and oncology in the areas of research
(basic, translational, clinical, and population science), education, clinical training, and guidelines
development, as a potential solution to unmet needs and advancement in patient care

investigators, professional societies, patients and advocacy groups, and government
and regulatory agencies (Fig. 13.1).

Research

In the research arena, the National Heart, Lung, and Blood Institute (NHLBI) and
the National Cancer Institute (NCI) convened a collaborative workshop entitled
"Cancer treatment-related cardiotoxicity: Understanding the current state of knowledge and developing future research priorities" in Bethesda, MD, that highlighted
scientific priorities regarding cancer treatment-related cardiotoxicity in 2013. This
meeting of experts recognized broad scientific efforts spanning basic science and
translational research studies, investigating mechanisms of disease and utilization
of biomarkers to improve upon CV risk stratification, to clinical trials evaluating the
effects of cardioprotective strategies and epidemiologic investigations into the
burden of this disease [4]. It also identified gaps and priorities for future research
with critical need to validate reported promising study findings in large clinical
models and translate the potential of recently elucidated mechanisms of
cardiotoxicity into tools for risk stratification, diagnosis, and treatment [4].

As one of the most important consequences of this meeting, new funding
opportunity announcements were released in November 2015 as a joint effort and

strategic priority of the NCI and the NHLBI to improve outcomes in cancer treatment-related cardiotoxicity (http://grants.nih.gov/grants/guide/pa-files/PA-16-035.html and http://grants.nih.gov/grants/guide/pa-files/PA-16-036.html). The institutes encouraged "collaborative applications that will contribute to the identi-fication and characterization of patients at risk" and emphasized mandatory collab-oration between oncology and cardiology specialties on all applications thus highlighting the critical importance of cross-disciplinary work that will continue to shape this field.

Recent exciting research in cardio-oncology has included presentations of inter-ventional prospective trials in breast cancer patients. Highly active targeted cancer therapeutics have revolutionized cancer care; however they also may introduce unexpected cardiovascular outcomes, and examination of these agents has intro-duced new paradigms in cancer and cardiovascular treatment. In the well-studied example of trastuzumab, after approval in the metastatic breast cancer setting, the anti-HER2 monoclonal antibody was introduced into clinical trials for early HER2-positive breast cancer. Given the known signal for cardiotoxicity observed in the metastatic setting, stringent cardiac criteria and monitoring schema were incorpo-rated into adjuvant trials, providing the ability to detect, but not prevent, cardiac toxicity [5, 6]. More recent clinical safety investigations are increasingly focused on primary cardiac prevention strategies aimed not only to prevent and/or reduce LV dysfunction but also to decrease clinically meaningful interruptions of trastuzumab treatment [7, 8]. Based on the knowledge of pathogenesis of heart failure, these investigations utilize neurohormonal cascade blocking agents such as beta-blockers, angiotensin-converting enzyme (ACE) inhibitors, and angiotensin receptor blockers (ARBs) concomitantly with anti-HER2 agents with a goal to prevent LV remodeling and LV dysfunction and importantly allow completion of HER2 therapy. Although relatively small in size, these randomized prospective trials represent a major step forward toward integration of cardiovascular safety into major oncology trials. Future confirmatory studies with validation of the initial findings will hopefully lead toward translation of these primary prevention strate-gies into clinical practice.

Professional Oversight

Professional medical societies have a long-standing legacy of improving patients' health by providing and developing education, training, clinical guidance, and research development for their members. In response to the growing member need, the American College of Cardiology (ACC) formed a Cardio-oncology Working Group in 2013 charged to explore existing cardio-oncology practices and identify areas of professional need. This group performed an environmental scan and a nationwide survey of cardio-oncology services and opinions among CV division chiefs and fellowship training directors that identified important challenges including the need for broader educational opportunities and training [1].

In consequence, the newly formed ACC Cardio-oncology Section and Council has set priorities to further develop and disseminate educational content using contemporary tools such as online cardiovascular websites and applications, CME courses, and integration with national and international conferences. In collaboration with the Annual Scientific Sessions 2015 (ACC.15) organizing committee, members designed Cardio-Oncology Intensive, a half-day program focused on highly relevant clinical questions in CV care of patients with cancer and cancer survivors (http://www.ajmc.com/journals/evidence-based-oncology/2015/june-2015/Advancing-Patient-Care-in-Cardio-Oncology-The-ACC15-Cardio-Oncology-Intensive). Growing educational opportunities come in the form of monthly webinars and annual meetings of the International Society of Cardioncology (ICOS), such as the 2015 Global Cardio-Oncology Summit (http://cardiac-safety.org/wp-content/uploads/2015/08/Global-Cardio-Oncology-Summit-Announcement.pdf), as well as MD Anderson's conferences and web-based series discussing topics relevant to heart disease in patients with cancer and cancer survivors.

Collaboration among professional cardiology and oncology societies offers unique opportunities for synergistic initiatives and advancement of the field. The ACC and American Society for Clinical Oncology (ASCO) convened a task group in 2014 that identified shared interest in broad areas including education and training, development of clinical guidance tools, and advancing research initiatives in the field of cardio-oncology. In addition to cardiovascular toxicity of cancer therapies, shared risk factors and etiologic commonalities between cancer, obesity, and cardiovascular disease have been recognized as an important area of need and potential for growth through professional collaboration. Among the proposed actions, joint development and dissemination of practice standards are most likely to critically influence the future of cardio-oncology and ultimately lead to effective incorporation of cardiovascular care into the continuum of cancer treatment, from diagnosis to survivorship (Fig. 13.1). Additional key areas for partnership among societies include shared use of registries, development of clinical practice toolkits, and joint educational and training activities.

Training

A national cardio-oncology survey, conducted among adult and pediatric cardiology division chiefs and cardiovascular training program directors, demonstrated that in the majority of centers (43 %), exposure to cardio-oncology occurs during regular clinical rotations with a small number of centers offering dedicated lectures as part of the core curriculum (11 %) [1]. Formal training in cardio-oncology for advanced cardiology fellows is currently limited to select few tertiary oncology centers, and cardio-oncology has not been included in previous versions of the Core Cardiovascular Training Symposium (COCATS) guidelines [9]. Development of cardio-oncology-specific competencies, training assessment tools, and curricular milestones is therefore of great interest as the first step toward standardization of training in cardio-oncology [10]. In this fashion, cardio-oncology will follow successful examples of other subspecialty content areas included in cardiovascular fellowship training recommendations such as cardiovascular prevention, vascular medicine, critical care cardiology, and others [9].

No formal training in cardio-oncology currently exists within the core curriculum of hematology/oncology fellowship programs. Therefore, exposure of medical oncology trainees to cardiac toxicities and complications of cancer therapy tends to be more anecdotal than structured. Creation of more formal exposure would likely be a component of a larger educational program in cancer survivorship.

Guidelines and Clinical Practice Standards

Development of clinical practice standards remains one of the most important endeavors of the cardio-oncology field. Joint publications by the American Society of Echocardiography (ASE) and European Association of Cardiovascular Imaging (EACVI) include expert consensus documents on multimodality imaging in evaluation of cardiovascular complications of radiotherapy [11] and in patients during and after cancer therapy [12]. The European Society for Medical Oncology (ESMO) has previously published clinical guidelines for risk prevention, assessment, monitoring, and management during anticancer treatment [13], and the American Heart Association (AHA) issued a scientific statement and summarized cardiotoxicity data after treatment of cancer in children, adolescents, and young adults. The European Society for Medical Oncology (ESMO) has previously published clinical guidelines for risk prevention, assessment, monitoring, and management during anticancer treatment [13], and the Heart Failure Association of the European Society of Cardiology (ESC) [14] and the American Heart Association (AHA) have issued position and scientific statements in cardio-oncology, respectively, with the latter focusing on cardiotoxicity after treatment of cancer in children, adolescents, and young adults [15]. The Society of Cardiac Angiography and Interventions (SCAI) has also published a consensus document on evaluation, management, and special considerations of cardio-oncology patients in the cardiac catheterization laboratory [16]. Despite a lack of data to support some of the recommendations, these guidelines and consensus statements do provide constructive insight into the immense knowledge gap in prevention, diagnosis, treatment, and management of heart disease in patients with cancer. Additionally, many of these statements do attempt to address the issue of screening for and diagnosing heart disease in the existing large and heterogeneous population of 13.7 million cancer survivors living in the United States. It is important to note objective challenges in developing clinical documents that need to meet strict evidence-based criteria required for guideline development. In 2005, for example, ASCO convened an expert panel for assessing cardiac and pulmonary late effects in asymptomatic cancer survivors; however the ASCO Board rejected the guideline due to the lack of direct and high-quality evidence regarding chemotherapy- and radiotherapy-induced cardiac and pulmonary late effects in cancer survivors in 2006 [17]. The panel was redirected to summarize the results of the systematic review of the literature and that was published in 2007 [18]. With growing evidence of the long-term adverse cancer treatment effects, closely linked to improved therapies and improved survival, the ASCO's Survivorship Guidelines Advisory Group has commissioned a new effort to develop a clinical guidance document expected to be released in 2016.

Conclusions

In summary, the landscape of cardio-oncology continues to develop with improved understanding of the mechanisms of cardiotoxicity, development and validation of tools for risk stratification, and novel paradigms in clinical trials and practices. Critical partnerships between cardiology and oncology providers, professional societies, and all stakeholders on broad platforms of education, research, clinical guidance, and training will shape the future clinical environment toward integrated and standardized cardio-oncology practices. It is hoped that continued development and recognition of the importance of multidisciplinary cardio-oncology care will support growth of this emerging field, ultimately leading to improved outcomes for patients with cancer and cancer survivors.

Acknowledgments Relevant disclosures and relationship with industry: Ana Barac has received research support from the NIH, research support and honoraria for lectures from Genentech Inc., and consultancy fees from Cell Therapeutics, Inc. Erica L. Mayer has received research support from Pfizer, Eisai, and Myriad.

References

1. Barac A, Murtagh G, Carver JR, Chen MH, Freeman AM, et al. Cardiovascular health of patients with cancer and cancer survivors: a roadmap to the next level. J Am Coll Cardiol. 2015;65:2739–46.
2. Yoon GJ, Telli ML, Kao DP, Matsuda KY, Carlson RW, Witteles RM. Left ventricular dysfunction in patients receiving cardiotoxic cancer therapies are clinicians responding optimally? J Am Coll Cardiol. 2010;56(20):1644–50. doi:10.1016/j.jacc.2010.07.023.
3. Ammon M, Arenja N, Leibundgut G, Buechel RR, Kuster GM, Kaufmann BA, Pfister O. Cardiovascular management of cancer patients with chemotherapy-associated left ventricular systolic dysfunction in real-world clinical practice. J Card Fail. 2013;19(9):629–34. doi:10.1016/j.cardfail.2013.07.007.
4. Shelburne N, Adhikari B, Brell J, Davis M, Desvigne-Nickens P, et al. Cancer treatment-related cardiotoxicity: current state of knowledge and future research priorities. J Natl Cancer Inst. 2014;106(9):pii: dju232.
5. Seidman A, Hudis C, Pierri MK, Shak S, Paton V, et al. Cardiac dysfunction in the trastuzumab clinical trials experience. J Clin Oncol. 2002;20:1215–21.
6. Slamon D, Eiermann W, Robert N, Pienkowski T, Martin M, et al. Adjuvant trastuzumab in HER2-positive breast cancer. N Engl J Med. 2011;365:1273–83.

7. Gulati G, Heck SL, Ree AH, Hoffmann P, Schulz-Menger J, Fagerland MW, Gravdehaug B, von Knobelsdorff-Brenkenhoff F, Bratland Å, Storås TH, Hagve TA, Røsjø H, Steine K, Geisler J, Omland T. Prevention of cardiac dysfunction during adjuvant breast cancer therapy (PRADA): a 2 × 2 factorial, randomized, placebo-controlled, double-blind clinical trial of candesartan and metoprolol. Eur Heart J. 2016;37(21):1671–80. doi:10.1093/eurheartj/ehw022.
8. Pituskin E, Mackey JR, Koshman S, Jassal DS, Pitz M, et al. Prophylactic beta blockade preserves left ventricular ejection fraction in HER2-overexpressing breast cancer patients receiving trastuzumab: Primary results of the MANTICORE randomized clinical trial. Proceedings of the 36th Annual CTRC-AACR San Antonio Breast Cancer Symposium Abstract (S1-05). 2015.
9. Williams ES, Halperin JL, Fuster V. ACC 2015 COre CArdiovascular Training Statement (COCATS 4) (Revision of COCATS 3). J Am Coll Cardiol. 2015;65(17):1721–3.
10. Lenihan DJ, Hartlage G, DeCara J, Blaes A, Finet JE, Lyon AR, Cornell RF, Moslehi J, Oliveira GH, Murtagh G, Fisch M, Zeevi G, Iakobishvili Z, Witteles R, Patel A, Harrison E, Fradley M, Curigliano G, Lenneman CG, Magalhaes A, Krone R, Porter C, Parasher S, Dent S, Douglas P, Carver J. Cardio-oncology training: a proposal from the International Cardioncology Society and Canadian Cardiac Oncology Network for a new multidisciplinary specialty. J Card Fail. 2016;22(6):465–71. doi:10.1016/j.cardfail.2016.03.012.
11. Lancellotti P, Nkomo VT, Badano LP, Bergler-Klein J, Bogaert J, et al. Expert consensus for multi-modality imaging evaluation of cardiovascular complications of radiotherapy in adults: a report from the European Association of Cardiovascular Imaging and the American Society of Echocardiography. J Am Soc Echocardiogr. 2013;26:1013–32.
12. Plana JC, Galderisi M, Barac A, Ewer MS, Ky B, et al. Expert consensus for multimodality imaging evaluation of adult patients during and after cancer therapy: a report from the American Society of Echocardiography and the European Association of Cardiovascular Imaging. J Am Soc Echocardiogr. 2014;27:911–39.
13. Curigliano G, Cardinale D, Suter T, Plataniotis G, de Azambuja E, et al. Cardiovascular toxicity induced by chemotherapy, targeted agents and radiotherapy: ESMO Clinical Practice Guidelines. Ann Oncol. 2012;23 Suppl 7:vii155–66.
14. Eschenhagen T, Force T, Ewer MS, de Keulenaer GW, Suter TM, et al. Cardiovascular side effects of cancer therapies: a position statement from the Heart Failure Association of the European Society of Cardiology. Eur J Heart Fail. 2011;13:1–10.
15. Lipshultz SE, Adams MJ, Colan SD, Constine LS, Herman EH, et al. Long-term cardiovascular toxicity in children, adolescents, and young adults who receive cancer therapy: pathophysiology, course, monitoring, management, prevention, and research directions: a scientific statement from the American Heart Association. Circulation. 2013;128:1927–95.
16. Iliescu C, Grines CL, Herrmann J, Yang EH, Cilingiroglu M, et al. SCAI expert consensus statement-executive summary evaluation, management, and special considerations of cardio-oncology patients in the cardiac catheterization laboratory. Catheter Cardiovasc Interv. 2015;87(5):895–9.
17. Carver JR, Shapiro CL, Ng A, Jacobs L, Schwartz C, Virgo KS, et al. ASCO clinical evidence review on the ongoing care of adult cancer survivors: cardiac and pulmonary late effects. J Oncol Pract. 2007;3:233–5.
18. Carver JR, Shapiro CL, Ng A, Jacobs L, Schwartz C, et al. American Society of Clinical Oncology clinical evidence review on the ongoing care of adult cancer survivors: cardiac and pulmonary late effects. J Clin Oncol. 2007;25:3991–4008.

Index